A Veterinary Technician's Guide to

Exotic
Animal Care

2nd Edition

Thomas N. Tully Jr.
DVM, MS, DABVP (Avian), DECZM (Avian)

Professor
Department of Veterinary Clinical Sciences
Louisiana State University—School of Veterinary Medicine
Baton Rouge, Louisiana

Mark A. Mitchell
DVM, MS, PhD, DECZM (Herpetology)

Professor
University of Illinois, College of Veterinary Medicine
Urbana, Illinois

AAHA
press

American Animal Hospital Association Press
12575 West Bayaud Avenue
Lakewood, Colorado 80228

ISBN: 978-1-58326-146-0

Library of Congress Cataloging-in-Publication Data

Tully, Thomas N.
  A veterinary technician's guide to exotic animal care / Thomas N. Tully Jr., Mark A. Mitchell. — 2nd ed.
     p. ; cm.
  Rev. ed. of: A technician's guide to exotic animal care / Thomas N. Tully Jr., Mark A. Mitchell. c2001.
  Includes bibliographical references and index.
  ISBN 978-1-58326-146-0 (pbk. : alk. paper)
  1. Exotic animals—Diseases. 2. Wildlife diseases. 3. Pet medicine. 4. Veterinary nursing. I. Mitchell, Mark A., 1967- II. Tully, Thomas N. Technician's guide to exotic animal care. III. American Animal Hospital Association. IV. Title.
  [DNLM: 1. Animal Diseases. 2. Animal Technicians. 3. Pets. 4. Veterinary Medicine—methods. SF 997.5.E95]
  SF997.5.E95T85 2012
  636.089'073—dc23
                          2012007076

Acquisitions Editor: Bess Maher
Cover design: Kimberly Lamb
Interior design: Jane Raese and Planet X Design
Cover photo © Getty Images/Stephan Hoerold

Printed in Canada
12 13 14 / 10 9 8 7 6 5 4 3 2 1

The authors would like to dedicate this book to veterinary technicians and nurses everywhere, who work hard to provide the best care for their avian and exotic animal patients.

Contents

CHAPTER 3. FERRETS   79

CHAPTER 4. RABBITS   107

List of Figures

CHAPTER 2. REPTILES AND AMPHIBIANS

CHAPTER 3. FERRETS

CHAPTER 4. RABBITS

CHAPTER 5. RODENTS: Guinea Pigs, Hamsters, Gerbils, Rats and Mice

CHAPTER 6. HEDGEHOGS

CHAPTER 7. SUGAR GLIDERS

CHAPTER 8. FISH

List of Tables

Foreword

As technicians, we are the first to have contact with clients and their animals. As with dogs and cats, it is important that we gather all necessary information in order to treat exotic animals. Often, we see clients who have acquired a new and exciting exotic species without having much knowledge about the husbandry, diet, and diseases associated with those animals. It is our role as technicians to provide that knowledge and guide our clients in the care of their new pet.

We can also help educate clients before they make the purchase of that exotic animal. Technicians need to know what questions to ask with regard to the nutrition, diet, and housing of the animal, and *A Veterinary Technician's Guide to Exotic Animal Care* provides that knowledge base in one convenient reference. *A Veterinary Technician's Guide to Exotic Animal Care* includes specifics on birds, reptiles, amphibians, rodents, fish, sugar gliders, rabbits, ferrets, and hedgehogs, all animals that have become very popular household pets in the last few years.

In addition to husbandry, diet, and disease information, this reference provides great infor-

mation on blood draw and injection sites for administering medications, parasites that are most common to the species, and anesthetics that are commonly used with the species.

I have been working with exotic animals for many years, and most of my knowledge on the subject of exotics has been gained through hands-on training and gleaning information from a variety of resources, each concentrating on one species. This book compiles in one reference information on all the common exotic pets seen in private practice. As a technician, I find this a valuable directory, which helps me either recall or learn new information about the species that I might encounter in the clinic.

The knowledge and information provided in this book is invaluable to our practice, as technicians work with veterinarians to expand their exotic animal clientele. I definitely recommend adding *A Veterinary Technician's Guide to Exotic Animal Care* to your reference library.

—Dianna Lydick, BS, RVT, CVT

Preface

This is a much-needed second edition of *A Veterinary Technician's Guide to Exotic Animal Care*. Over the past 10 years there has continued to be an evolving body of knowledge as to the proper care and treatment of avian and exotic animal species. While maintaining the foundation of information regarding birds, reptiles, ferrets, rabbits, rodents, hedgehogs, sugar gliders, and fish found in the first edition, this edition expands in critical areas to elevate the reader's understanding of these diverse animal groups. This continues to be a basic text covering the most common exotic animal species treated in small-animal hospitals. The chapters cover important information required by owners, while focusing on the skills needed by the veterinary technician/nurse (hereafter veterinary technician) who works with these animals.

Today's pet owners demand quality care for their animals and expect both veterinarians and veterinary technicians to have basic knowledge of handling, diseases, husbandry, and nutrition. This text provides the essential information in a systematic formula that covers the basic responsibilities of veterinary technicians; and full-color photos and line drawings improve understanding of educational and technical concepts.

Exotic companion-animal owners should be encouraged to seek veterinary care for their animals when first purchased and, at least, on a yearly basis for health examinations. The initial visit helps prevent one of the most common causes of death in pet exotic animals: improper husbandry/nutrition. Examination of the patient and, more importantly, education of the owner are the primary objectives of the first visit. The education process, which often is the responsibility of the veterinary technician, may include handouts, educational video, and recommended Internet websites.

Veterinarians actively seek technicians who have an interest in working with exotic animal species. To gain clinical confidence, veterinary technicians must initially be motivated to become experienced in handling and collecting diagnostic samples from the animals mentioned in this text. Basic knowledge learned about dogs and cats will serve the interested exotic animal technician well, with confidence quickly growing in proportion to the number of animals treated.

As mentioned, this second edition is more detailed and up-to-date and provides a significantly increased number of full-color figures, line drawings, and tables. Each chapter covers the following main topics: husbandry, nutrition, restraint, physical examination, diagnostic sampling, therapeutics, and disease. There are references at the end of each chapter for individuals who seek more detailed information on a particular topic. For the reader's benefit, some products, medications, and manufacturers are listed in the text. These recommendations are based on what the authors have found to work best, but are not meant to endorse a particular company. Occasionally, manufacturers aren'tmentioned because a drug is generic and produced by many companies. This edition continues to provide the basic guidelines veterinary technicians need to perform quality exotic animal pet care.

What has not changed since the first edition was published is that veterinary practices have a continuing demand for interested and qualified technicians in the area of avian/exotic animal medicine. The authors continue to encourage veterinary technicians to get involved in this exciting, growing, and challenging field of veterinary medicine.

Acknowledgments

The authors gratefully acknowledge the assistance of Mr. Michael Broussard. We would also like to thank Ms. Bess Maher at AAHA Press for her patience and support in successfully guiding this much-needed text to completion. Thanks to Susie Tully, Claudia Rose Tully, Fiona Elizabeth Tully, Lorrie Hale Mitchell, Mary Mitchell, and R. J. Mitchell for providing moral support and putting up with the authors' constant emotional demands while working on this project.

The authors would like to thank the reviewers of the current edition: J. Jill Heatley, DVM, MS, Dipl. ABVP (Avian), Dipl. ACZM; Dianna Lydick, BS, RVT, CVT; and Tiffany Wolf, DVM.

Many thanks also go to the First Edition Advisory Group: Dr. Laurel Collins, ABVP, Dr. Richard Goebel, Dr. Charles Hickey, Dr. Clayton McKinnon, and Dr. Hal Taylor.

CHAPTER 1

Avian

INTRODUCTION

There are close to 9,000 different avian species worldwide. These are not different breeds of the same species, like dogs and cats, but are, in fact, entirely different animals within the class Aves. Upon first learning of this difference, it would seem impossible to become qualified to treat so many different types of birds. With this in mind, a technician must learn and become knowledgeable about basic avian husbandry, diagnostic sampling, and patient care. Most veterinary practices see only companion avian species (e.g., parrots, macaws, and cockatiels) and caged birds (e.g., finches and canaries). These are the species that technicians need to become familiar with and comfortable handling and treating. Through experience and modification of technical skills, the transition between avian species is easy to make, if needed, for wildlife or zoological avian species (e.g., toucans, flamingos, penguins, and ostriches). Companion avian species need to be examined yearly, groomed regularly, and vaccinated on a regular schedule. As with other exotic species, the presentation of the patient in the exam room allows the technician to provide husbandry and nutritional information to the client. Captive-reared companion avian species are excellent pets, with each species having advantages and disadvantages to ownership—similar to the physical and personality differences observed in cat and dog breeds. If placed on a proper diet and maintained on that nutritional regimen, most pet birds live long, healthy lives.

HUSBANDRY

Environmental Concerns

Many new pet bird owners purchase their pets with a few preconceived ideas that have been learned from a lifetime of misinformation. One of these misconceptions is that birds are sensitive to cold and drafts. In reality, avian species are much more sensitive to heat than they are to cold or drafts. Birds have an ability to acclimatize to almost any environment over time, especially cooler weather. Although many birds come from arid, tropical, and subtropical regions of the world, there are microenvironments within these areas that provide protection from the oppressive heat. Many of these microenvironments range from 75° to 85°F. If parrots are allowed to stay outside in a protected cage against the prevailing wind with a roof and nest box, they will acclimatize to temperatures that drop into the lower 30°F range (Figure 1.1). If temperatures drop lower than freezing, owners should be advised to provide a heat lamp for temperature regulation.

Birds will respond to indoor temperatures much the same as they do to outside seasonal variations. They will molt feathers in the spring as the hotter summer months approach and will molt and produce more down feathers in the autumn as the cooler winter months approach. Although owners might complain about the extra feather loss in the spring and autumn, this is not an unusual finding. Even with air-conditioning, the ambient tempera-

ture of a house rises and falls with the seasons of the year. Birds should not be moved from an air-conditioned environment into an outdoor flight during the peak months of summer or winter, because they are not acclimatized to the environment. Placing a bird near an air-conditioner's vent is also not advised, because air near a vent is considerably cooler/warmer than the surrounding air temperature, which creates added physical stress on the bird to compensate for the constant change in temperature that occurs as the system shuts off and on to maintain the thermostat setting. It is best to place the cage in a room in which there is interaction with the other family members, away from direct vent airflow.

Interaction with members of the family is important, but also normal sleep can have as much or more impact on a bird's psychological well-being. If a psittacine species (e.g., parrot) is housed in a room in which lights and conversation occur well past dusk, a separate cage should be placed in a quiet part of the house for sleeping. On most days psittacine species should be allowed sleep time that corresponds to the number of nighttime hours. Inconsistent sleep time has been associated with psychological disorders in parrots, including feather picking.

Cage design has been elevated to an art. Many different cage designs are manufactured from different products, ranging from brass wire to Plexiglas (Figures 1.2 and 1.3). Most cages are designed for indoor use only, and most, if not all, commercial cages should be used only indoors. Owners usually buy cages for indoor use based on individual taste, the ability of the cage to reduce spread of litter and dust into the surrounding environment, and how well the cage blends with the interior design of their house. The only requirement from a health point of view is that the cage be of appropriate size for the bird(s) that it will

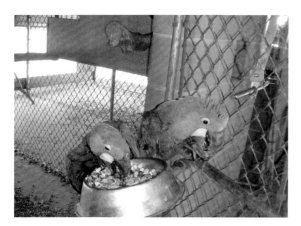

Figure 1.1 *A typical flight cage used for a breeding pair of parrots.*

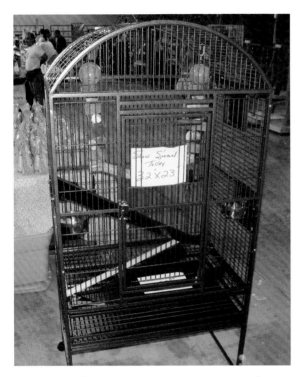

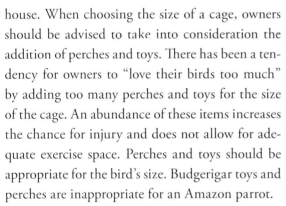

Figure 1.2 *Parrot cages come in many sizes and colors.*

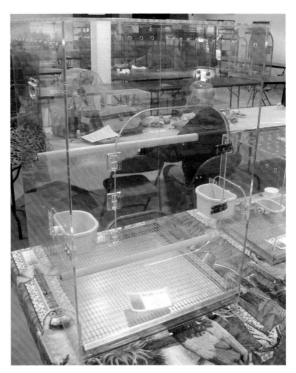

Figure 1.3 *Plexiglas cages make good transport carriers and reduce the incidence of cage litter falling on the floor.*

house. When choosing the size of a cage, owners should be advised to take into consideration the addition of perches and toys. There has been a tendency for owners to "love their birds too much" by adding too many perches and toys for the size of the cage. An abundance of these items increases the chance for injury and does not allow for adequate exercise space. Perches and toys should be appropriate for the bird's size. Budgerigar toys and perches are inappropriate for an Amazon parrot.

Natural wood perches, cut from hardwood trees (e.g., oak, maple, or hickory), are recommended for pet birds (Figure 1.4). The natural wood can be readily replaced, and it also provides a variable diameter and foot surface for the birds to use, which helps to exercise their feet. Tell your clients never to use sandpaper on the perches, because this causes irritation to the foot area that comes

into contact with this abrasive surface. Abrasive perches for larger birds (e.g., scored cement, terracotta) can dull the tip of the claw, but again, the soft weight-bearing part of the bird's foot is against the rough surface. If an abrasive perch is used for a parrot species, only one of the rough perches should be in the cage, with the majority of roosting areas made of natural wood branches.

Newspaper is the substrate of choice to line the cage bottom. This substrate is cheap and allows the owner to observe the bird's fecal material, thereby monitoring the pet's eating habits and gastrointestinal system. Newspaper also gets dirty, making it readily apparent to the owner that routine cleaning of the cage is required. Although newspaper is a great substrate in a cage, newspaper with colored inks can be toxic and therefore should be separated from the bird via a grate. Other substances

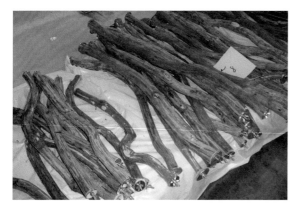

Figure 1.4 *Natural wood perches are recommended for their differing diameters and surface structure.*

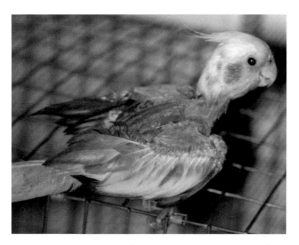

Figure 1.5 *Many outdoor cages are made from galvanized wire and held together with J-clips.*

(e.g., ground walnut shells and corncobs) used as birdcage substrate dry out fecal material and hide excreta from the owner, giving him or her the impression that the cage is "clean." There have also been instances of birds ingesting their substrate.

Most pet birds maintained inside do not need grit to aid in digestion. These birds shell their seed and, for the most part, grind the kernel, forgoing the need for grit. If an owner insists on using grit, crushed oyster shell or eggshell is recommended not only as a mechanical means to grind the food in the ventriculus, but also as a dietary

calcium source. The anti-mite tin that contains an insecticide disk to be placed on the outside of the cage is also not recommended. Pet birds that are housed inside do not come into contact with lice or mites, and the insecticide they contain will not affect the mites that are commonly diagnosed as infesting budgerigars. Sandpaper perches, grit, and anti-mite devices are a waste of money for pet bird owners and, in many cases, will contribute to health problems.

Outdoor flights are uniformly manufactured through private companies or owners using different gauges of hardware cloth and J-clips (Figure 1.5). The outdoor flights are built according to the bird's size and the breeding requirements of the particular species. The main requirements for outdoor flights are appropriate size and wire gauge, flight maintained off the ground, proper nest box structure, roof or partial roof, prevailing wind protection (especially in the winter), and heat lamp, when applicable. Predator control is essential in outdoor flights and large aviary buildings; there have been a number of tragic cases of predators (especially raccoons) attacking birds housed outdoors. In addition, opossums can excrete a parasite in their feces, *Sarcocystis* spp., which is eaten by cockroaches and deposited (by way of feces) in the bird food. It is very difficult, but vital, to control vermin and insects in complex aviary structures, because these pests can carry a number of bacterial and parasitic diseases. Any predator-, insect-, or vermin-control program must take into account bird exposure to the agent being used for eradication of these pests.

Nutrition

This area of companion avian medicine has been one of the most active in advancing the health of companion birds. Twenty years ago the only commercially available feed for parrots was seed.

Of course, if an owner has another species of bird (e.g., pigeons, peafowl, waterfowl, and ratites), the commercially available feed is recommended.

For companion avian species, which include parrots, macaws, and caged songbirds, advances in nutrition have been made in the form of pellets (Figure 1.6). These pelleted bird diets are manufactured by a number of companies and come in many shapes, sizes, and flavors. The secret to getting a bird transitioned from a seed diet to a pelleted diet is to start young and, if possible, to allow the bird to see other birds eating the pellets. There are also commercially manufactured seed cakes and seed balls that will aid the transition from loose seed to pellets (Figures 1.7 and 1.8). It is much easier to convert a group of birds from a seed diet to a pelleted diet than a single bird. Single cockatiels, one of the most popular pet birds, might be the most difficult bird to transition to a pelleted diet. A bird that is being transitioned to a pelleted diet should be weighed every two to three days. If there is a consistent weight loss, the seed diet should be resumed and another method used for pellet acceptance. Some birds will not accept a pellet diet, but this is rare. If the pellets are colored, some birds will eat only specific colors, which can change the color of the fecal material and promote food waste. This does not cause any health problems, but does assure the owner that the bird is eating the pellets and not just crushing them in its beak.

Although some feed manufacturers promote pelleted diets as containing all of the required nutrients for a complete diet, a diversified diet with pellets as the foundation is recommended. This diversified diet should contain seeds, vegetables, possibly cheese and cooked eggs, and a small amount of fruit (Figure 1.9). Some pet bird species that have fruit as a large part of their diet (e.g., lories) require a greater percentage of fruit and

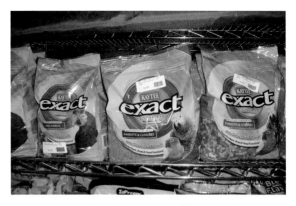

Figure 1.6 *Pelleted diets are readily available in pet stores.*

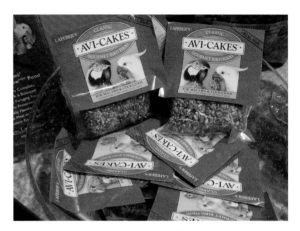

Figure 1.7 *Many companies offer trial sizes that can be provided to avian clients.*

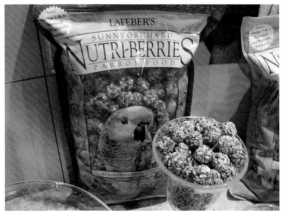

Figure 1.8 *Compacted seed treats often help birds transition from a primary seed diet to pellets.*

nectar. As always, it is up to the owner to research the nutritional requirements of his or her pet and make sure to provide a proper diet. The diversified diet not only supplements a variety of nutritional components, it also psychologically stimulates the bird with different sizes and textures of the food-stuffs that it eats.

Foraging is another form of feeding a bird in a stimulating manner. A number of foraging devices have been manufactured in recent years to challenge parrots to work for their food (Figure 1.10). A significant amount of highly recommended information exists for owners and technicians in the form of articles and electronic media on the advantages of providing a foraging environment for companion avian species. A psychologically stimulated bird is a happy bird that might exhibit fewer vices, such as feather picking and stimulated reproductive activity.

Anorexic birds can be fed using a "ball-tipped" gavage needle. The stainless steel gavage needle can be easily disinfected but is unyielding when passed down the esophagus into the crop. It is very important that one becomes experienced using a "ball-tipped" gavage needle before using it to administer food or medicine to a bird (Figure 1.11).

Pet owners should be guided to make fresh water available at all times. They should also be aware that water containers should be cleaned daily and refilled with a fresh supply. To prevent "poop soup," sipper bottles that attach to the side of the cage are recommended for parrot species (Figure 1.12). The birds cannot dump the container in the bottom of the cage or defecate in their water. Tell owners to touch the bird's beak and tongue to the tip of the sipper tube when it is first introduced to make sure the animal knows that water is available at the end of this strange stainless steel device.

Tell owners that they may provide stick treats, but the stick and wire must be removed from the cage after the bird has finished eating the attached seeds. Spray millet, millet on the natural seed head, is a welcome treat for smaller psittacine species, such as lovebirds and cockatiels.

Make your pet owners aware that calcium supplementation (Figures 1.13A and 1.13B) is a must, and for smaller birds, a cuttlebone will provide the source. The soft side faces the bird, and the bird eats the bone, as calcium is required in the diet. These are not beak-sharpening devices, but calcium sources. For larger birds, a mineral block will provide the calcium supplement, because they

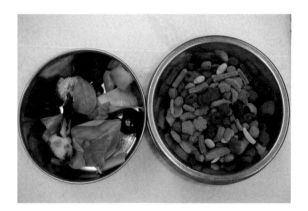

Figure 1.9 *For many parrot species a diversified diet is recommended.*

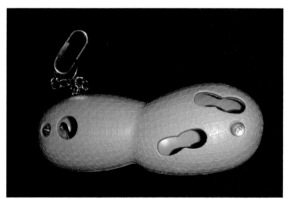

Figure 1.10 *Foraging "toys" are psychologically stimulating for caged birds.*

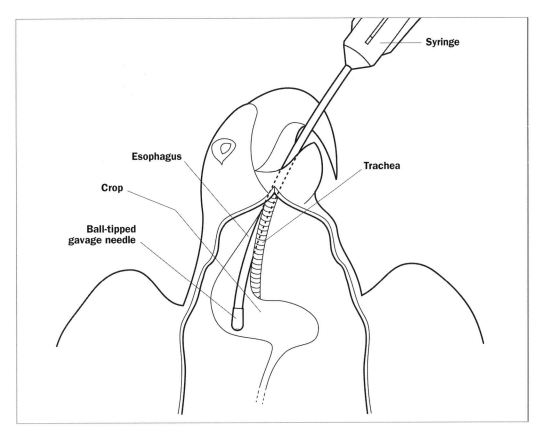

Figure 1.11 *Proper placement of a gavage feeding tube in a parrot. Illustration by Michael L. Broussard.*

can crush a cuttlebone in seconds. If your owners want to place a vitamin or mineral supplement in the water or on the bird's food, guide them to strictly follow the instructions provided with the product. Often, birds will not drink or eat substances that have been tainted, which can reduce the required nutritional intake of these animals. If the bird does drink the water and eat the food with the supplement, both containers need to be cleaned daily because of vitamin degradation and predisposition to bacterial growth.

Transport

Bird owners should be reminded always to transport their animal(s) to the veterinary clinic in their cage, transport cage, or plastic pet carrier. If the cage is small enough and easily carried, this is the best method to transport the bird. Having the bird in its own environment creates a sense of familiarity and allows the veterinary technician an opportunity to evaluate the enclosure. Transportation of the cage in which a bird lives applies to birds that weigh <150 grams (e.g. finches, canaries, budgerigars, cockatiels). A transport cage or plastic pet carrier is recommended for larger birds (e.g., parrots, macaws). A plastic pet carrier can be modified by attaching a wooden dowel or branch across the bottom half of the carrier as a perch (Figure 1.14). Newspaper should be placed on the bottom of a transport

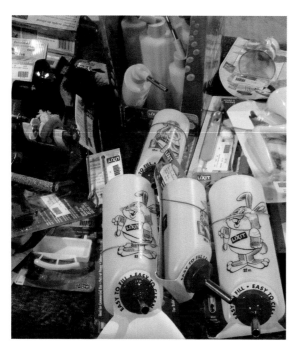

Figure 1.12 *Sipper water bottles that hang on the outside of a cage prevent "poop soup" when used as the source of a bird's drinking water.*

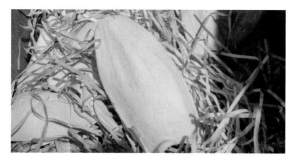

Figure 1.13A *A cuttlebone provides a calcium source for smaller birds.*

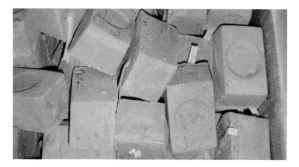

Figure 1.13B *A mineral block is a calcium source for larger birds.*

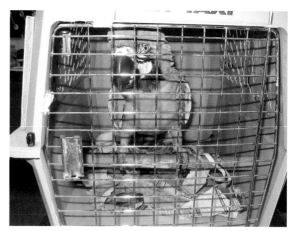

Figure 1.14 *Companion birds should be transported to the veterinary hospital in a modified pet carrier.*

cage or pet carrier for easy cleaning and to evaluate/collect fecal samples.

Grooming

Bird owners are constantly seeking quality health care for their birds. This health care includes professional grooming services. For many veterinary practices, this is understood for dogs and to a lesser extent cats, but not for avian species. One of the most common companion bird presentations to veterinary clinics is for grooming services. Grooming birds includes beak, feather, and nail trims.

Parrots have a natural overbite, which owners might consider to be overgrowth. The clinic should have a book or reference guide that shows normal birds, giving the groomer an idea of proper beak length. Malocclusion of the beak from trauma, parasites, or developmental abnormalities will cause the beak to grow off center, predisposing the structure to become overgrown. Using a motor-driven hobby tool, one can shape the beak back into a normal appearance. The final result of the beak trim will depend on the anatomy one has to work with, based on the patient's history. Normally, the beak will grow from the underlying germinal epithelium covering the bone that provides the beak its foundation. As the beak epithelium grows out, it might do so in an irregular pattern, which, although normal, might not give the surface a smooth character that is desirable to the owner. Carefully applying the stone bit of the motor tool over the irregular areas will smooth out the beak. If the groomer puts too much pressure on the beak, the underlying vascular layer will be compromised and bleeding will occur. To smooth the lower beak, place the tip of the upper beak into the lower beak. Apply mineral oil to shine and moisten the beak surface, which provides a nice presentation for the owner. Practice and experience will help to improve beak-grooming techniques, especially on larger parrots and macaws.

Nail trimming is usually done upon owner request and not necessarily needed to provide good health maintenance. Bird nails can become very sharp, enabling a bird to hold on to the perch. Some birds, such as cockatoo species, have quick-growing nails that curl around, becoming entangled in the cage bars (Figure 1.15). The nails should be bluntly trimmed to the level of the plantar surface of the foot with a motor-driven hobby tool (Figures 1.16 and 1.17). If bleeding continues after the trim, silver nitrate–tipped wooden applicator sticks are recommended for hemostasis. Young birds' nails have a tendency to bleed more often than older birds' nails. The nails should be trimmed when the bird is hurting the owner or when there is excessive overgrowth. For small birds (e.g., <150 grams) electrocautery units can be used to reduce the length while providing hemostasis (Figure 1.18).

Blood feathers are new growing feathers ensheathed and engorged with blood that is carrying nutrient to the developing structure (Figure 1.19). If a primary or secondary blood feather is

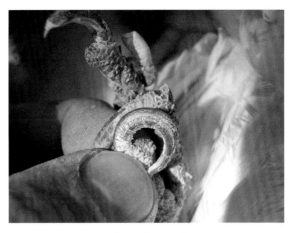

Figure 1.15 *Long claws that need trimming on a cockatoo.*

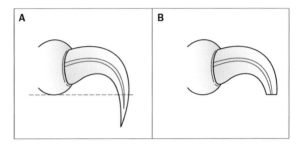

Figure 1.16 *Recommended length to trim a parrot's claw. Illustration by Michael L. Broussard.*

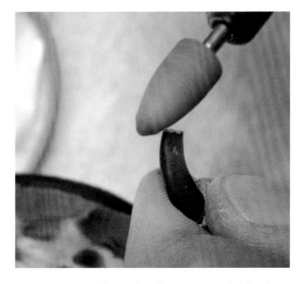

Figure 1.17 *A Dremel tool is recommended for claw trimming on larger parrot species.*

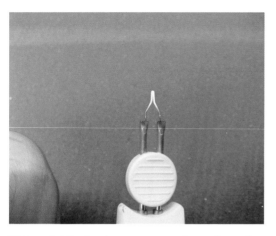

Figure 1.18 *An electrocautery unit can be used to trim claws on birds that weigh <150 grams.*

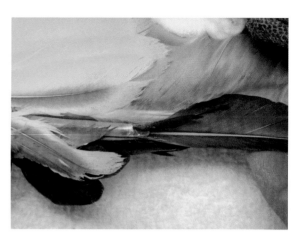

Figure 1.19 *A blood feather. The feather extending out of the sheath can be safely trimmed.*

cut or broken, grasp the base of the feather with hemostats and pull straight out. Digital pressure should be applied to the feather follicle for 2 to 3 minutes to aid in hemostasis.

Owners might have many reasons for wanting their bird's wing feathers trimmed. The main reason is to restrict flight capabilities, thereby preventing an unwanted escape. Often, birds that are flighted will be more independent, spending less quality time with the owner and increasing the possibility of flying into walls, ceiling fans, and glass doors. The owner should always be cautioned that trimming a bird's wing feathers will restrict flight, but will not prevent it. Precautions against flight should always be maintained when the bird is outdoors. In recent years, body harnesses have been made for pet birds, and these should be placed on a bird at an early age to expedite recognition and acceptance of these devices. The groomer should ask how the owner would like the wing feathers trimmed and what he or she wants to accomplish with the restricted flight. The more restrictions an owner places on a non-flighted bird, the greater the number of feathers

that will need to be trimmed. The main feathers to be trimmed are the primary flight feathers on both wings and, to a lesser extent, the secondary flight feathers (Figure 1.20). The feathers should be trimmed under the dorsal covert feathers so the cut feather cannot be seen when the wing is in the normal position. Adequate flight restriction can be obtained in short, fat birds (e.g., Amazon parrots, African gray parrots) with bilateral trimming of the primary flight feathers. In young African gray parrots, this is extremely important, because they often fall and cut open their chest over the keel bone. Many Amazon parrots have pretty orange secondary flight feathers that owners like to keep. Long, thin birds (e.g., cockatiels and conures) need to have their primary and secondary flight feathers trimmed to achieve adequate flight restriction. Many companion avian species need their wings trimmed twice a year.

Bird Bands and Microchipping

Companion birds are required to be identified, as stated by the Wild Bird Conservation Act. The most common method of identifying pet

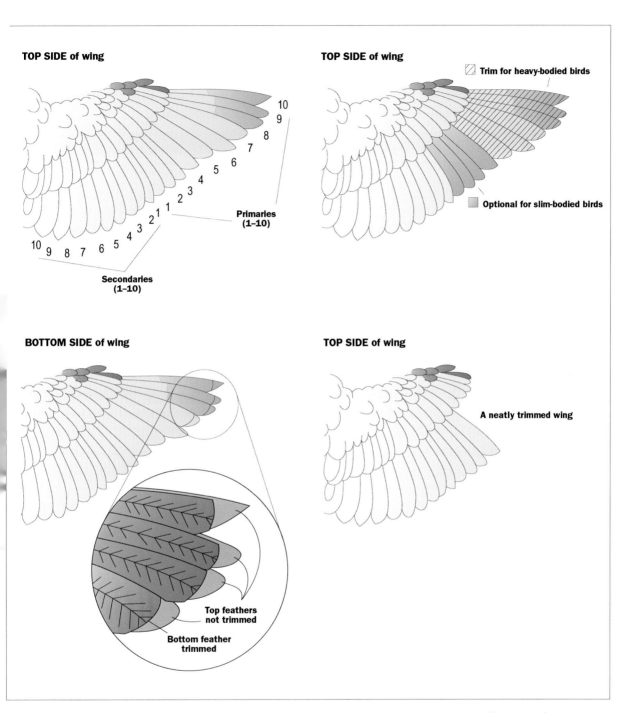

Figure 1.20 *A recommended method for trimming wing feathers on companion avian species. Illustration by Michael L. Broussard.*

and cage birds is by leg bands. Unfortunately, leg bands often become entangled in cage structures and toys. A safer option is removing the band and inserting a microchip into the pectoral muscle. This protects against leg injury or possible death, and the bird can still be identified.

HISTORY

As with other animal species, it is very important to get a thorough history from the owner prior to examining the avian patient. Identification is the first important information that the technician needs to obtain from the owner. Identification includes the name of the patient, species of bird, and the age (if known). Birds can be obtained from a number of sources, so it is important to know how long the animal has been at that particular house and where it was acquired in order to determine the overall patient health. Find out whether the owner can provide a vaccination history, when the bird last molted, and the character of feces. Most birds coming into the clinic will be companion animals, but some are breeding birds that are seldom, if ever, handled. Ask the owner if the bird is a pet bird or a breeding bird and how often it is taken out of the cage. Most breeding birds are housed in outdoor flights, but a specific understanding of where the bird is maintained is needed to determine if there has been possible exposure to wild avian species or vermin. Because most owners will bring the patient in a plastic pet carrier, the history should include the type and size of cage, substrate, toys and perches, disinfectants used, and regularity of cleaning the cage.

Once the environment has been determined, nutrition is the next major area of questioning. The specific brand, type, and amount of food, as well as how much the bird eats on a daily basis

(prior to the presenting problem and since it has been ill), must be determined. If there are any supplements or treats offered, this should be noted on the form. It is important to ask the owner how often the water is changed and the source of the water. There have been cases of embryonic and neonatal deaths that were caused by well water and automatic watering systems that contained bacteria.

A review of the total pet household, including other birds, must be noted in the history. This information would incorporate birds that are housed together, new bird additions to the aviary or household, recent attendance by the owner at bird shows/fairs, and quarantine procedures.

Once you have the information about the environment and history, you should review the patient's past and current health problems. If the bird was recently purchased, the new owner might not know the entire patient disease history. An investigative phone call to the previous owner can give you or the veterinarian important information that could help make a final diagnosis.

Before an avian patient is restrained to perform a physical exam, the technician determines an overview of the animal's general disposition from a distance. The bird should be examined for perching ability, ease of breathing, awareness of the surroundings, and stool characteristics. It is common for birds to have a very liquid stool when excited or in unfamiliar surroundings. The owner should be asked about any abnormalities in the patient's fecal color and consistency. Often a bird is presented in the cage in which it is housed and a number of droppings are on the paper substrate at the bottom for the veterinarian or technician to evaluate. If possible, this "hands-off" evaluation is best achieved when looking through a one-way mirror or a small window in the exam room door.

The bird will act more natural when it is alone in the room with the owner, rather than with someone it does not trust. Any abnormalities should be noted in the patient's record.

RESTRAINT

One of the greatest causes of anxiety for many veterinarians and veterinary technicians in this field is the capture and restraint of either a small bird or a large parrot. When catching a small bird, many are afraid of causing a sudden unexplained death; on the other hand, handlers of large parrots usually have a fear of personal injury. However, it is important to emphasize that it is the rare avian patient that dies from a "heart attack" or fear associated with the capture event. The technician must remember that sick birds are being presented to the veterinary clinic for care and treatment. During the initial assessment and history evaluation, one must decide if the patient is in a condition to be handled for further examination.

When an avian patient, or any exotic animal patient, is so ill that capture and restraint might cause death, the owner needs to be fully informed of the possible consequences. To reduce stress on small birds during capture, the overhead light should be turned off after the technician has established the location of the bird. In the dark, birds do not often move or see the hand prior to capture. The lighting of the room should be returned to normal once the patient is in the technician's hands. This method of capture works extremely well when a bird is free-flying in the room or with large, difficult-to-catch parrots. Small birds (<120 grams) can be held in one hand. The head is maintained between the forefinger and middle finger, as the bird rests in dorsal recumbency in the palm of the hand, with the thumb, ring finger, and pinkie loosely holding the body (Figure 1.21).

When working with large parrots, experience and the use of proper capture techniques help alleviate the fear of having fingers crushed by a large parrot's beak. Most injuries occur when the person trying to capture a large parrot is distracted or hesitates and is not concentrating on the primary goal of properly restraining the patient. For companion birds, capture should always be achieved through the use of a towel, which allows you to hide your hand as you maneuver it around the back of a bird's neck. If the bird has never been captured with a towel or is friendly, the towel should be presented from the front of the animal. The frontal presentation will not scare the bird, will allow it to see the towel during capture, and might prevent the bird from developing a fear of capture. If the bird is difficult to capture, it is recommended that you quickly grasp the back of the bird's neck with a toweled hand while the bird is biting the side of the transport carrier. Large birds

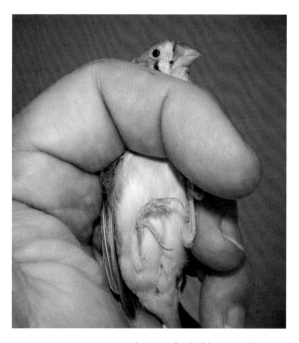

Figure 1.21 *Proper technique for holding small caged bird.*

should be held in an Elizabethan grip around the neck, with the thumb and forefinger touching and pressing up against the mandible, the other hand holding the feet. With the bird's head and feet restrained, the bird is held against the handler's body, thereby restricting one wing, while the other wing is held in place by the index and little finger of the hand holding the head. A towel can also be used to restrict the wings while restraining the avian patient (Figure 1.22). The Elizabethan grip does not damage the bird's face and gives the handler more control over the beak.

Once the patient has been captured with a towel (or in the case of breeder birds, with a net or gloves), it can be placed in an avian restraint device for examination or diagnostic testing (e.g., radiographs; Figure 1.23). This Plexiglas board can restrain birds from the size of a budgerigar to a hyacinth macaw. Typically, birds that are placed in the device are less stressed than ones held by veterinary technicians. The veterinary technician should loosely hold the bird's wings against its body to prevent the wings from flapping, potentially causing injury to the patient, while it is being placed in the restraint board. Birds in the restraint device can be examined and diagnostic samples obtained, including blood and choanal and cloacal cultures.

There are many different species of birds that might present to a veterinary clinic, each of which provides different obstacles and dangers to the person trying to capture the patient. If you are not sure how to capture and restrain an animal, please ask someone who knows the proper technique. This will help protect you and the patient from serious injury. Owls, eagles, and hawks have powerful sharp talons that can cause serious puncture wounds. Raptors need to be captured using leather gloves, and their feet should be taped prior to an examination. Herons, cranes, and egrets have long

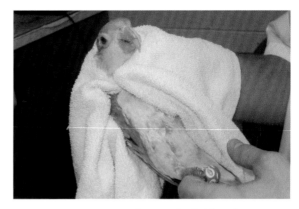

Figure 1.22 *Proper technique for holding larger parrot species.*

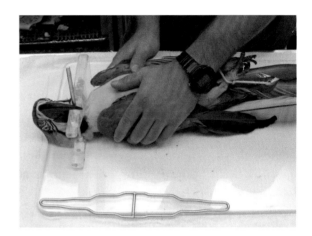

Figure 1.23 *A Plexiglas restraint board can be used for examination or positioning of patients for diagnostic imaging.*

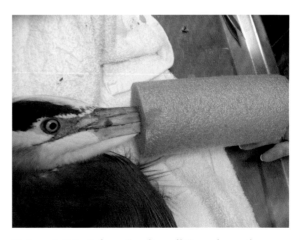

Figure 1.24 *A foam "pool noodle" can be used to reduce the "stabbing" danger from long, sharp beaks.*

sharp beaks, which they routinely thrust toward the eyes of someone they perceive as a threat to their well-being (Figure 1.24). These birds should be captured and restrained by someone who is wearing protective eyewear. Again, if you are not sure how to capture and restrain an avian patient, please ask an experienced veterinary technician or veterinarian.

PHYSICAL EXAMINATION

The first and most important information the veterinarian will obtain about the avian patient is the body weight. All exotic animal patients must be weighed on a digital gram scale that measures in 1-gram increments. Tame birds can be placed on a perch that is attached to the base of the scale with Velcro strips. Untamed birds can be weighed in a container or in the restraint device (Figure 1.25).

Once the bird has been examined prior to capture and it has been determined that the patient is in a condition to be restrained, the veterinarian will perform a hands-on physical examination. The feather quality is the first feature that is examined on the bird. Feathers are examined for abnormal molting, development, damage, abnormal color, ectoparasites, and feather loss (Figures 1.26 and 1.27). Next, the veterinarian will start at the head and look straight at the bird, analyzing the beak and eyes for asymmetry, and the beak for abnormal wear. The nares are examined next for any nasal discharge or intranasal growths associated with granulomas.

Ocular examinations are very important, especially on older birds and injured raptor species. The typical ophthalmology assessment includes looking for ocular discharge and eyelid, conjunctival, corneal, anterior chamber, and lens health. The foregoing parameters can be examined without using any equipment, including a small

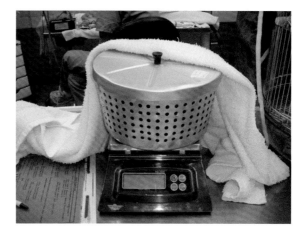

Figure 1.25 *Smaller birds can be weighed in a container.*

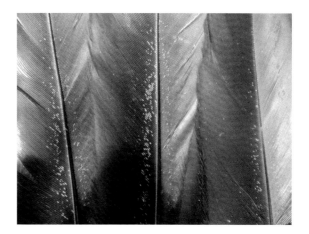

Figure 1.26 *Lice eggs (nits) on the feathers of an avian patient.*

animal ophthalmoscope. To examine the posterior chamber and retina, a more detailed ocular investigation is required. The more detailed ophthalmology examinations are required for raptors and pet birds that present with head trauma.

Using a beak speculum (Figure 1.28), the veterinarian will observe the oral cavity, including the choanal slit. The terminus of the upper respiratory system, the choanal slit, is lined with epithelial projections called papilla (Figure 1.29). The papilla readily sloughs in the presence of an

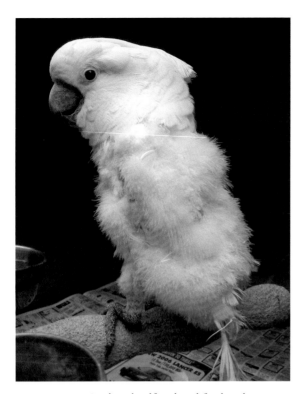

Figure 1.27 *Bird with self-induced feather damage.*

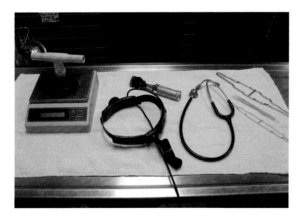

Figure 1.28 *Instruments and equipment used to properly examine a bird.*

upper respiratory infection. Evidence of a chronic upper respiratory infection includes sloughed papilla and a swollen, inflamed choanal slit. The oral cavity should be free of any abscesses, plaques, or necrotic

tissue. The glottis is located at the base of the tongue and should also be free of abscesses or epithelial plaques.

Most pet bird species have a dry oral cavity, which makes it difficult to determine hydration status in these species. Hydration status in avian species should be determined by assessing corneal moisture, globe position in the orbit, skin elasticity through skin tenting, cloacal mucosal moisture, and packed cell volume.

The crop, or ingluvies, is positioned at the level of the thoracic inlet. Crop stasis, or a large doughy feel to the crop because of undigested food, is often a sign of bacterial ingluvitis. Foreign bodies or trauma associated with hand-feeding might be noted as bruising in this area or by confirmation of a presentation history provided by the owner. If the owner feeds food that is too hot, bruising can occur; or if presentation of the patient is delayed after the thermal burn, necrosis of the crop and skin might be observed (Figure 1.30). A fistula can form at the location of the thoracic inlet, with the crop adhering to the surface epithelium—causing ingested food to dribble out onto the feathers. In this case, owners might complain of "food coming out of the bird's chest."

The keel bone is the modified sternum of flighted birds and is the location of the major pectoral muscles. The pectoral muscles on flighted birds can account for up to 20% of the total body weight. By palpating the pectoral muscles, one can determine the general body condition of a companion avian patient. The pectoral muscles should fill the entire space provided by the keel. If the keel is prominent, the bird is considered underweight (Figure 1.31).

In the caudal areas of a bird's body, very few diagnostic observations can be made because of the large surface area of the keel bone. Palpation of the

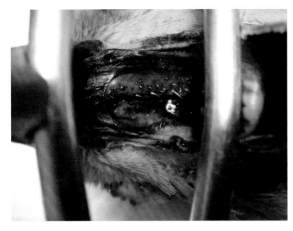

Figure 1.29 *Using an avian beak speculum to examine the choana.*

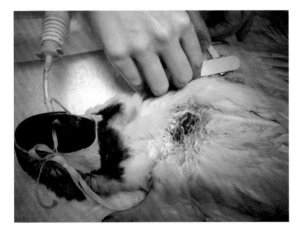

Figure 1.30 *Thermal trauma to the crop and surface epithelium due to feeding of overheated formula.*

caudal coelomic cavity behind the keel bone might reveal hepatomegaly associated with a tumor, an egg in the reproductive tract, or ascites resulting from internal ovulation. Cranial to the insertion of the tail feathers on the dorsal midline is the location of the uropygial, or preen gland (Figure 1.32). The uropygial gland is absent in some companion avian species, for example the Amazon parrot, but well developed in waterfowl. The gland is typically a bilobed structure with a papilla emanating from the center that might include a tuft of feath-

ers. Any bleeding, inflammation, or asymmetry of this gland is abnormal.

Most birds project their waste from the body; therefore, the feathers around the vent are normally clean. Any soiling or pasting of waste noted around the vent should be considered abnormal. The vent and cloaca are examined for papillomas (cloacal warts), especially in larger parrots and macaws. A cotton-tipped applicator can be placed in the cloaca, carefully everting the structure to observe the mucocutaneous junction. The normal appearance should be smooth, but if any roughness is observed on the tissue surface, further testing is required. Using 5% acetic acid (vinegar) applied to a cotton-tipped applicator and placing the solution on the questionable surface, one can obtain a tentative diagnosis. If the mucous surface of the cloaca is intact, the vinegar will not adhere, but if the surface is compromised by papillomas, the surface will turn white.

Birds' lungs are located on the ventral aspect of the thoracic vertebrae. By locating the head of the stethoscope on the dorsal body wall in this area, one may listen for any abnormal respiratory sounds. It is also very important to listen for abnormal respiratory sounds from the air sacs. A bird's body cavity is composed of four paired and one unpaired air sac. Coelomic fluid and space-occupying masses (e.g., tumors) can adversely affect airflow. Therefore, any sound noted when listening to the air sacs along the lateral body wall should be considered abnormal. The heart is best auscultated on the left lateral body wall under the wing in the axillary region. Auscultated heart murmurs in companion avian species, especially cockatoos, have been diagnosed with ventricular septal defects.

The wings and legs are the last body structures to be examined after the bird is auscultated. The wings and legs are examined for fractures, joint integrity,

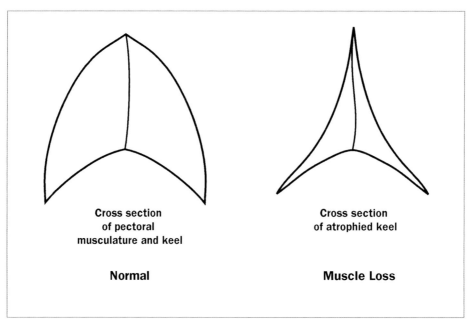

Figure 1.31 *Normal keel versus thin keel. Pectoral musculature helps determine the body condition of an avian patient. A full-bodied bird with a well-developed pectoral mass usually indicates good health. Illustration by Michael L. Broussard.*

and range of motion. The nails and plantar surface of the feet are the final areas that are assessed for any abnormal physical characteristics.

As with other animals, after the examination is complete, any abnormal findings are recorded and a list of differential diagnoses is established. Based on the top differential diagnoses, diagnostic tests are prioritized to confirm a diagnosis or to determine the severity of disease.

"Put It Down"
If the bird has an increased respiratory rate, excessive vocalization, or difficulty breathing during the physical examination, you might have to "put it down" until it is able to withstand the rigors of the evaluation process.

Use the following criteria to decide whether to put off evaluating an avian patient until a later time:[1]

- If the bird is panting or breathing rapidly, first alter your grip on its head, so the head is free to move. The bird should immediately begin to turn its head in search of something to bite. If it does not, PUT IT DOWN.
- A paper towel, or a corner of the towel being used to restrain the bird, can be placed into its mouth. It should immediately begin to bite at this, demonstrating that it has sufficient oxygen reserves to do so. If it lets the material lie lamely in its mouth, PUT IT DOWN.
- Have the bird grasp your hand or finger with both of its feet. (This should be part of the physical

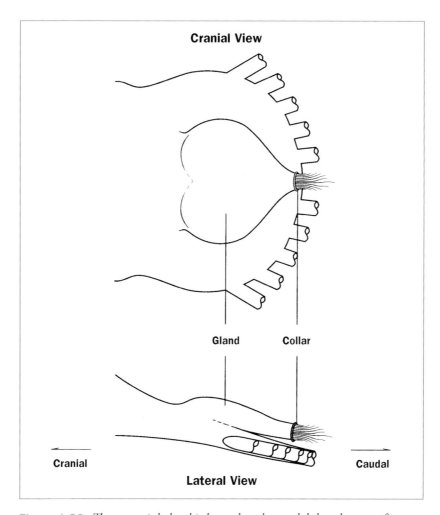

Figure 1.32 *The uropygial gland is located at the caudal dorsal aspect of many avian species. This gland aids in feather grooming and waterproofing. It is very well developed in aquatic avian species. Illustration by Michael L. Broussard.*

examination, to determine symmetry and strength of grip.) If the bird's grip is weak or nonexistent, PUT IT DOWN.

- If the bird's eyes close during the physical examination, PUT IT DOWN. Conversely, do not be reassured if the bird has its eyes open— many birds hold their eyes open as they draw their last breath.
- If in doubt, PUT IT DOWN. Return the bird to the location (cage, owner) where it is most

comfortable and observe it while discussing possible etiologies for the bird's decreased respiratory capacity with the owner.

DIAGNOSTIC SAMPLING

Blood Collection

Many veterinarians and veterinary technicians think that it is nearly impossible to obtain any usable quantity of blood from an avian patient

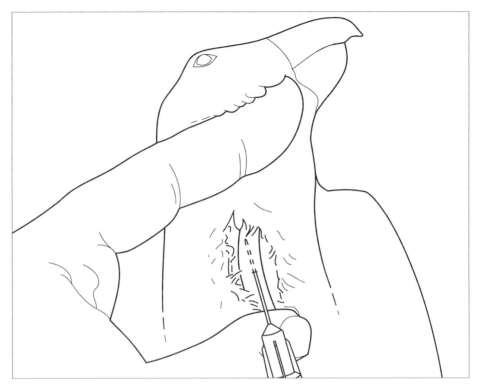

Figure 1.33 *Proper technique for collecting blood from a bird's jugular vein. Illustration by Michael L. Broussard.*

without compromising its health or killing the bird. (See Chapter 2 for additional information on preparation of blood smear, estimate of white blood count, and determination of differential cell count.) This is a totally false assumption that has been perpetuated within the profession. With the technology available today, blood samples can be easily obtained (even from the smallest avian patient) that will provide usable diagnostic information. Approximately 1% of the bird's blood volume can be taken safely for diagnostic testing, or 1 ml/100 grams of body weight.

Each particular avian species has a vein that is recommended as the choice site for blood collection. In companion avian species, this is the right jugular vein (Figure 1.33). Birds do have a left jugular vein, but it is less developed than the right.

Other veins or venous sinuses that can be used for blood collection in avian patients are the basilic vein (Figure 1.34), the median metatarsal vein, or the occipital venous sinus. Blood collection techniques used for other animals should be followed with avian patients. The right jugular vein can be observed in a featherless tract of epithelium in the right lateral cervical region. A 3 cc syringe with a 26-gauge needle is recommended as the instrument of choice for birds weighing more than 30 grams and less than 2 kilograms. For birds less than 30 grams, a 1 cc syringe is recommended, because of the low volume of blood that can be safely removed from the patient. Unless the patient is extremely fractious, no general anesthesia is required when drawing blood. Once the blood has been retrieved in the syringe, it should be placed

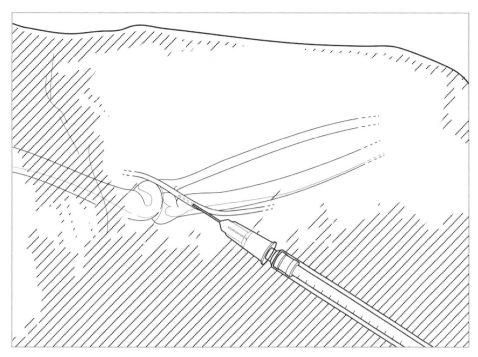

Figure 1.34 *Location of the basilic vein for blood collection and intravenous administration of therapeutic agents. Illustration by Michael L. Broussard.*

in a Microtainer tube (Becton Dickinson Microbiology Systems, Cockeysville, MD) and gently agitated to allow exposure to the anticoagulant. This procedure needs to be performed quickly because avian blood has a tendency to coagulate rapidly. Table 1.1 lists the hematological reference ranges for parrot species, and Table 1.2 lists the plasma biochemical reference ranges for common parrot species. For hematological testing or complete blood counts, a purple top Microtainer tube is recommended, and for plasma biochemistries, a green top Microtainer tube should be used.[2]

Bone Marrow Aspiration

The site of choice in avian patients for bone marrow aspiration is the proximal tibiotarsal bone. A 22-gauge, 1.5" spinal needle is placed at the lateral aspect of the proximal tibiotarsal bone of an anesthetized patient (Figure 1.35). The needle is slowly rotated with gentle pressure toward the medullary cavity. When a sudden reduction of pressure is felt, the medullary cavity has been reached, and the technician then removes the stylet of the spinal needle. A 6 cc syringe is placed on the needle, and bone marrow is drawn into the needle with short quick pulls on the plunger. In birds the common amount of bone marrow aspirated will fill the hub of the needle. Pressure is released off the plunger, and the needle removed from the bone. Remove the needle from the syringe and draw about 4–5 cc of air into the syringe, place the needle back on the syringe, and eject needle contents on a clean microscope slide.

Microbiology

Microbiological sampling techniques that are used on other animals can be applied to the avian

Table 1.1 Avian Hematological Reference Ranges[2]

VALUE	AFRICAN GRAY PARROT	AMAZON PARROT	BUDGERIGAR	COCKATIEL	COCKATOO	CONURE	ECLECTUS PARROT	LOVEBIRD	MACAW	PIONUS	QUAKER PARROT
Hematocrit (%)	42–53	43–49	44–54	43–58	42–51	43–56	43–50	43–55	43–54	43–54	n/a
Red Blood Cells ($\times 10^6$/ml)	2.80–3.36	2.33–2.95	3.90–4.70	3.8–4.58	2.50–2.95	3.13–3.94	2.7–3.1	2.63–3.50	n/a	2.7–3.5	n/a
Hemoglobin (g/d)	15.1–16.9	14.4–16.7	13.4–15.3	12.1–14.6	12.0–14.8	12.1–14.8	14.1–16.0	11.9–15.1	n/a	14.2–15.5	n/a
Mean Corpuscular Volume (fl)	143–155	163–170	115–124	128–142	154–170	135–147	157–170	155–166	n/a	154–164	n/a
Mean Corpuscular Hemoglobin (g/dl)	32.3–45.6	49.8–58.2	25.9–30.9	24.9–36.0	45.0–55.5	30.0–40.1	51.3–54.2	40–48	n/a	41.4–46.0	n/a
Mean Corpuscular Hb Concentration (g/dl)	23.16–31.78	32.8–35.31	19.80–26.75	18.91–25.61	24.12–32.91	23.5–28.6	31.2–34.0	21.9–29.3	n/a	25.8–28.7	n/a
White Blood Cells ($\times 10^3$/ml)	6.0–13.0	5.0–12.5	3.0–8.0	5.0–9.0	5.0–12.0	4.0–9.0	9.0–15.0	3.0–8.0	7.0–12.0	5.0–13.0	8.0–17.0
Heterophils (%)	45–72	32–71	41–67	47–72	45–72	45–72	46–70	41–71	48–72	55–74	47–70
Lymphocytes (%)	25–50	20–65	22–58	27–58	20–50	22–49	23–57	28–52	18–52	19–70	20–63
Monocytes (%)	0–1	0–1	0–2	0–1	0–1	0–1	0–1	0–1	0–1	0–1	0–4
Eosinophils (%)	0–1	0–0.05	0–0.05	0–2	0–2	0–1	0–1	0–1	0–1	0–1	0–4

Table 1.2 Avian Plasma Biochemical Reference Ranges[2]

VALUE	AFRICAN GRAY PARROT	AMAZON PARROT	BUDGERIGAR	COCKATIEL	COCKATOO	CONURE	ECLECTUS PARROT	LOVEBIRD	MACAW
Albumin (g/dl)	0.2–2.4	0.3–2.4	0.9–1.2	0.8–1.8	0.3–0.9	0.3–0.9	1.1–2	0.3–0.9	0.3–2.4
Alkaline Phosphate (U/L)	12.0–92.0	8.0–100.0	24.0–96.0	12.0–100.0	24.0–104.0	24.0–104.0	32.0–111.0	n/a	12.0–100.0
Amylase (U/L)	415–626	184–478	302–560	113–870	288–876	192–954	562–684	n/a	239–564
Aspartate Aminotransferase [AST] (U/L)	112–339	155–380	160–372	130–390	145–346	147–360	144–339	130–343	60–165
Bile Acids (mol/L)	12.0–85.0	35.0–144.0	35.0–110.0	45.0–105.0	37.0–98.0	35.0–90.0	30.0–110.0	34.0–88.0	30.0–80.0
Calcium (mg/dl)	8.3–11.7	8.5–13.0	8.5–11.0	8.3–10.9	8.4–11.0	8.4–11.0	8.1–11.9	8.6–11.5	8.3–11.0
Cholesterol (mg/dl)	100–250	150–220	120–220	90–195	90–200	83–190	100–261	125–195	96–264
Creatine Kinase [CK] (U/L)	120–410	120–410	120–360	167–420	150–400	140–397	132–410	160–320	90–360
Creatinine (mg/dl)	0.1–0.5	n/a	n/a	0.1–0.5	0.1–0.8	0.1–0.8	n/a	0.1–0.8	0.1–0.7
Globulin (g/dl)	1.2–3.6	1.6–3.7	1.1–1.7	2.5–3.8	2.5–3.8	2.5–3.8	2.0–3.32	2.5–3.8	2.1–3.8
Phosphorus (mg/dl)	3.5–6.9	n/a	3.7–7.1	4.0–7.7	4.2–7.8	4.0–7.9	n/a	n/a	4.0–7.8
Protein, Plasma (g/dl)	2.7–4.4	2.6–4.5	2.1–4.3	2.1–4.8	2.6–2.8	2.4–4.9	3.2–4.3	1.8–3.7	2.4–4.4
Uric Acid (mg/dl)	1.9–9.7	2.3–9.8	4.0–12.2	3.5–10.4	3.6–10.7	2.7–10.2	2.0–11.0	3.2–10.2	1.5–11.0

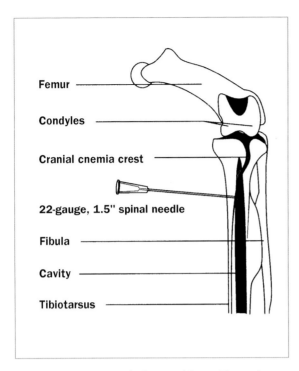

Figure 1.35 *Proximal tibiotarsal bone. This is the site of choice for bone marrow aspiration. Illustration by Michael L. Broussard.*

patient. Regular and mini-tipped culturettes are used, depending on the size of the orifice being sampled. Larger culturettes are recommended whenever possible, to increase the chances of isolating a pathogenic organism. Common sites cultured in avian patients include the choana, crop, and cloaca (terminus of the digestive tract). Cultures are also taken of internal lesions through an endoscopic cannula or biopsy samples of abnormal tissue.

Most of the organisms associated with avian disease are aerobic, and this is the most common diagnostic growth test. If there is a possibility of an anaerobic organism causing disease in the patient, inform laboratory personnel about the differential diagnosis, so they can properly prepare the sample for isolation of that class of bacteria. The same

protocol should be followed for fungal and mycobacterium isolation and identification.

Common pathogenic bacterial isolates in companion avian species include some *E. coli* and *Enterobacter* spp., *Pseudomonas* spp., *Klebsiella* spp., and in some cases *Mycobacterium avium*. *Aspergillus* spp. are often diagnosed in raptors and waterfowl that are stressed through rehabilitation or oil spill cleanup procedures. Common fungal infections in companion avian species also include *Aspergillus* spp. (especially African gray parrots) and *Candida albicans* (especially in young hand-fed birds). The first diagnostic test that might be performed is a Gram's stain on the fecal material. The Gram's staining of fecal material or crop contents will help the veterinarian assess gastrointestinal health through determination of current flora within the digestive system. Companion avian species should have a majority of Gram-positive rods and very few, if any, *Candida albicans* organisms (oval-shaped Gram-positive organisms). If any Gram-negative rods are noted on the stain, a total evaluation of the patient will be performed to determine the significance of the finding. A patient with diarrhea or that is anorexic upon presentation could be affected by the abnormal percentage of Gram-negative organisms and further testing will be initiated. Birds showing no abnormal signs usually are not affected by an abnormal bacterial population, but should be monitored and tested to establish baseline data.

Radiology

Companion avian species, in most cases, should be radiographed under general anesthesia on an avian restraint board, using isoflurane or sevoflurane, in order to increase the chances of obtaining quality radiographs with minimal stress to the bird. Proper assessment of the patient is required to determine the animal's ability to withstand this procedure. Common presentations that require radiographs include trauma, fractures, heavy metal toxicosis, respiratory distress, gastrointestinal stasis (proventricular dilatation disease), swallowing a foreign body, and nonspecific neurologic signs. Digital radiographic units are recommended, but if not available, high-detail film is a must when radiographing any small exotic animal species, especially birds. The same radiology techniques used for other companion animals need to be followed with avian species. This would include always getting two views, on perpendicular planes, of the desired area of interest. Closing the pop-off valve and maintaining the patient in an inflated state when the radiographic image is acquired will increase the contrast of internal organs and body systems.

Other Diagnostic Imaging Modalities

In recent years there has been an increased usage of ultrasound (US), computed tomography (CT), and magnetic resonance imaging (MRI) on avian species. As with traditional radiographic imaging, it is recommended that the avian patient be placed under general anesthesia for these alternative diagnostic imaging procedures. Because of the air sac system of birds' lower respiratory tract, US images are difficult to obtain within the body cavity. The liver and heart can be imaged through ultrasonography, because there is a continuous tissue window caudal to the keel through the liver into the heart. Because the window is very small, heart assessment using echocardiography is limited. CT and MRI procedures can be performed on birds and offer a significant amount of information in cases for which these diagnostic modalities are recommended. Preparation of the patient prior to the MRI and CT procedures is important because of machine platform movement, cool air temperatures within the room where the machines

are located, length of procedure (particularly for MRI), and the need to monitor the patient from outside the room when the images are obtained. It is always recommended that you use diagnostic imaging personnel who are familiar with performing examinations on avian patients and interpreting those results.

Parasitology

External Parasites

As discussed earlier, many new bird owners believe that all avian species commonly have external parasites, particularly lice. It is important that veterinary clinic personnel inform these owners that it is rare for pet avian species to become infested with any type of external parasite. Caged birds are seldom exposed to environments where they would contact the parasites that live on the skin or feathers. Outdoor aviaries, where people breed parrot species, might provide the opportunity for the transmission of lice or mites from infested native birds. Raptors, waterfowl, and other fowl will commonly present with ectoparasites, at which time the owner should be guided to initiate treatment of the bird and environment. Most of the external parasites that are mentioned in this section can be treated with ivermectin, with the recommended dose being 0.2 mg/kg orally or subcutaneously for 2 to 3 treatments, 14 days apart (Ivomec, Merck AgVet Division, Rahway, NJ), or fipronil, spraying on the skin under the wings and repeating in 30 days (Frontline, Merial, Duluth, GA).[3]

If birds are maintained indoors, there is very little chance of exposure to external parasites. Aviary birds and other avian species that are maintained in flights have a better chance of being diagnosed with parasitic arthropods. There are two common ectoparasites that infest caged birds: *Sternostoma tracheacolum* and *Knemidokoptes* spp. *Sternostoma*

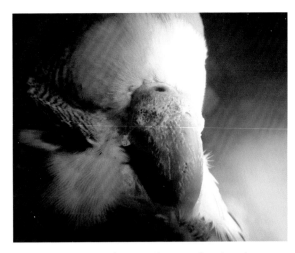

Figure 1.36A *Budgerigar that is infested with* Knemidokoptes *spp. mites.*

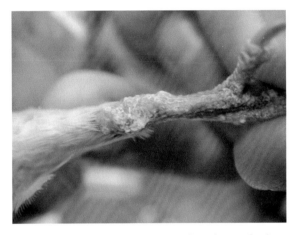

Figure 1.36B *This mite species affects the nonfeathered areas of the bird.*

tracheacolum is also known as the tracheal/air sac mite, and it mainly affects canaries and finches. Birds diagnosed with the tracheal mite show signs of respiratory distress and make a clicking sound when breathing. Ivermectin is the treatment of choice for birds infested with *Sternostoma tracheacolum*.

Knemidokoptes spp. lives in the featherless areas around the face and legs (Figures 1.36A and 1.36B). Common names for these arthropod parasites are scaly face and scaly leg mites.

The names are derived from the irritation of the surface epithelium that causes a hyperkeratosis of the affected skin and beak. Budgerigars are the most common pet birds to be diagnosed with *Knemidokoptes* spp., although other species can be susceptible, particularly eclectus parrots and canaries. As with tracheal mites, ivermectin is the treatment of choice for *Knemidokoptes* spp.

Chewing lice of the order Mallophaga and domestic poultry mites, *Dermanyssus gallinae* and *Ornithodoros sylviarum*, can affect parrot species that live outdoors in breeding flights. Environmental cleaning is very important in the prevention of reinfestation of the lice and mites. A 5% carbaryl powder can be used in conjunction with ivermectin therapy to treat infested birds.

Internal Parasites

As with external parasites, internal parasites are uncommon in companion birds that are hand-raised and maintained indoors. Birds that live in breeding flights, and especially birds that have access to the ground, have a better chance of exposure to internal parasite eggs and larvae. All birds should have direct fecal and fecal flotation examinations as part of a complete health check. Psittacine species infected with the protozoan parasite *Giardia psittaci* will present with chronic to intermittent watery diarrhea and with loose, malodorous mucoid stools.[3] Another protozoan parasite that is diagnosed in avian patients (particularly doves, pigeons, and raptors) is *Trichomonas gallinae*. Whereas giardiasis is associated with the intestinal tract, trichomoniasis is found as white plaques or necrotic masses in the mouth and esophagus.[4] Metronidazole (Flagyl, G. D. Searle Co., Chicago, IL; this is a generic product sold by many companies) can be used to treat both *Giardia psittaci* and *Trichomonas gallinae*.

Two coccidian parasites can be diagnosed in caged birds. *Atoxoplasma* spp. organisms are diagnosed in canaries, finches, and mynah birds. The diagnosis is usually made during a pathology examination of a dead juvenile bird that has died shortly after appearing depressed and fluffed. *Atoxoplasma* spp. organisms are shed in the feces of adults that show no signs of infection. Treatment of any coccidian disease is difficult; often the best outcome is a reduction of shedding and exposure to unaffected birds. Trimethoprim/sulfadiazine (Roche Pharmaceuticals, Nutley, NJ; this is a generic product sold by many companies) is the recommended treatment for avian coccidian parasitic diseases. *Sarcocystis falcatula* is the other coccidian parasite diagnosed in companion avian species. This parasite usually affects aviary birds housed outdoors in breeding flights. The life cycle of *Sarcocystis falcatula* involves the opossum (*Didelphis virginiana*) and cockroaches. As with *Atoxoplasma* spp., *Sarcocystis falcatula* is usually diagnosed during a pathology examination of a dead bird. The extensive life cycle requirements of the parasite make environmental management extremely important if the owner wants to prevent exposure and infection within an aviary.

Hemoproteus spp., *Plasmodium* spp., and *Leukocytozoon* spp. are parasites that might be noted in red blood cells of wild-caught psittacine species, raptors, doves, and pigeons. These parasites are transmitted through the bite of infected arthropods. Unless there is an overwhelming infestation of these parasites, treatment is not recommended.

Before the Wild Bird Conservation Act was passed in the early 1990s, a vast number of large psittacine species were being imported into the United States. Wild-caught cockatoo species and African gray parrots were often diagnosed with tapeworms. With the passage of the conservation act, the number of these species being diagnosed with cestodes has diminished. Treatment of cestode infestations can be accomplished with praziquantel (Droncit, Haver/Diamond Scientific, Shawnee, KS; this is a generic product sold by many companies).

Nematodes, as with most of the parasites that affect avian species, commonly affect birds that live in outdoor environments. Ascarids have a direct life cycle, in which simply ingesting eggs can infect a bird, whereas *Capillaria* spp. and *Syngamus trachea* need earthworms as an intermediate host. Ascarids and *Capillaria* spp. live in the intestinal tract, and *Syngamus trachea* are found in the oral cavity and esophagus. Birds infested with intestinal parasites will be depressed and emaciated. In most cases, nematode eggs are shed in the feces and can be seen in a fecal flotation exam. It is important to treat the bird and, if possible, the environment.

SURGICAL AND ANESTHETIC ASSISTANCE

Surgical preparation techniques for birds are similar to those for other species treated at a small-animal hospital. There are a few main differences regarding avian species, and they will be covered in this section. The normal body temperature for birds ranges from 103° to 105°F. To maintain this high body temperature, birds eat often, and the food rapidly passes through the digestive tract. For this reason, fasting is recommended only for 2 hours prior to surgery. For isoflurane or sevoflurane anesthesia, birds are induced via a face mask and then intubated with a noncuffed endotracheal tube (Figure 1.37). A noncuffed endotracheal tube is recommended because most avian species have complete tracheal rings and an inflated cuff could induce pressure necrosis on the epithelium lining of the trachea. The glottis is readily observed at the base of the tongue once this anatomical structure is extended using hemostats (Figure 1.38). The neck should be extended when placing the endotracheal tube

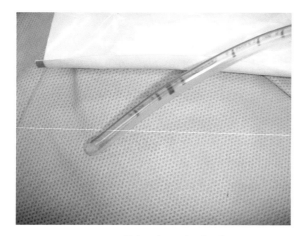

Figure 1.37 *Noncuffed endotracheal tube, recommended for avian species.*

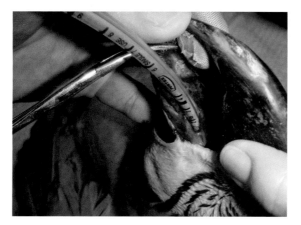

Figure 1.38 *Endotracheal tube in place on a blue and gold macaw.*

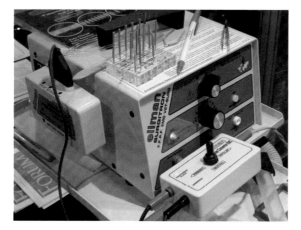

Figure 1.39 *A radiosurgery unit is an essential piece of equipment for an avian/exotic animal practice.*

into the recommended position, about the mid-cervical region. It must be remembered that the syrinx, or voice box, of avian species is located at the tracheal bifurcation. With the syrinx located at this level in the respiratory tract, a patient can still vocalize—even with proper placement of the endotracheal tube. If head surgery needs to be performed or if there is a blockage of the trachea, an air sac cannulation can take place to provide oxygen or anesthesia into the respiratory system. Isoflurane anesthesia has a side effect of respiratory depression; therefore, bagging the patient 2 to 3 times a minute will help offset any problems caused by the anesthetic gas.

The surgical plane of anesthesia and patient status can be monitored by the palpebral and pedal reflexes, heart and respiration rate, and plucking feathers. To prepare a surgical site on the body, feathers must be plucked in the direction opposite of the way they lie (against the grain). A wide area must be plucked and feathers removed from the surgical field with a handheld vacuum device. Feathers have the amazing tendency to reappear in the surgical field if not properly removed. Once feathers are removed from the surgical site, the skin is well exposed for the procedure. Site preparation is much less involved for birds than for mammalian species that have been clipped. Surgical scrub should involve two scrubs, using a commercial surgical scrub product and sterile saline. Often radiosurgical units are used in avian surgical procedures (Figure 1.39). If alcohol is used as part of the scrub procedure, the bird will be in flames when the surgeon initiates the incision. Alcohol also contributes to hypothermia in the patient, increasing surgical complications for the anesthetist. To monitor body temperature, an esophageal thermometer works much better than a cloacal probe. To maintain heat, a veterinary conductive fabric warming unit (Hot Dog,

Augustine Biomedical & Design, Eden Prairie, MN) is placed under the patient and a convective air heating device placed around the patient (Bair Hugger Arizant Health Care, Eden Prairie, MN) (Figures 1.40 and 1.41).

Clear plastic drapes help the anesthetist monitor the patient during surgery. The plastic drapes help in observing the bird's respiration, but could contribute to hyperthermia. Any change in the patient's temperature is best monitored with a thermometer, and actions should be quickly taken to stabilize the body temperature into the normal range. A respiratory monitor that is attached to the tracheal tube and the tube extending from the anesthesia machine will put out sounds with each breath. These monitors can be used on birds that are as small as budgerigars to birds that are as large as ostriches. The respiratory monitor will help the anesthetist determine if the bird is going into a deeper plane of anesthesia or is becoming "light." Recent years have seen significant advances in surgical monitoring devices that allow patient assessment while under general anesthesia (DVM Solutions, San Antonio, TX). These new monitoring devices can measure respiration, heart rate, body temperature, and exhaled CO_2, among other parameters (Figure 1.42).

Birds should recover quickly from gas anesthesia. Once the vaporizer is turned off, oxygen should be administered until the patient shows signs of recovery. During recovery, the bird must be maintained in a critical care unit to help with body temperature stabilization (Figure 1.43).

HEALTH MAINTENANCE AND DISEASE

Respiratory and Gastrointestinal Bacterial/Fungal Infections

Birds have a well-developed respiratory system that is composed of 4 paired and 1 unpaired air

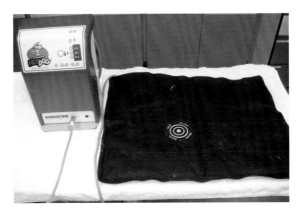

Figure 1.40 *Conductive thermal heating blankets have replaced the traditional warm water blanket.*

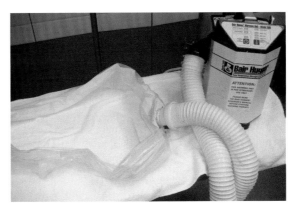

Figure 1.41 *Convective heating units help stabilize a bird's body temperature during surgery and critical presentations.*

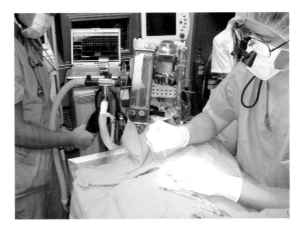

Figure 1.42 *It is very important to use magnification and monitoring equipment when performing avian surgery.*

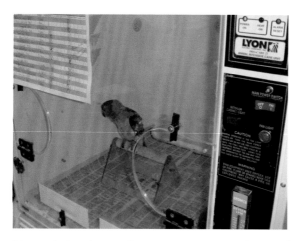

Figure 1.43 *A critical care unit is an essential piece of equipment for clinics that treat avian patients.*

sac(s) and an extensive upper respiratory sinus (infraorbital) (Figure 1.44). Most people assume that the only diet a bird should eat is seed. As a result, many pet birds are fed a diet deficient in vitamins, especially vitamin A. Because vitamin A is an integral component of epithelial health, a companion bird that is suffering from hypovitaminosis A will have a compromised respiratory and gastrointestinal epithelium. The compromised epithelial surface provides an environment for microorganisms to adhere to and infect the bird. External stress factors affect the immune system of birds, which reduces their internal ability to fight the infection or aid antibiotic treatment. Birds that are immature, old, being transported, quarantined, or in shows are the most susceptible to bacterial and fungal infections. Some avian species are able to handle external stresses better than others. The gyrfalcon and red-tailed hawk commonly become infected with *Aspergillus* spp.

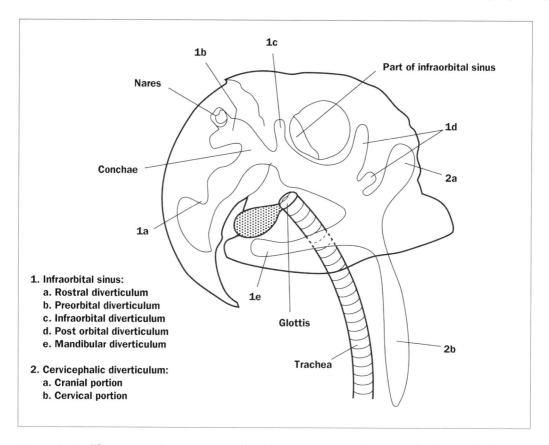

Figure 1.44 *The upper respiratory system of birds is very extensive. Illustration by Michael L. Broussard.*

infections, whereas other raptors are less susceptible to this often-fatal fungal infection.

It is essential to identify the organism and find out what drug(s) will effectively treat bacterial and fungal infections (Figure 1.45). Stabilization of the patient and boosting its physiologic status through supportive care will aid in the successful treatment of these cases. If birds are not diagnosed or treated properly for the appropriate length of time, the bacterial and fungal infections can kill them or cause irreversible anatomic damage.

Feather Picking and Feather Loss

One of the most frustrating avian case presentations for veterinarians to treat is a bird suffering from feather loss or self-inflicted feather picking. If the head feathers are intact, this usually means that the animal is pulling or traumatizing its own feathers. If the head feathers are also affected, this often indicates a generalized health problem. The veterinarian will give a bird with feather loss a complete physical examination, incorporating a good owner history, to make sure there are no treatable medical problems before making a diagnosis of psychological feather picking.

A number of parasitic, infectious, and noninfectious diseases can initiate and perpetuate feather loss in a pet bird. It is only through the thorough and diligent understanding of a case that the correct treatment can be provided to the patient. If it is determined that the problem is psychological, environmental and nutritional changes can be recommended to the owner for a possible resolution of the problem. If the initial recommendations are unsuccessful, veterinarians can prescribe psychotropic, antidepressant, or antihistamine drugs. Researchers are investigating the possibility of hypersensitivity reactions in pet birds and agents that might cause allergic reactions.

Elizabethan collars have been used with some success in preventing birds from pulling feathers. An alternative to Elizbethan collars are "neck stretchers" that are made out of foam "pool noodles" or hexalite cast material (Figures 1.46A and 1.46B). Though helpful, both of these alternatives are just physical barriers and do not actually treat the underlying cause of feather picking. The primary cause should be identified and treated for long-lasting resolution of this frustrating disease.

Trauma

There are many situations in which birds can become injured through traumatic accidents. Flying into ceiling fans, sliding glass doors, walls, and cars; getting burned in water or being burned by hand-feeding formula; and being bitten by a cagemate (or other animal such as a dog or cat) are the most common causes of traumatic injury to avian patients. Upon presentation, a traumatized patient should be quickly assessed and stabilized. Only when the patient is stabilized should extensive treatment or diagnostics take place. Maintaining hydration status and treating

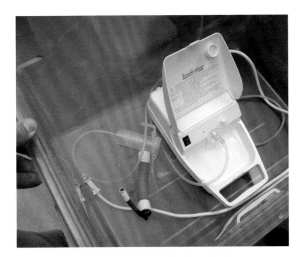

Figure 1.45 *Components needed to nebulize avian patients.*

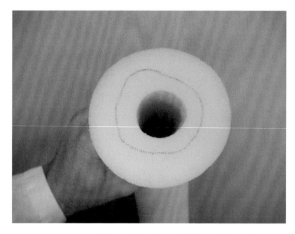

Figure 1.46A *A foam "pool noodle" can be used to make a neck extender.*

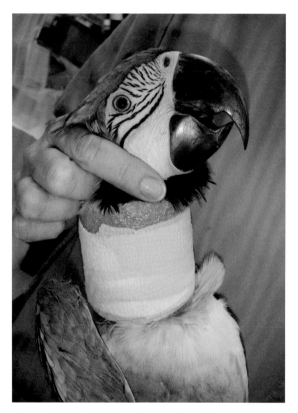

Figure 1.46B *Pool noodles can be used to prevent self-trauma.*

shock, parasites, and infection are required for serious injuries (Figure 1.47). Educating owners about common household hazards and trimming a bird's wings will reduce the incidence of traumatic injury.

Egg-Binding

Dystocia, or egg-binding, is the inability of a hen to complete the process of laying an egg. The egg usually is caught in the shell gland of the oviduct and needs to be removed by the veterinarian. Cockatiels are one of the most common pet bird species that present with this problem. Treatment for egg-binding includes heat, humidity, calcium, oxytocin, and propulcid. After the hen has been stabilized and the therapeutic agents have been given an appropriate length of time to take effect, a slow, gentle push on the egg toward the cloaca often aids in its expulsion from the vent, usually with the bird under general anesthesia for increased relaxation of the abdominal muscles and cloaca. Aspiration of the egg contents and subsequent collapse of the shell might aid in the passage of misshapen or abnormally large eggs. In birds that have a history of egg-binding or laying a large number of eggs, a salpingectomy is advised to prevent a possible future life-threatening condition.

Heavy Metal Toxicosis

Lead and zinc are the most common heavy metal toxins that affect pet birds. Companion birds come into contact with lead from peeling paint, weights, toys, solder, wine caps, and lead-headed nails. Zinc exposure is usually through galvanized wire and containers and toys. If a bird presents with neurologic signs, a heavy metal screen should be performed. Zinc toxicity is more nonspecific, usually presenting as gastroenteritis. Radiographs

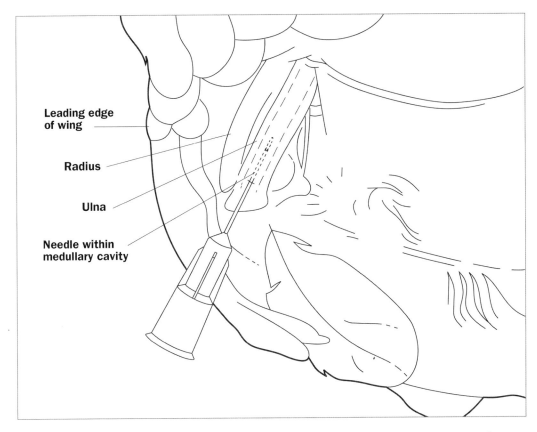

Figure 1.47 *Proper placement of an intraosseus catheter. Illustration by Michael L. Broussard.*

often identify heavy metal foreign bodies within the gastrointestinal tract. Chelation therapy can be initiated immediately if heavy metal toxicosis is suspected. The use of calcium disodium ethylene-diaminetetraacetate should be carefully monitored, because it has been reported to cause gastrointestinal and renal toxicosis.[5] Removal of the foreign body(ies) through the use of laxatives or surgery will accelerate the treatment process. Uptake of the serologic heavy metal by bone tissue will often cause a relapse of the disease after the initial treatment, because the body will absorb the dead bone cells containing the material. The relapse condition must be mentioned to the owner—noting that periodic rechecks and blood testing will monitor the patient's condition until the danger is over, which is often more than a six-month period.

Other Diseases

There are many other diseases that infect companion avian species. Common viral diseases include polyoma virus, psittacine beak, and feather disease. It is believed that bornavirus might be associated with proventricular dilatation disease. A herpesvirus may be the underlying etiologic agent responsible for causing papillomatosis in large parrot species and macaws, an idea not universally accepted. Reputable diagnostic laboratories have tests to identify polyoma virus, psittacine beak and feather disease, and bornavirus. A vaccine for polyoma virus is available to protect birds from this devastating disease. It is important to vaccinate both young and older birds to maintain aviary health and protect the reputation of bird breeders.

ZOONOTIC DISEASES

The primary zoonotic disease associated with pet birds is *Chlamydia psittaci*. Avian chlamydiosis is an intracellular bacterium that presents as a number of disease conditions in birds, but is a respiratory condition in humans. The organism is spread through respiratory secretions and fecal material from infected birds. If an owner develops spiking temperature episodes and a chronic respiratory condition, a physician must be notified of the ownership of birds. *The Compendium of Measures to Control* Chlamydophila psittaci *Infection Among Humans (Psittacosis) and Pet Birds (Avian Chlamydiosis)*, 2010, is published by the public health veterinarians in conjunction with the Centers for Disease Control and Prevention, and outlines human and avian disease conditions, diagnostic methods, and treatment regimes.[6]

SELF-STUDY QUESTIONS

1. Describe basic husbandry recommendations for a pet bird. Include cage size, location, cage environment, and recommended ambient temperature of the area in which the cage is placed.

2. Describe the recommended diet for most companion avian species.

3. What is the recommended technique for capturing and restraining a large parrot? A canary?

4. How is the hydration status of a bird evaluated?

5. Describe the proper method of performing a physical examination on an avian patient.

6. For most pet birds, how is the body condition evaluated?

7. If a bird gets stressed during the physical examination, what are the five criteria used to "put it down" and place it in a critical care unit?

8. How much blood can be safely collected from an avian patient?

9. Describe blood collection techniques used for avian patients.

10. What common anatomical sites are bacterial cultures collected from and what pathogenic organisms are often isolated?

11. Describe the common diagnostic imaging modalities used for avian species. List advantages and disadvantages of each regarding avian patients.

12. Describe how to intubate a bird.

13. How do you assess depth of anesthesia in an avian patient?

14. Describe grooming techniques used for birds.

15. What methods are used to individually identify birds?

16. What are common disease presentations in avian patients?

17. What is avian chlamydiosis and what are the consequences if humans are infected by the bacterial organism?

REFERENCES

1. Lightfoot T. Avoiding disaster in the critical patient. Proceedings of the Annual Conference, Association of Avian Veterinarians, 1998:265–71.
2. Altman RB, Clubb SL, and Dorrestein GM. Hematologic and plasma biochemical reference ranges of common psittacine species. In: Quesenberry KE, ed. *Avian medicine and surgery*. Philadelphia: WB Saunders; 1997:1005–7.
3. Carpenter JW. *Exotic animal formulary,* 3rd ed. St. Louis, MO: Elsevier/Saunders; 2003:564.
4. Clyde VL, and Patton S. Diagnosis, treatment, and control of common parasites in companion and aviary birds. *Seminar in Avian and Exotic Pet Medicine* 1996;5(2): 52–64.
5. McDonald SE. Lead poisoning in psittacine birds. In: Kirk RW, ed. *Current veterinary therapy IX, small animal practice*, Philadelphia: WB Saunders; 1988:713–18.
6. Centers for Disease Control and Prevention. Compendium of measures to control *Chlamydophila psittaci* infection among humans (psittacosis) and pet birds (avian chlamydiosis); 2010.

FURTHER READING

Gage LJ, and Duerr RS. *Hand-rearing birds.* Ames, IA: Blackwell Publishing; 2007.
Tully TN, Dorrestein GM, and Jones AK. *Handbook of avian medicine,* 2nd ed. Oxford, UK: Saunders/Elsevier; 2009.

Reptiles and Amphibians

CHAPTER 2

INTRODUCTION

For the past decade, reptiles and amphibians have been considered one of the fastest-growing segments of the pet trade. Those that have a fear of these animals might find this hard to believe, but the numbers don't lie. The most recent American Veterinary Medical Association pet survey statistics suggest that there was a 25.5% increase in the number of reptiles being kept as pets in the United States between 2001 and 2007. This increased number of animals being maintained in captivity has expanded the need for qualified veterinarians and veterinary technicians to provide the quality medical and surgical care that pet owners have come to expect from our profession. A certified veterinary technician with experience in working with these animals will prove to be valuable in the employment market.

Taxonomy

Proper identification of a reptile or amphibian is essential to case management. As a veterinary technician, you might be expected to provide your client with information about the natural history of an animal and to make suggestions regarding the environmental and nutritional needs of that animal. Unfortunately, many reptiles and amphibians have been assigned 3 to 4 different common names, depending on who collected or sold a particular animal. It is not uncommon to enter different pet stores and find the same species being sold under different names. Clients can become frustrated while researching the particular needs of an animal if they are searching for literature under an uncommon (nonscientific) name. The scientific classification of animals (taxonomy: genus and species) is an important tool that can be used to determine the needs of a particular animal, because it provides a "real identity" to the animal. Of course, with more than 8,000 different species of reptiles and 5,000 species of amphibians, learning all of these scientific names would be impossible. Fortunately, the number of reptiles and amphibians available through the pet trade is closer to 200, and most pet retailers carry only 15 to 30 different species. Because the actual number of reptiles and amphibians that are likely to present to a veterinary hospital is not overwhelming, it should be possible for individuals working with these animals to develop a resource library to become familiar with both their scientific and common names. The scientific classification of animals is dynamic and can change, so keeping up with new and updated literature is recommended. A list of scientific and common names can be found in Table 2.1.

HUSBANDRY

Environmental Concerns

It is interesting that reptiles and amphibians have been marketed as first pets for children. There are two primary reasons this should be discontinued. First, reptiles and amphibians can harbor potentially zoonotic pathogens (e.g., *Salmonella* spp.) as a component of their indigenous intestinal microflora. Fortunately, the potential for exposure to these pathogens can be minimized by practicing standard disinfection (e.g., hand washing after handling the animal or working in its environment); this might be beyond the scope of young children and explains why these animals don't make good first pets. The other reason is that pet reptiles and amphibians require significantly more attention regarding their husbandry and management than do other pets, such as birds, dogs, and cats. Many of the successes and failures experienced by your clients are directly related to their ability to accommodate their pet reptile's nutritional, psychological, and environmental requirements.

The single most important factor in maintaining a healthy reptile or amphibian in captivity is providing an appropriate environmental temperature range (ETR). Reptiles and amphibians are ectotherms and depend on their environmental temperature to regulate their core body temperature. Establishing an appropriate ETR for a reptile or amphibian requires knowledge of the animal's native environment and living habits.

Reptile and amphibian species are found throughout much of the world's temperate and tropical climates. To survive within these climates, reptiles and amphibians have adapted to specific niches. An arboreal lizard (such as a green iguana) and a burrowing lizard (such as a skink) from Central America might be found in the same geographic location, but they are exposed to different ETRs because of their different behavioral patterns. A green iguana might experience temperatures greater than 100°F in the trees and 85°–90°F in the shade, whereas a subterranean animal might experience temperatures less than 85°F in its burrow. Researching the origin and specific needs of a reptile will improve one's ability to care for these animals in captivity. Providing an appropriate ETR for a reptile or amphibian can be accomplished using a number of commercially available products. Recommendations for heating products should be based on the

Table 2.1 **Reptile and Amphibian Taxonomy**

CLASS REPTILIA

Order Crocodylia
(Alligators, Caimans, Crocodilians, Gharials)

American Alligator	*Alligator mississipiensis*
American Crocodile	*Crocodylus acutus*
Speckled Caiman	*Caiman crododilus*

Order Chelonia
(Turtles, Tortoises, and Terrapins)

Box Turtle	*Terrapene carolina*
Red-Ear Slider	*Trachemys scripta elegans*
Gopher Tortoise	*Gopherus polyphemus*
Desert Tortoise	*Gopherus agassizii*
Leopard Tortoise	*Geochelone pardalis*
Mata-Mata	*Chelus fimbriatus*
Red-Footed Tortoise	*Geochelone carbonaria*
Snapping Turtle	*Chelydra serpentina*
Sulcatta Tortoise	*Geochelone sulcatta*

Order Squamata
(Lizards and Snakes)

Lizards

Bearded Dragon	*Pogona vitticeps*
Bosc's (Savannah) Monitor	*Varanus exanthematicus*
Chinese Water Dragon	*Physignathus cocincinus*
Green Anole	*Anolis carolinensis*
Green Iguana	*Iguana iguana*
Green Plumed Basilisk	*Basiliscus plumifrons*
Jackson's Chameleon	*Chamaeleo jacksonii*
Leopard Gecko	*Eublepharis macularius*
Panther Chameleon	*Furcifer pardalis*
Prehensile-Tailed Skink	*Corucia zebrata*
Veiled Chameleon	*Chamaeleo calyptratus*

Snakes

Ball Python	*Python regius*
Boa Constrictor	*Boa constrictor constrictor*
Burmese Python	*Python molurus bivittatus*
Corn Snake	*Pantherophis guttata guttata*
Garter Snake	*Thamnophis spp.*
King Snake	*Lampropeltis getulus*
Reticulated Python	*Python reticulatus*

CLASS AMPHIBIA

Order Anura
(Frogs and Toads)

African Clawed Frog	*Xenopus laevis*
American Bullfrog	*Lithobates catesbeiana*
Argentine Horned Frog	*Ceratophrys ornata*
Cane Toad	*Anaxyrus marinus*
Leopard Frog	*Lithobates pipiens*
Poison-Arrow Frog	*Phyllobate* spp., *Dendrobates* spp.

Order Gymnophiona
(Caecilians)

Aquatic Caecilian	*Typhlonectes natans*
Indonesian Caecilian	*Ichthyophis kohtaoensis*

Order Urodela
(Salamanders and Newts)

Axolotl	*Ambystoma mexicanum*
Hellbender	*Cryptobranchus* spp.
Mudpuppy	*Necturus maculatus*
Tiger Salamander	*Ambystoma tigrinum*

anatomy and natural behaviors of the reptile or amphibian. For example, the large surface area of the turtle's carapace serves as a heat collection device when the animal basks under radiant light. Therefore, the use of substrate heat sources (e.g., hot rocks and undertank heating pads) will be of limited value.

The preferred method of providing heat for reptiles and amphibians is radiant light. Reptiles and amphibians naturally bask under the radiant light of the sun to store heat, which serves to maintain their core body temperature. Variable-wattage incandescent bulbs can be used to provide an appropriate ETR (Figure 2.1), and although reptiles and amphibians both regulate their core body temperatures from their environmental temperature, amphibians do not require the higher temperature sought by reptiles and thus require lower-wattage bulbs to set their temperatures. Always provide a barrier between the light source and the animal to prevent contact with the heat source. Thermometers should be used to measure the temperature and ensure that the ETR is appropriate for that particular species. The best types of thermom-

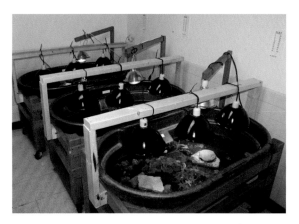

Figure 2.1 *Variable-wattage incandescent lighting can be used to provide an appropriate ETR for any reptile. Typically, a higher-wattage bulb will be placed on one side, with a lower-wattage bulb on the other. A thermometer is essential to confirm the temperature range.*

eters are those that have a thermal probe that can be moved within the vivarium to assess temperature. The "stick-on" thermometers commonly used for aquariums are not recommended because they provide only limited information regarding the temperature in a limited area within the vivarium.

Historically, "hot rocks" have been recommended for reptiles; however, these heating elements have been associated with severe thermal burns and are not typically recommended. In many cases, the hot rock was the only source of heat for the reptile in its enclosure. Reptiles will gravitate to environmental heat to regulate their core temperature. Many hot rocks can generate excessively high temperatures (>110°F) or "hot spots" that can severely burn an animal. Large reptiles that can actually cover a hot rock can trap the heat and develop a significant burn. This problem is not exclusive to hot rocks. Snakes given direct contact with an incandescent bulb (e.g., radiant heat) in an environment where the temperature is not regulated have also been known to wrap themselves around the bulb and severely burn themselves. The veterinary technician should be able to make recommendations for clients that would prevent these disasters from occurring. Newer-generation hot rocks are offered for sale and claim not to generate the excessive temperatures observed in the past. Another disadvantage of the hot rock is that it provides only a single point source of heat. Hot rocks have been used successfully with other heat sources (e.g., radiant light) to provide a basking area for "sun-loving" species. Hot rocks should be used only for basking lizards that do not "cover up" the hot rock, and the surface temperature of the hot rock should be monitored closely. Burying the hot rock in the substrate within the vivarium can also minimize any potential complications. Hot rocks should never be recommended for amphibians.

Undertank heating pads are commonly used for snakes and lizards. Undertank heating sources can be placed on one side of an animal's enclosure, leaving the other area unheated. This will effectively provide the animal with an appropriate ETR. When these devices are placed under a glass enclosure, the heat generated can be much higher than on the pad's surface, leading to burns. The temperatures generated by these heating devices should be monitored closely.

The reptile's and amphibian's metabolism, immune system, and behavior are directly related to their ability to maintain their core body temperature. A reptile or amphibian maintained at an inappropriate ETR will become hypothermic and have a decreased metabolism, resulting in inactivity and limited growth. A reptile or amphibian with decreased immune function will be unable to mount an effective immune response against bacterial, viral, and fungal pathogens. Many of these animals are classified as "poor-doers." Successful treatment (e.g., antibiotics) of infectious diseases in reptiles requires that the animal be maintained at an appropriate ETR for their metabolism to effectively distribute the medication to the target tissues.

Recommendations for providing a reptile or amphibian with an appropriate ETR will depend on the species, so it is important to research the specific needs of an animal to ensure the most appropriate recommendation is being made. In general, temperate species of reptiles and amphibians thrive at temperature ranges between 75° and 85°F and 70° and 78°F, respectively; tropical species of reptiles and amphibians at 78° to 90°F and 74° to 80°F, respectively; and desert species of reptiles at 85° to 95°F. Radiant light (e.g., incandescent lamps or ceramic heat emitters) most closely resembles the radiant heat generated by the sun that reptiles and amphibians encounter in the wild, and is the preferred method for providing heat for these animals in captivity.

Full-spectrum lighting has received a great deal of attention in the reptile and amphibian literature because of its role as an "artificial sun" in the management of captive animals. Captive reptiles and amphibians are typically housed indoors, which limits the benefits they can obtain from the sun. For this reason, it is important that they have an artificial source of "sunlight." It is important to note that not all forms of artificial light are similar. Veterinary personnel working with reptile and amphibian patients need to develop a working understanding of the important components of sunlight and the types of artificial lights that are best for these animals, to ensure that technicians can make the appropriate recommendations to their clients regarding the care of their pets.

Reptiles and amphibians depend on the sun to provide them with three different sources of radiation: ultraviolet (290–400 nm), visible (400–700 nm), and infrared (>700 nm). Visible light is important because it amplifies the colors that reptiles and amphibians see, which can have an effect on feeding behaviors and reproduction. The quality of visible light varies among different types of lightbulbs. For example, fluorescent bulbs typically produce a better-quality visible light than incandescent bulbs. Infrared radiation generates the "environmental heat" that is important to ectothermic reptiles and amphibians. Incandescent and metal halide bulbs are typically the best at generating infrared radiation.

Ultraviolet radiation can be divided into ultraviolet A (320–400 nm), ultraviolet B (290–320 nm), and ultraviolet C (<290 nm) wavelengths. Ultraviolet A has been associated with managing different behaviors in reptiles and amphibians; however, there is much we still don't know about it. Ultraviolet C is a potent form of irradiation.

It does not play a direct role in the management of captive reptiles and amphibians, but is used in ultraviolet sterilizers (germicidal) for aquatic systems. Ultraviolet B (UVB) plays an important role in the endogenous synthesis of vitamin D in vertebrates that possess the photochemical structures in their skin capable of initiating the process.

Not all vertebrates have the ability to do this. Cats, for example, do not synthesize vitamin D using this process, but instead acquire their vitamin D through the consumption of prey. It has been speculated that carnivorous reptiles must do the same, but some researchers have shown that "meat-eating" reptiles have the capacity to synthesize vitamin D when exposed to UVB radiation.[1,2] An animal that derives its vitamin D from photochemical synthesis requires regular exposure to UVB radiation to ensure that it will synthesize adequate levels of vitamin D.

Vitamin D serves several functions in the body, including the absorption of calcium at the level of the intestine and maintaining cardiovascular health. To date, there has been limited research to assess the role of UVB in the endogenous synthesis of vitamin D in reptiles (e.g., <15 species studied out of >3,000 species) and amphibians; therefore, it is best to assume that reptiles and amphibians require exposure to UVB radiation to synthesize vitamin D and provide it to them.

To ensure that a captive reptile or amphibian is provided the maximal UVB radiation, the bulb should be positioned within 12–18 inches of the animal and not directed through glass. Glass refracts short-wavelength light, effectively inhibiting UVB radiation penetration. Reptiles should be provided a 12-hour light, 12-hour darkness cycle under normal conditions; however, individuals interested in breeding these animals should establish photoperiods that mimic natural seasonal cycles. Full-spectrum lightbulbs should

be replaced every 9–12 months because they lose their effectiveness over time. It is important to research the different bulbs available commercially, because the quality of the bulbs can vary. The bulbs that typically produce UVB include fluorescent tubes, compact fluorescent bulbs, and metal halide bulbs.

Environmental humidity is often overlooked by pet reptile owners. Most recommendations for relative humidity in captive settings are based on the climate that an animal originates from: tropical 80%–95%, temperate 60%–70%, and desert 40%–50%.[3] Many reptiles are dependent on environmental moisture to aid with shedding and to maintain hydration. When animals are predisposed to low relative humidity, they are prone to dysecdysis (difficulty shedding), dehydration, respiratory infections, and behavioral anomalies. Humidity can be maintained or increased in an enclosure by using large-surface-area water bowls, bubbling or heating water in a mason jar, covering the enclosure lid with a plastic sheet, and routine misting. A hygrometer should be placed in the cage to closely monitor the relative humidity. Environmental humidity levels are considered more important in amphibians because they are more susceptible to desiccation than reptiles. Humidity levels for temperate and tropical amphibians should be maintained between 60% and 80% and 70% and 90%, respectively.

Reptiles and amphibians have developed various behaviors that enable them to fill a certain niche in their environment. Attempts should be made to provide the animal with "cage furniture" that encourages these behaviors. For example, green iguanas are arboreal (tree-climbing) animals that naturally climb into tree branches to bask under radiant sunlight. When these animals are placed in an enclosure that does not contain branches, they are more likely to be stressed. Stress can initiate a cascade of physiologic changes in the body that can affect metabolism and immune function. Pet owners should be made aware of the importance of fully researching the specific needs of their new pet and providing them a suitable captive environment. Cage furniture should be safe, noningestible, and easy to clean.

There are a number of different substrates available in the pet retail market. Every substrate has potential advantages and disadvantages related to its use (Table 2.2). Recommendations to the owner should always include providing the pet with a substrate that is safe, easy to clean, and aesthetic (Figure 2.2). Substrates should be cleaned regularly; all fecal material and urates should be removed daily to prevent possible contact dermatitis.

Nutrition

In the wild, reptiles and amphibians have the opportunity to select from a diverse array of food items in their environment to meet their daily needs, but with more than 12,500 species of reptiles and amphibians in the world, it can be difficult to re-create these diets in captivity. By researching the specific dietary requirements

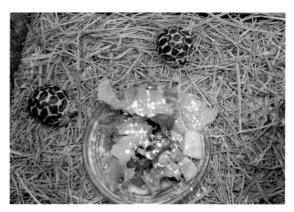

Figure 2.2 *There are many different types of substrate available for reptiles and amphibians. Substrate selection should be based on the specific animal's needs. In most cases, reading up about its life history can provide insight on what would be best (e.g., grass hay for tortoises).*

of reptiles and amphibians and having an understanding of the nutritional value of commercially available foods, a technician can educate clients and ensure their success with managing their pet reptile or amphibian.

Reptiles can be classified into one of three dietary categories: carnivores, omnivores, and herbivores. Adult amphibians are all carnivorous, whereas larval forms might be carnivorous

Table 2.2 **Substrates Commonly Recommended for Reptiles and Amphibians**

SUBSTRATE	ADVANTAGES	DISADVANTAGES
Newspaper	Inexpensive	Aesthetically unpleasing
	Easy to clean	Affords no cover to reptile
	Easy to monitor feces, urine	
Orchid Bark	Aesthetically pleasing	Predisposes to foreign body
	Natural	Reduces relative humidity
		Dusty (respiratory signs)
Calcium Carbonate Sand	Aesthetically pleasing	Costly
	Easy to clean	Foreign bodies in eye, mouth, GI tract
Aspen Wood Shavings	Aesthetically pleasing	Reduces relative humidity
	Easy to clean	Splinters/foreign bodies

(e.g., salamanders) or herbivorous (e.g., tadpoles). Carnivores are the easiest animals to accommodate, because they will accept whole prey such as other reptiles, amphibians, birds, and mammals, which are a nutritionally balanced food resource. A common mistake that pet owners make when feeding carnivores is to offer live prey. When a reptile or amphibian is not hungry, it will rarely kill the prey item. If left unattended, the prey could become hungry and feed on the reptile or amphibian, which could prove fatal. To prevent this from occurring, recommend to your clients that they offer only prey items that are not alive. Snake owners are the most likely to complain that their snake won't feed on prekilled prey; however, because snakes use olfaction to detect their prey items they can be trained to eat prekilled prey.

Another common group of carnivores—the insectivores—feed exclusively on invertebrates. Six invertebrates are commercially available, including the domestic cricket (*Acheta domestica*), mealworm (*Tenebrio molitor*), superworm (*Zoophobias morio*), earthworm (*Lumbricus terrestris*), greater wax moth larva (*Galleria mellonella*), and soldier fly larva (*Hermetia illucens*). These invertebrates are often offered for sale without having been nutritionally prepared. All living creatures require energy, and if feeder invertebrates are not offered food, they will provide little nutritional value to the reptile or amphibian they are fed to. Commercially available invertebrates are adequate in protein and fat, but are deficient in specific amino acids, vitamins, and minerals (especially calcium). One exception is soldier fly larvae, which have more than adequate calcium levels. Unfortunately, if the reptile or amphibian eating them doesn't penetrate their cuticle, they won't gain access to any real nutrition and will tend to pass the dead larvae intact. The most common nutritional disorder observed in insectivores is secondary nutritional hyperpara-

thyroidism. A rapidly growing insectivore, such as a leopard gecko, will develop muscle tremors and seizures and possibly die when offered a calcium-deficient diet. This problem can be prevented by properly preparing the feeder invertebrate. Many pet retailers offer invertebrates apples or potatoes, believing that they are providing the prey items a balanced diet; however, these foods provide little more than carbohydrates and moisture and do not correct the mineral deficiency. A solution to this problem is to offer a balanced commercial invertebrate diet. Research evaluating these diets has proven that they can significantly improve the nutritional value of the prey item.[4] Recommend that your clients offer the commercial diet for a minimum of 24 hours prior to feeding the prey items to the reptile or amphibian (Figure 2.3). This should ensure that the invertebrate will be "gut-loaded." There are also mineral supplements that can be used to "dust" the prey items and increase their nutritional value. These mineral supplements should be used according to label recommendations.

Herbivores are the hardest group of reptiles to accommodate in captivity because of the limited availability of quality vegetables and fruits. In the wild, herbivorous reptiles select their diet from a variety of available resources, whereas in captivity they are limited to what is available.

Romaine lettuce and mustard and collard greens are most frequently recommended as the base diet for captive herbivores. Other plant products, such as spinach, broccoli, green beans, kale, squash, dandelion leaves, and other dark leafy vegetables, can be used to further diversify the diet. Certain plant products, such as kale and spinach, should be limited in the diet because they contain oxalates and can bind valuable dietary calcium in the digestive tract and increase the likelihood of a mineral deficiency.[5] Other plant products, such as

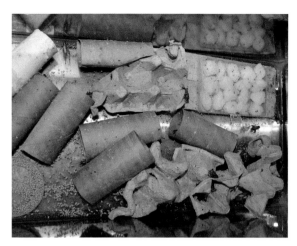

Figure 2.3 *Live foods should be provided appropriate nutrition prior to offering them to a reptile or amphibian. These crickets are being fed a commercial cricket chow.*

broccoli, contain goitrogens, which can alter thyroid metabolism and should likewise be limited. The key to success with herbivore diets is to provide a diverse selection of food products to increase the nutritional value offered to the animal. Fruits should not constitute more than 10%–15% of the animal's diet, because they are devoid of protein and essential minerals.

In recent years, commercial herbivore diets have been manufactured that improve our ability to provide a more balanced diet. Many of these diets are marketed as complete and recommended as a sole source of nutrition; however, little is known about reptile nutrition and a more diverse diet should be recommended. A diet that combines a commercial product (25%–40%) with high-quality plant sources, such as romaine lettuce and mustard and collard greens, may be used.

There are a number of commercially available nutritional supplements for reptiles and amphibians. The available supplements might contain calcium, calcium and phosphorus, vitamins, amino acids, or a combination of these nutrients.

As noted, little is known about the specific dietary requirements of reptiles and amphibians. In the past, many of the nutritional problems diagnosed in reptiles and amphibians were associated with vitamin and mineral deficiencies and the need for supplements was apparent. More recently, diseases associated with excessive vitamin and mineral supplements have been reported and a concern has arisen regarding how much of these supplements to provide.[6] Clients should be made aware of the risks of vitamin and mineral oversupplementation. Veterinary personnel should make specific dietary recommendations based on the reptile's or amphibian's age and physiological status (e.g., gravid).

Transport

Reptiles can elicit quite an array of emotions in people. Clients with dogs or cats might not appreciate sharing a waiting room with a large reptile. To prevent potential disaster in your veterinary hospital, recommend that reptile and amphibian owners transport their pets in a closed, secured enclosure. Snakes and lizards travel well in ventilated burlap or cotton bags (e.g., pillow cases). Larger snakes, lizards, and tortoises may be transported in large plastic boxes or garbage cans with airholes. Semiaquatic reptiles (e.g., red-eared slider turtles) and amphibians (e.g., bullfrog) should be transported in a plastic box (with airholes) with a level of water that covers the animal's feet. Semiaquatic animals maintained in deep water for transport are prone to drowning. Totally aquatic amphibians (e.g., Surinam frog) should be transported in a plastic enclosure with sufficient dechlorinated water to cover the animal. Recommend to your clients that they not change the bedding of the enclosure before transporting the animal, so that the veterinary technician can examine the fecal and urine material.

Grooming

There are rarely situations in which reptiles are groomed. But in some cases with lizard species, owners may complain about sharp claws that cause painful scratches. Lizard (e.g., green iguana) claws can be blunted with similar techniques described for bird claws/nails, that of using a Dremel® tool or the tip of an electrocautery unit. An alternative to trimming the claws is to use plastic nail caps for dogs and cats.

HISTORY

A thorough history is essential to making an appropriate diagnosis for any exotic animal case, because many of the problems identified in exotic animals are directly related to inappropriate husbandry. A veterinary technician should first collect the signalment, including age, breed, and sex, if they are known. Knowledge of the animal's age and sex can be useful when developing a differential diagnosis list. For example, an adult, intact female green iguana with a history of weakness and lethargy during the months of December through March might be suffering from a reproductive problem (e.g., follicular stasis or dystocia), whereas an adult male would not.

After collecting the signalment, focus on background information, including where the animal was acquired, length of time owned, if the client has other pets or reptiles/amphibians, if he or she recently acquired another animal, and the interaction between the owner and the pet (e.g., frequency of handling). This information should provide the technician with an initial understanding of the client's knowledge of the pet reptile or amphibian.

The next set of questions should focus on how the animal is managed at home (husbandry), including whether the animal is housed indoors or outdoors; if it has supervised or unsupervised run of the house; the cage size and material; the cage location in the house; temperature, humidity, lighting, light cycle, and substrate used in the cage; types of cage furniture; if the reptile/amphibian is housed with another animal; and how often the cage is cleaned and type of disinfectant used. Questions about the animal's nutrition are also important and should include type of food (natural or commercial), amount offered daily, frequency, supplements, water source, and how often the food and water are changed.

Finally, the questions should focus on the animal's health status, including medical history, current presenting problem, and duration of the complaint. Although it is natural to want to focus on the presenting problem first, a great deal of information could be lost if the animal's history is not collected using a systematic approach.

RESTRAINT

Using appropriate techniques for handling an animal for an examination is essential to protect the technician, the veterinarian, the client, and the patient. A working knowledge of the animal's anatomy and physiology is an important consideration. First, determine what weapons the animal might use to defend itself. For example, a green iguana might use its tail to "whip" the technician, use its teeth to bite, or use its claws to climb away or on the technician. Identifying these weapons prior to restraining the animal will reduce the likelihood of injury for both the technician and the patient. Reptiles and amphibians lack a diaphragm, and if they are grasped tightly around the rib cage, they could literally suffocate. Chelonians should never be held upside down for extended periods, because the viscera can place extra pressure on the lungs, again leading to difficulty breathing. Appropriate training and practice will enable a technician to safely manage a wide range of nonvenomous reptiles.

LIZARDS

For small specimens, place your thumb and index finger on either side of the ramus (mandible), allowing the animal's body to rest in the palm of your hand. Never constrict the animal's body when you are restraining it, because reptiles, except crocodilians, lack a diaphragm and you can suffocate them. For larger specimens, again place your index finger and thumb on the corners of the mandible and use your second hand to hold the rear legs against the animal's tail (Figure 2.4). Never grab a lizard by the tail. Some species (e.g., green iguana) have the ability to "drop" their tail (tail autotomy) as a defense mechanism that allows the animal to avoid capture by a predator. Clients are not impressed when their pet lizard's tail is broken because of poor restraint technique.

SNAKES

Place your index finger and thumb under the mandible and use your other hand to support the snake's body (Figure 2.5). One person is required for every 2–3 feet of snake. Large constrictor species should never be handled without assistance. Although it is rare, these large, powerful snakes are capable of seriously injuring a careless individual. Only trained professionals should handle venomous snakes, and access to antivenom should be arranged at a local hospital.

CHELONIANS

Most chelonians can be handled by grasping the middle of the shell (Figure 2.6). Many of the biting turtles (e.g., snapping turtles) should be grasped at the rear of the shell. For a physical examination, the head and neck can be gently withdrawn from

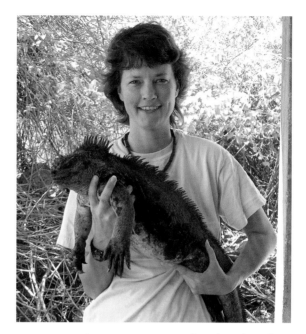

Figure 2.4 *Appropriate restraint for a large lizard.*

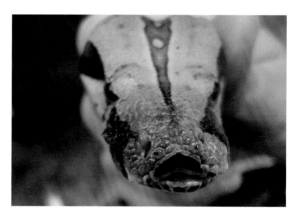

Figure 2.5 *Appropriate head restraint for a snake.*

the shell (Figure 2.7). Do not exert excessive force when restraining chelonians, because you could easily damage their cervical spine. In those cases when the animal cannot be physically managed, the veterinarian can provide an appropriate sedative or anesthetic.

CROCODILIANS

Crocodilians are lightning-fast and can inflict a nasty bite. They can also use their tail as a weapon.

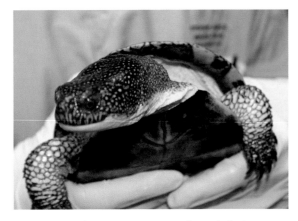

Figure 2.6 *Appropriate restraint for a chelonian.*

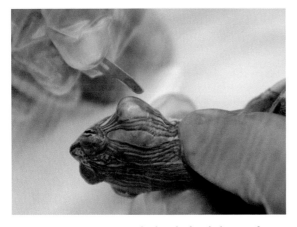

Figure 2.7 *Restraining the head of a chelonian for examination. This animal has an aural abscess.*

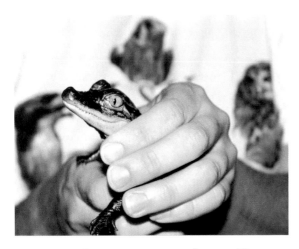

Figure 2.8 *Appropriate restraint of a crocodilian.*

Crocodilians should be restrained only by experienced professionals. Getting control of the mouth is important when restraining a crocodilian. The muscles used to close a crocodilian's jaws are very powerful, whereas the muscles used to open the jaws are not as powerful. Therefore, once the mouth of a crocodilian is closed it can be held securely with minimal effort. When restraining a crocodilian, first grasp the head at the base of the skull. Once that is done, pressure can be placed on the upper jaw to close the mouth. The mouth can then be held closed and taped (e.g., with duct tape) to keep it closed. Be careful not to wrap the tape around the nares when securing the jaws. Once the mouth is appropriately restricted, a crocodilian can be restrained in a manner similar to that described for large lizard specimens (Figure 2.8).

AMPHIBIANS

Amphibians have a very delicate and sensitive integument. The epidermis is covered by a protective mucous barrier, similar to that of fish, which protects these animals against pathogens. There are also amphibians, such as poison-dart frogs, that produce toxins in these mucous secretions. To prevent danger to yourself and the animal, wear a pair of examination gloves that have been moistened with dechlorinated water or distilled water to prevent both damage to the animal's protective mucous barrier and toxic exposure to the handler. Large amphibians (e.g., Argentine horned frogs and hellbenders) can inflict a nasty bite, and precautions should be taken when managing these large specimens. Most amphibians can be grasped in the palm of the hand and examined. Anurans can be restrained by grasping them with your index finger and thumb in the axillary region. Some salamanders can detach their tail, as described with lizards and, therefore, should never be grasped by the tail.

PHYSICAL EXAMINATION

The physical examination of a reptile or amphibian will relay a great deal of information to the veterinarian and direct the selection of diagnostic tests and initial treatment options. Reptiles and amphibians have evolved to mask their illnesses to prevent predation. Therefore, the veterinarian will perform a hands-off examination of the animal in its enclosure before a routine hands-on examination. The veterinarian will closely observe the animal's general disposition, respiratory rate, and locomotion and record his or her findings before proceeding to a hands-on examination.

The veterinarian will always perform a hands-on physical examination in a thorough and consistent manner. Some prefer to start at the head and work their way back, whereas others start from the tail and work to the head. A basic understanding of what is normal for that animal is also an important prerequisite. For example, chameleons typically have bright yellow mucous membranes. If this was not known, one might misclassify the animal as being icteric. It is important to maintain a resource library that will allow identification of specific differences among species.

An animal's eyes should be clear and free of discharge. The nares and external ears (tympanum in chelonians, lizards, and amphibians; absent in snakes) should be free of discharge and ectoparasites (e.g., ticks and mites). Some reptiles possess salt glands in the nares that can produce a clear, crystalline secretion.

The oral cavity should be opened with care, because aggressive manipulation can lead to broken teeth or tomia (chelonians) or damage to the mucous membranes. A rubber spatula or folded piece of radiographic film can be gently inserted into the mouth of a lizard or snake to aid in viewing the oral cavity. A paper clip can be used to gently pry open a chelonian's jaws. Aggressive reptiles might gape as a defensive or offensive measure, which facilitates examination of the oral cavity. The oral cavity should be clear and free of discharge, parasites, and abscesses. The mucous membranes should be moist and pale pink. The glottis (airway) should be free of discharge and parasites.

The skin should be clean and free of defects. Imported animals are often covered with ectoparasites and the veterinarian will examine them closely, especially in the gular fold (under the chin), mouth, and around the eyes. The limbs will be evaluated for range of motion and palpated for any skeletal deformities. The veterinarian will palpate the coelomic cavity and assess it for pain and abnormal masses. The internal organs of reptiles and amphibians are consistent across species, and a basic understanding of reptilian and amphibian anatomy is necessary to interpret abnormal findings (Figures 2.9A and 2.9B). Reptiles (e.g., leopard geckos) and amphibians (e.g., frogs) with white or light pigmented ventrums can be further examined using a transilluminator. Placing the light source along the lateral body wall of the animal will help outline several internal organs. Cystic calculi and gastrointestinal foreign bodies in reptiles and amphibians have been diagnosed using this technique.

A physical examination should include auscultation of the animal's heart and lungs. Auscultation in reptiles is especially difficult because the scales or carapace can inhibit one's ability to fully assess the heart and lung fields. A thin, damp paper towel can be placed on the animal's skin to reduce friction between the bell of the stethoscope and the scales. The veterinarian might not be able to hear the heart and lungs, even when using this technique. Nevertheless, when a pathology (e.g., pneumonia, pulmonary edema) is diagnosed,

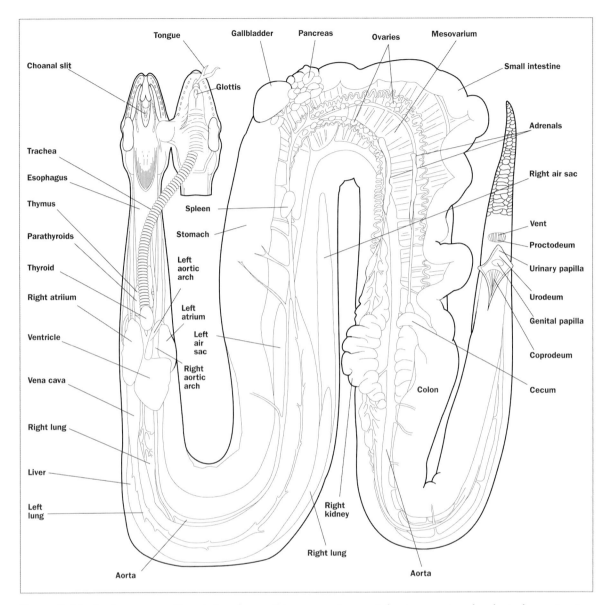

Figure 2.9A *Snake anatomy. Knowledge of a reptile's anatomy is essential to interpreting the physical examination findings. Illustration by Michael L. Broussard. Illustration adapted from Reptile Medicine and Surgery (Elsevier 2005).*

it helps direct additional testing. Although reptiles are difficult to auscult, it is important to be thorough and consistent with every patient and perform this assessment.

An ultrasonic Doppler is the best way to measure heart rate in reptiles and amphibians. The heart of most reptiles and amphibians is located within the pectoral girdle. For lizards, salamanders, and frogs/toads, the Doppler should be placed in the axillary region and directed medially. Monitor lizards are an exception; their heart is located more distally in the chest. A snake

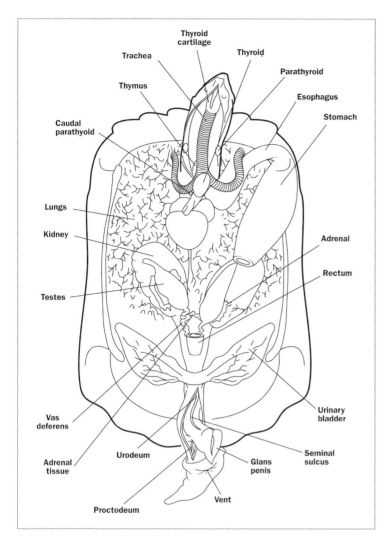

Figure 2.9B *Chelonian anatomy. Illustration by Michael L. Broussard. Illustration adapted from Reptile Medicine and Surgery (Elsevier 2005).*

Attempts to determine the sex of the reptile should also be made during the physical examination. Some reptiles are sexually dimorphic (e.g., have physical characteristics that help determine sex), whereas others are not. For example, some lizards, such as green iguanas (Figure 2.10) and bearded dragons, have pores on the ventrum of their legs (thighs only in iguanas; thighs and ventral pelvis in bearded dragons) that can be used to determine their sex. The pores are larger in the males than in females. Terrestrial chelonians can often be sexed by looking at their plastron (ventral shell). Males have an indentation (concavity) that allows them to mount the female. Aquatic chelonians do not have this same structure, although they might have others. For example, female red-eared slider turtles (*Trachemys scripta elegans*) are larger than males, and the males have longer front claws. Sex determination in snakes is best done by probing the base of the tail for the presence/absence of hemipenes (Figure 2.11).

DIAGNOSTIC SAMPLING

Veterinarians use the information gathered from a detailed history and thorough physical examination to develop a list of differential diagnoses. The veterinarian will then use available diagnostic tests—such as hematology, plasma chemistry analysis, radiographs, microbiological isolation, cytologic

heart is typically found one-third to one-quarter the distance from its head. When a snake is placed in dorsal recumbency, its heartbeat can be visually observed. A Doppler probe placed over a snake heart allows for not only measuring the heart rate, but also listening for abnormal heart sounds (murmurs). The chelonian heart is located in the proximal third of the coelomic cavity. To listen to its heart, place the Doppler probe in the area between the head and forelimb (right or left) and direct it caudally.

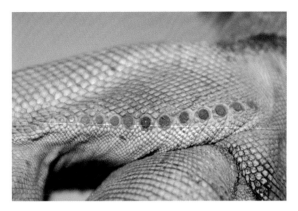

Figure 2.10 *Femoral pores on the ventral thigh of a male green iguana.*

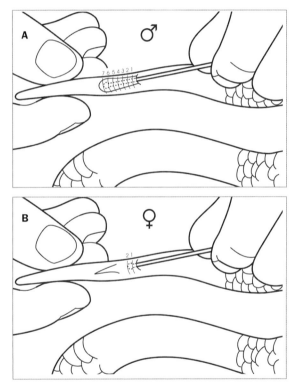

Figure 2.11 *Probing snakes is the best method for determining the sex of these animals. Stainless steel probes with a blunt end or round tip are preferred. The probe should be lubed with an appropriate gel to minimize tissue trauma. The probe is inserted slightly lateral and caudal to the vent (A). If the probe can be inserted for >5–7 scales, it is a male, confirming the presence of a hemipenis (B). If the probe is inserted <2–4 scales, it is a female.*

examination, and parasitologic examination—to determine the cause of the animal's illness.

Blood Collection (and Interpretation)
Reptiles and Amphibians

Reptiles and amphibians mask their illnesses, making diagnosis difficult. Hematologic sampling provides a veterinarian with insight into possible physiologic changes and the disease status of an animal. Samples are routinely collected and submitted to evaluate the red and white blood cells (complete blood count), plasma enzymes, and electrolytes. The volume of blood that can be safely collected from a reptile is 0.5%–0.8% of its body weight or 0.5–0.8 ml/100 g body weight.[7] It is important to consider the animal's history and physical examination when determining the volume of blood that can be collected. An animal that has experienced an acute blood loss (e.g., trauma) cannot afford to have large volumes of blood collected. Fortunately, most laboratories can perform a complete blood count (CBC) and a plasma chemistry analysis on ≤1 ml of blood.

Blood samples should be placed in appropriate collection tubes immediately after collection. Microtainers (Becton Dickinson, Franklin Lakes, NJ) are useful for this purpose, because they use dry anticoagulants, which are less likely to dilute small-volume samples. Laboratories vary in their preference for type of collection tubes, so it is important to contact them prior to submitting samples. It used to be thought that some anticoagulants were more apt than others to cause erythrocyte or leukocyte lysis; however, more recent work suggests that this is not necessarily the case. In general, blood being used for CBC should be mixed with ethylenediaminetetraacetic (EDTA) acid purple top tube or lithium heparin (green top tube). Blood samples for plasma chemistries should also be placed in lithium heparin. When dealing with small blood volumes, lithium heparin might be the best choice, because it can be used to store the sample for both a CBC and plasma chemistry analysis. If serum is to be used for the chemistry analysis, no anticoagulant is needed.

Red blood cell estimates are not typically done for reptiles and amphibians unless there is a problem. This is because manual counts need to be performed and standard hematologic machines cannot count nucleated erythrocytes. Fortunately, most veterinarians are comfortable reviewing packed cell volume (PCV) to get an appreciation of the erythrocyte numbers; PCV values for reptiles and amphibians are typically between 20% and 40%. When veterinary technicians read manual differentials for white blood cell counts, they should note what they see with the erythrocytes. Immature erythrocytes in reptiles and amphibians, as with those of fish and birds, are smaller, have a higher nuclear to cytoplasmic ratio, and have a basophilic cytoplasm, compared with mature erythrocytes. It is important to document and consider large differences (3–4+) that are noted in color (polychromasia) or size (anisocytosis) of erythrocytes when interpreting the overall erythrocyte status of a patient.

CBC in reptiles and amphibians requires special care. Because all of the blood cells are nucleated in reptiles and amphibians, standard hematologic equipment cannot be used. Instead, manual counts must be done. To perform a manual count in these animals, start by making a high-quality blood smear, using standard microscope slides or coverslips. Blood cells from reptiles and amphibians are more fragile than those of mammals; therefore, it is important to use caution when making blood smears to minimize the likelihood of cell rupture ("smudgeocytes"). Premixing a blood sample with 22% bovine albumin (Gamma Biologics, Houston, TX) can stabilize the cells

and minimize "smudgeocytes." To do this, add 1 drop of bovine albumin and 5 drops of whole blood into a test tube. Mix the solution by gently rotating/rocking it. Once the solution is mixed, use a hematocrit tube to collect some blood from the tube and make your smears using standard glass microscope slides. Blood smears can also be made using coverslips (without bovine albumin). In reptiles, there has been no significant difference in the number of "smudgeocytes" noted between samples premixed with albumin and made with slides and those made with coverslips, although both techniques had significantly fewer "smudgeocytes" than smears made using glass slides that were not pretreated with albumin.[8]

Once the slides/coverslips are made, the simplest way to estimate the white blood cell (WBC) count is the following:

1. Count the number of WBCs on 10 fields at 400× (10× eyepiece and 40× objective). The fields should represent a section of the blood smear where the cells fill (but don't overfill) the slide and are evenly distributed.

2. Take the total number of WBCs counted and divide that number by 10 to get an average number of cells per field.

3. Take the average number of cells per field and multiply that by 2,000 to get an estimated WBC count.

After the WBC estimate has been completed, perform a differential to determine the representative WBCs. The WBC types found in reptiles include the heterophil and monocyte (Figure 2.12A), and lymphocyte (Figure 2.12B), eosinophil, and basophil. The azurophil is an azure staining cell that is within the monocyte lineage. With the exception of the heterophil, the reptilian and amphibian WBCs are similar in appearance and function to mammalian WBCs. The heterophil is considered analogous to the mammalian neutrophil; however, its appearance and function are slightly different. The reptilian and amphibian heterophil has a round to oval nucleus and red-orange, rod-shaped granules. Beginners often misinterpret a heterophil as an eosinophil. The following is a standard method for performing a differential count in reptiles and amphibians.

Perform a 100- or 200-cell differential to determine the proportions of WBCs. The more cells counted (200 vs. 100), the tighter the results will be. These proportions can then be multiplied by the estimated WBC count (see 3, estimated white blood cell count, above) to estimate absolute values of the different cell types.

heterophil % × WBC estimate =
estimated absolute heterophil count

lymphocyte % × WBC estimate =
estimated absolute lymphocyte count

eosinophil % × WBC estimate =
estimated absolute eosinophil count

monocyte/azurophil % × WBC estimate = ##
estimated absolute monocyte/azurophil count

basophil % × WBC estimate =
estimated absolute basophil count

Lizards

Blood samples are routinely collected from the ventral coccygeal vein or jugular vein in lizards. The ventral tail vein is located on the ventral midline of the tail. The blood sample should be collected from within the proximal one-quarter of the tail. When a sample from an adult male

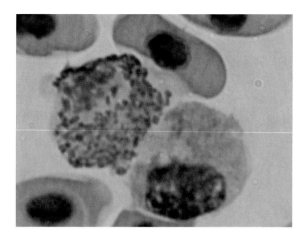

Figure 2.12A *Blood cells from a green iguana: heterophil (red) and monocyte (blue).*

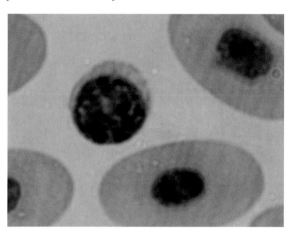

Figure 2.12B *Blood cells from a green iguana: lymphocyte.*

animal is required, one should avoid the hemipenes by collecting the sample distal to the hemipenal bulges. Clean the venipuncture site with an appropriate disinfectant (e.g., betadine or chlorhexidine) to remove any excess organic debris. A 22- to 25-gauge needle fastened to a 3 ml syringe should be used to collect the sample. For large animals, a longer needle (1.5–2") might be required to collect the sample. The needle should be inserted perpendicular to the skin and to the point of the caudal vertebrae (Figure 2.13). Gently apply negative pressure as the needle-syringe is withdrawn off the caudal vertebrae. In some cases, the venipuncturist must "walk the bone" to identify the blood vessel. Always be conscientious of your patient when collecting a sample and be as "quick and kind" as possible. Some lizard species use tail autotomy as a defense mechanism against predators and will drop their tail if handled inappropriately.

The jugular vein is an excellent site for collecting larger volumes of blood from lizards. The jugular vein of lizards, like that of birds, is located on the lateral aspect of the neck. The jugular vein is not typically visible in a lizard, but knowing the landmarks will help ensure success with collecting blood from this site. The primary landmarks to use for jugular venipuncture are the tympanum

(ear) and shoulder. The jugular vein can typically be found along an imaginary line drawn between those two sites. The vessel is generally shallow, 3–6 mm in depth from the surface of the skin. Again, clean the venipuncture site with an appropriate disinfectant to remove any excess organic debris. A 22- to 25-gauge needle fastened to a 3 ml syringe should be used to collect the sample. The needle should be inserted parallel to the skin (Figure 2.14).

The ventral abdominal vein is a vessel still used by some veterinary personnel to collect blood samples from lizards, but it is more difficult to sample from and generally provides smaller sample volumes than the jugular or ventral tail veins. The ventral abdominal vein is located on the ventral midline within the body cavity. The site should

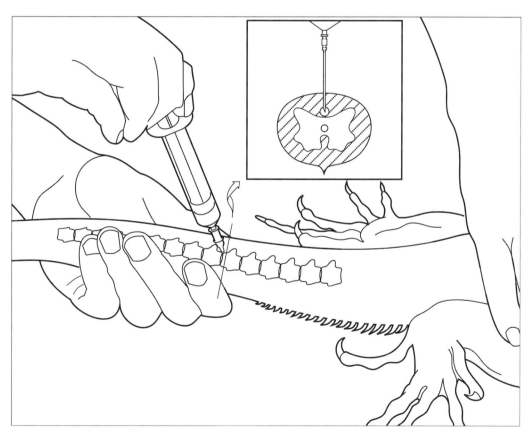

Figure 2.13 *Blood collection in a green iguana via the ventral tail vein. Illustration by Michael L. Broussard.*

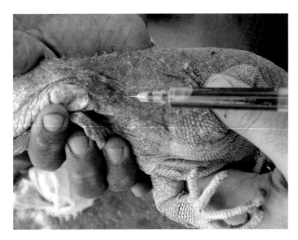

Figure 2.14 *Blood collection in a green iguana via the jugular vein.*

be aseptically prepared. Again, a 22- to 25-gauge needle fastened to a 3 ml syringe should be used. The bevel of the needle should face up, and the needle inserted at an approximately 15°–30° angle, practically parallel to the body wall. Negative pressure should be applied once the needle is inserted. Do not "fish around" when performing this technique; being overly aggressive can lead to visceral damage.

There has been some discussion over the value of collecting blood samples for diagnostic testing from toenail clips. Many do not recommend this procedure because it produces longer-term pain than simple needle insertion, can affect behavior (e.g., animals that dig might not do so because of pain), and, most importantly, can affect sample quality. Blood collected from toenail trims is diluted with lymph, which can affect biochemistry values and WBC parameters. Because it is not possible to know to what extent the lymph dilution affects the quality of the samples, it is impossible to interpret the value of the samples.

Chelonians

Blood samples are routinely collected from the jugular vein, subcarapacial vein, ventral and dorsal coccygeal veins, femoral vein, and brachial vein. The preferred site for blood collection in chelonians is the jugular vein, because the other sites have higher likelihoods of providing lymph-diluted samples. Lymph-diluted samples will have a watery appearance. Holding the sample for 2–3 minutes will help determine whether there is lymph dilution, because an "oil and vinegar" appearance to the sample will develop (clear fluid over cells). If a lymph-diluted sample is suspected, it should be discarded, because it will be impossible to interpet. Blood collection in chelonians might require sedation if the animal does not tolerate restraint of its head or limbs. Placing excess strain on the neck or limbs during restraint can lead to broken cervical vertebrae or limbs. A 22- to 25-gauge needle fastened to a 3 ml syringe can be used to collect blood samples at any of the prescribed sites. The venipuncture sites should be aseptically prepared to remove any excess organic debris. The right jugular vein is generally more prominent than the left and is located on the lateral aspect of the neck, approximately at the level of the tympanum. The technician should gently retract the head to facilitate exposure. An index finger should be placed on the neck to assist with jugular vein visualization. In some cases, the jugular vein cannot be seen and a "blind-stick" needs to be attempted.

The subcarapacial vein (azygous vein) is located dorsal to the cervical vertebrae. This vein/sinus is an excellent site for collecting blood samples, although there is a higher likelihood of lymph dilution than there is when drawing from the jugular vein. Needle selection for this technique will vary based on the size of the chelonian. A 25-gauge, 5/8" needle is generally sufficient for chelonians <500 grams, whereas a 22-gauge, 1.5" needle will be needed for larger animals. The needle should be inserted at a 45° angle over the head of the chelonian (Figure 2.15). The technician can

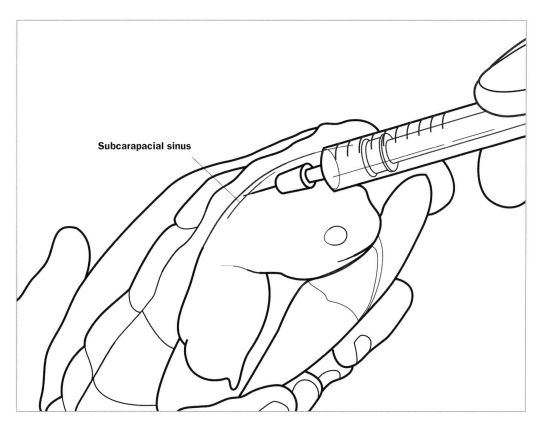

Subcarapacial sinus

Figure 2.15 *Blood collection from the subcarapacial vein of a chelonian. Illustration by Michael L. Broussard.*

place a finger or spatula/tongue depressor over the head of the animal to hold it in place if it is not holding still. The technician should apply negative pressure as he or she inserts the needle and should monitor the hub of the needle closely. If a clear fluid enters the hub, lymph is being collected. In this case, replace the needle and start again. Because there are a number of spinal nerves and soft tissues and the spinal cord in the vicinity of the subcarapacial vein, the technician should use caution when inserting and redirecting the needle.

The brachial vein is located on the posterior aspect of the forelimb. This venipuncture site has been used with great success with tortoises, especially the giant tortoises, and collection can be performed without sedation. The technician should withdraw the leg and place one or more fingers proximal to the elbow to facilitate exposure. The needle should be inserted perpendicular to the posterior aspect of the biceps tendon and negative pressure applied immediately after penetrating the skin. This venipuncture site is a "blind-stick." One drawback of this site is that the brachial vein is closely associated with lymph, and if a diluted or "mixed" sample is collected, it cannot be used for hematologic evaluation. The femoral vein is located on the ventral surface of the thigh. This vessel is often accessible in tortoises that have pulled into their shell. A 22- to 25-gauge needle of varying length (depending on the size of the animal) can be used to collect the sample. The site should be prepared using standard asepsis. The needle should be inserted perpendicular to the thigh over the femur. Once inserted, the needle might need to be "walked" over the femur to locate the vessel. If the blood that is collected is bright red, the sample likely came from the femoral artery. If this is the case, apply direct pressure to the injection site for 2 minutes to ensure proper hemostasis is achieved.

The dorsal coccygeal vein is located on the dorsal midline of the tail. The tail should be extended and a 25-gauge needle inserted on the dorsal midline in a cranial direction. Again, this site is closely associated with lymph, and a mixed sample could be collected. The ventral coccygeal vein can be approached using the same strategy outlined in the lizard section.

Snakes

Blood samples are routinely collected from the heart, ventral coccygeal vein, and jugular vein of snakes. Cardiocentesis is the preferred method and provides large volumes of blood if necessary. The heart is located approximately one-third to one-quarter the distance from the head. This procedure is routinely performed on snakes weighing more than 200 grams without sedation. It is essential that there be enough assistance to restrain the snake during the procedure to prevent injury to the animal and the handlers. The animal should be positioned on its dorsum and the heart localized by visual inspection or palpation. Snakes are quite capable of moving their heart cranially or caudally, so it is important to "immobilize" the heart by inserting an index finger cranial to the heart, and the thumb caudal to the heart. A 22- to 25-gauge needle of variable length, based on the size of the snake, should be inserted under the scale at the most distal point of the beating heart (ventricle) (Figure 2.16). Apply negative pressure once the needle is inserted. The blood will literally be pumped into the syringe with each heartbeat. If a blood sample is not collected after inserting the needle, it is important to withdraw the needle and start over. Do not be overly aggressive when collecting a blood sample from the heart, because it is possible to lacerate the heart or large vessels and cause significant bleeding or death.

The ventral coccygeal vein is located on the ventral midline of the tail. Collection of blood from this site is usually possible only in larger snakes (>1 meter). The snake's body should be supported by a set of hands every 3–4 feet of body length. The tail should be grasped by the individual collecting the sample. The sample should be collected in the proximal one-third of the tail. Care should be taken not to damage the hemipenes of a male by staying on the midline. A 22- to 25-gauge needle should be inserted at a 45° angle under a ventral scale and advanced to the caudal vertebrae. Negative pressure should be applied and the needle retracted until blood is visualized in the hub of the needle.

Jugular veins are typically recommended only as sites for intravenous (IV) catheterization in snakes; however, some have found that these vessels can also be used for venipuncture. The landmarks for the jugular veins are the interior edges of the right or left ribs approximately 6–9 (ventral) scales cranial to the heart. The venipuncture site should be prepared using standard asepsis. A 25-gauge needle can be used to collect the sample.

The palatine vessels are often identified as potential venipuncture sites in snakes; however, experienced phlebotomists do not use them because sample volumes are typically small, there is potential for accidental bites, and it is possible to damage the oral cavity of the snake when collecting from them. Rottweilers have large lingual vessels that can be used for blood collection, but technicians don't use that site for the same reasons that were just mentioned.

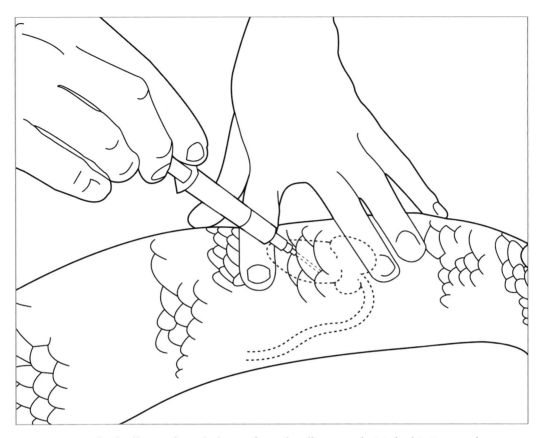

Figure 2.16 *Blood collection from the heart of a snake. Illustration by Michael L. Broussard.*

More on Amphibians

Blood samples can be collected in amphibians from the ventral abdominal vein, ventral coccygeal vein (salamanders, newts, caecilians, and tadpoles), heart, femoral vein, and lingual plexus. Restraining an amphibian for blood collection can be tricky because the animals can be quite slippery. Everyone involved in collecting the samples should wear moistened examination gloves to prevent damaging the animal's skin. Anesthesia (tricaine methane sulfonate; MS-222) might be required to sedate the animal for venipuncture. A 25- to 27-gauge needle fastened to a 3 ml syringe should be used for blood collection in amphibians. One should expect increased cellular destruction using the smaller-gauge needle. It is a good idea to heparinize the needle prior to blood collection to prevent clotting.

The ventral abdominal vein is often readily visible in larger amphibians by direct viewing or through transillumination of the body wall (e.g., placing a transilluminator/penlight near the lateral body wall). Blood collection techniques are similar to those described for lizards.

Blood can be collected from the ventral coccygeal vein in larger salamanders and newts, caecilians, and tadpoles (Figure 2.17). The approach to this vein is similar to that described for lizards. Some salamanders and newts, like lizards, have tail autotomy and can drop their tail as a natural defense mechanism if handled inappropriately.

Cardiocentesis should be used with caution in amphibians. There are some reports of animals dying after having blood collected from their heart. Some veterinarians have had good experience using cardiocentesis in amphibians; however, a rare death has been known to be associated with the procedure. The heart of most amphibians is located within the pectoral girdle; therefore, the needle should be directed medially through the axillary region to collect the sample (Figure 2.18). A 25- to 27-gauge needle should be used to collect the sample. No more than one to two attempts should be made using this technique, to limit the likelihood of inducing pathology. Some suggest using this method of venipuncture only as a last resort.

The femoral vein can be used to collect samples from larger frogs and toads. The technique used to collect blood from this site is similar to that described for chelonians.

The lingual plexus can be used for larger amphibians. The lingual plexus is a complex of blood vessels located under the fleshy tongue. A soft, rubber speculum should be used to gently open the animal's mouth. The skeletons of these animals are fragile in comparison with those of reptiles, and special care should be taken to prevent fractures. Once the mouth is open, a cotton-tipped applicator can be used to displace the tongue and facilitate exposure to the venous plexus. A needle (with no syringe attached) can be inserted into the venous plexus, and blood can be collected out of the hub of the needle using a microhematocrit tube. Sample contamination from saliva and food material in the oral cavity is likely when using this technique.[9]

Microbiology

Bacteria are ubiquitous in the environment. These organisms are commonly differentiated by staining characteristics using a Gram stain (positive or

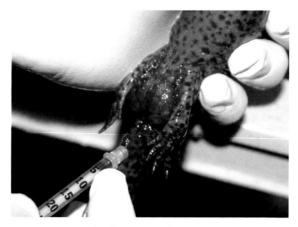

Figure 2.17 *Blood collection from the ventral coccygeal vein of an axolotl.*

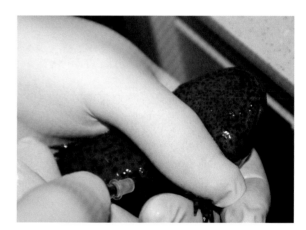

Figure 2.18 *Blood collection from the heart of an axolotl.*

negative) and can be further differentiated based on their biochemical needs: aerobic or anaerobic, lactose fermenting or nonlactose fermenting, and so on. Both Gram-positive and Gram-negative bacteria have been associated with infections in reptiles and amphibians, although opportunistic Gram-negative bacteria are more commonly isolated.

Reptiles and amphibians are ectotherms, and their core body temperature is regulated based on the environmental temperature and their behavioral activities (e.g., basking). Most commercial microbiologic incubators are set at 37°C because they were developed to grow pathogenic bacteria from humans. Because reptile core body temperatures can vary from this standard (37°C), it has been suggested that different temperatures be used to isolate bacteria from reptiles and amphibians. Unfortunately, establishing an incubator temperature that parallels a reptile's or amphibian's body temperature would be difficult. One possible solution would be to place one sample in a 37°C incubator and another at the animal's body temperature to accommodate organisms that thrive at lower temperatures. Regardless of the technique selected, one should always consider a negative culture from a contaminated wound the possible result of human inability to provide the organism an appropriate temperature.

Radiology

Radiographs serve as an important diagnostic tool in reptile and amphibian medicine. Radiographs are routinely used to assess a variety of health conditions in these animals, including reproductive (e.g., dystocia), skeletal (e.g., fracture), gastrointestinal (e.g., foreign body), renal (e.g., renomegaly), and respiratory (e.g., pneumonia) problems. Standard safety protocols should be employed when radiographing reptiles and amphibians. The animal might need to be anesthetized for the procedure, although some animals will remain still if placed in a darkened room, given blinders, or placed in a tube (e.g., snakes).

A radiographic technique chart should be established based on the capacity of a facility's radiographic machine. A high-capacity radiographic unit capable of producing 300-milliampere exposures at times of at least 1/60th of a second is recommended. The kVp settings should be adjustable by increments of two to provide finite detail. A thorough understanding of reptile and amphibian anatomy is essential to radiographic interpretation. Dental radiographs can be used to collect images of small reptiles and most amphibians. The introduction of digital radiography has simplified collecting images for reptiles and amphibians, allowing multiple images to be taken and processed in seconds to minutes. Individuals with this capacity can use this method to take as many images as are necessary in a short period of time to obtain the information they need to direct their cases.

It is important always to collect at least two radiographic images when evaluating a reptile or amphibian patient. This will help to resolve the fact that these animals are three-dimensional and that the images are each only two-dimensional. The most common radiographic images taken are via the dorsoventral (ventrodorsal) and lateral approaches. In chelonians, a third image, the anterior-posterior or cranial-caudal approach, should also be collected. This allows for independent review of the lungs, which is especially important in chelonian cases with suspected pneumonia.

Parasitology
External Parasites

Imported reptiles routinely have ectoparasites, such as mites, ticks, and leeches. These parasites survive by ingesting blood from their host. Heavily parasitized juvenile animals can develop life-threatening anemia. Many of these ectoparasites also serve as vectors for other diseases, including bacterial and possibly viral infections.[10] The diagnosis of an ectoparasite infestation can be made during a thorough physical examination. Leeches are readily identifiable on aquatic reptiles and amphibians. These large ectoparasites should be grasped with forceps and gently separated from the host. The open lesion where the leech was attached should be cleaned and disinfected (e.g., 0.5% chlorhexidine).

Ticks are typically not as large as leeches, but are readily identified on external examination. There are three primary life stages of the tick: larva, nymph, and adult. The nymphal and adult stages are differentiated from the larval stages based on the number of appendages (larval: 6; nymphal and adult: 8). The tick burrows its mouthparts into the host to facilitate feeding. Tick removal can be accomplished by grasping the mouthparts where they insert into the host and pulling them out perpendicular to the reptile's skin. Once the parasite is removed it should be properly disposed of.

Mites are the smallest of the ectoparasites (1–2 mm) and can be easily overlooked; a magnifying glass or loupe might be helpful in some cases to spot the mites. Mites can be found anywhere on the reptile host, although they tend to accumulate around the eyes, mouth, and gular fold (snakes). A cotton-tipped applicator soaked in mineral oil can be used to remove a mite to confirm the diagnosis. The treatment protocols for ectoparasites vary (Table 2.3). Neither ivermectin nor its derivatives should be given to chelonians, as it may be fatal.

Internal Parasites

Endoparasites are common in reptiles and amphibians. The same groups of endoparasites commonly identified in domestic species are also routinely identified in reptiles and amphibians, including protozoa, nematodes, trematodes, and cestodes. Many reptiles presented to veterinary hospitals are imported and should be assumed to have parasites until proven otherwise. It is also important to consider that many captive-born reptiles are also infested with parasites, because of the methods used for raising these animals. Most of the popular captive-raised reptiles are held under high densities with limited/no quarantine, a perfect situation for the dissemination of parasites.

Animals and parasites have evolved to "live together," even though the parasite steals nutrition from the host. In captivity, when a reptile or amphibian is exposed to the stress of an inadequate environment and diet, parasites can become more problematic. Parasites will continue to acquire energy from the host, regardless of the host's change in appetite. In these cases, the parasites can become life-threatening. A fecal examination should be performed to identify potential parasites so that an appropriate treatment can be initiated. A fecal saline direct smear and a fecal flotation should be performed on all fecal samples. The direct smear will enable the reviewer to identify bacteria and protozoa, and the fecal float is used to identify larger parasite ova (e.g., roundworms). A fecal examination should always be repeated in 2 weeks, and again in 4 weeks, to determine if the animal is really negative (because shedding can be transient). There are a number of treatment protocols that have been established for treating parasites in reptiles and amphibians (Table 2.3).

THERAPEUTICS

There are no approved therapeutics for reptiles in the United States. Routes of administration for therapeutics and fluids include per os (PO), subcutaneous (SC), intramuscular (IM), intraosseus (IO), intracoelomic (ICO), and intravenous (IV). Animals that are in critical condition require routes of administration that provide rapid drug delivery, such as IM, IO, or IV, whereas less critical animals can be given therapeutics PO or SC.

IV injections should be administered through an IV catheter. The preferred site for IV catheterization in chelonians, lizards, and snakes is the jugular vein. The cephalic vein can also be used in lizards. IO catheters can be placed in the femur or tibia of lizards. Some veterinarians pre-

Table 2.3 **Antiparasitic Agents Used in Reptiles and Amphibians**

DRUG	DOSE	COMMENTS
Fenbendazole	25–100 mg/kg PO Repeat in 7–14 prn	Nematodes[21]
Ivermectin	0.2 mg/kg IM, SC	Nematodes[22] NEVER USE IN CHELONIANS
	5 mg/L Water	Topical spray to treat mites[23]
Levamisole	10–20 mg/kg	Nematodes[24]
Metronidazole	25–100 mg/kg PO Repeat in 2 weeks	Protozoa[22] Uracoan rattler, milk snakes, tricolor king snakes, and indigo snakes at 40 mg/kg
Praziquantel	5–8 mg/kg IM, SC	Cestodes and trematodes[25]

fer using the tibia for this procedure. The catheter can be inserted on the tibial plateau. The gular scutes are a good site for IO catheter placement in chelonians.

IM injections are routinely administered into the epaxial muscles along the spine or in the large muscle groups in the front limbs. Reptiles and amphibians have a renal portal system that can be affected by drug administration in the tail or rear limbs. To avoid these complications, always administer medications in the cranial one-half of the body. The muscle masses of reptile and amphibian limbs are relatively small compared with those of mammals; therefore, injections should be performed sparingly and injection sites (e.g., right leg, left leg) should be alternated.

Reptiles and amphibians are difficult to pill. Fortunately, there are a number of commercial compounding pharmacies that can compound a therapeutic into a liquid and simplify administration. Administering oral medications is a straightforward process for reptiles. The glottis is located at the base of the tongue, and it is easily seen and therefore easy to avoid when dosing with a syringe or passing a tube.

SURGICAL AND ANESTHETIC ASSISTANCE

Anesthesia and analgesia are relatively new concepts in reptile and amphibian medicine. Only a decade or so ago, individuals "anesthetized" reptiles by placing them in a refrigerator or freezer to severely restrict their metabolism. This technique should never be used because it does not provide the animal consistent anesthesia or analgesia and can prove fatal. Prior to any anesthetic procedure, the animal should be assessed and determined to be stable. Basic health monitoring should include evaluating the hydration status, heart and respiratory rates, and baseline blood work.

Tricaine methane sulfonate (MS-222) and clove oil are commonly used anesthetics for amphibians. These compounds can be delievered through an immersion/bath. The water used for the bath should come from the animal's enclosure to minimize changes in water quality. The water depth for the bath should be set to the level of the elbow of the patient. If kept in deep water, the amphibian could drown. These compounds are absorbed via the skin, primarily through the ventral abdominal patch, or gills (e.g., axolotls). Both anesthestics have been found to provide general anesthesia; however, MS-222 is considered to be safer and provides a longer duration of anesthesia. Doses for MS-222 in amphibians can vary depending on whether the animal is terrestrial (0.5–2 g/L) or aquatic (100–500 mg/L), and whether it has gills (100–200 mg/L) or not.

The anesthetics and analgesics used for domestic species (e.g., dogs and cats) are routinely used in reptiles and amphibians, including the dissociatives, propofol, and inhalant anesthetics. The most common dissociatives used in reptile and amphibian anesthesia are ketamine and tiletamine plus zolazepam. Ketamine has been used successfully in reptiles and amphibians. Recommended doses vary with reptile and amphibian order, health status, and size of the animal. A dose of 5–10 mg/kg ketamine can be given for short painless procedures or as a preanesthetic to facilitate intubation; a slightly higher dose might be needed for chelonians: 10–20 mg/kg. In most species, the animals will be induced within 10–20 minutes. Ketamine provides little to no visceral analgesia; therefore a preoperative and postoperative analgesic should be considered for painful procedures. A dose of 55–88 mg/kg has been recommended for surgical anesthesia, but ketamine alone should not be considered an adequate surgical anesthetic in these species.[11] There have been a number of side effects reported with ketamine use, including respiratory arrest, bradycardia, and prolonged recovery (1–4 days). Many of these side effects are associated with the administration of high doses (>100 mg/kg), but they can also occur at lower doses. Many anesthetic complications can be prevented by properly evaluating the animal prior to a procedure and monitoring the animal closely during the procedure. Tiletamine is a more potent dissociative agent that is combined with zolazepam to provide sedation and is an anticonvulsant. Tiletamine has been used in snakes and crocodilians with some success, but recoveries are still prolonged. Tiletamine, like ketamine, should not be used for surgical anesthesia in reptiles, but as an induction agent in combination with an inhalant anesthetic. A dose of 3–5 mg/kg is routinely used with good results.

The alpha-2 agonists, such as medetomidine and dexmedetomidine, are also routinely used for reptiles and amphibians. These drugs can be used with the dissociative anesthetics to provide a more "complete" anesthesia. The alpha-2 agonists provide visceral analgesia and muscle relaxation, which complement the dissociatives. These anesthetic agents can cause cardiopulmonary depression, so it is important to monitor animals closely during their anesthetic procedure. Doses can vary by species and whether they are used in combination with other anesthetics. Typically, medetomidine doses are 0.025–0.1 mg/kg and dexmedetomidine doses are 0.01–0.05 mg/kg.

Propofol has gained in popularity with veterinarians because it provides general anesthesia with a rapid recovery. The primary disadvantage of propofol is that it must be administered intravenously or intraosseously, which can be difficult in smaller patients. An IV butterfly catheter can be used to administer boluses to an animal as the procedure warrants. A dose of 10–14 mg/kg IV in lizards and snakes provides reasonable general anesthesia for 15–30 minutes. A dose of 12–15 mg/kg IV is recommended for chelonians.[12] This anesthetic has been used in amphibians with success, too. Intracoelomic injections of propofol (35–45 mg/kg) have been found to provide sedation to surgical anesthesia in frogs and salamanders.

Inhalant anesthetics have reduced many of the risks associated with injectable anesthetics. Unlike injectable anesthetics (e.g., ketamine), which cannot be controlled once administered, delivery of an inhalant anesthetic through a precision vaporizer can be controlled based on need. Animals under general inhalant anesthetics should be intubated. Endotracheal tubes ensure that the appropriate anesthetic and oxygen rates are being administered. Endotracheal tube size will vary with the order and size of the animal. Chelonians and crocodilians have closed tracheal rings, like birds, and should not have their endotracheal cuff inflated. The majority of reptile and amphibian cases presented in private practice are animals under 5 kg and can be maintained using a non-rebreathing system. When a procedure on a larger animal (>5 kg) is required, a circle system, similar to that used in dogs, can be used.

The most common inhalants used in veterinary practice are isoflurane and sevoflurane, and both of these anesthetics have been used successfully in reptiles and amphibians. Our knowledge about the metabolism of these gases in reptiles and amphibians is limited and often related to our knowledge of it in mammals. The elimination of isoflurane and sevoflurane is exclusively through the respiratory system. There are two trains of thought about anesthetizing an exotic animal: "full-throttle" and incremental anesthesia.

The "full-throttle" approach is based on the desire to deliver a high percentage of anesthetic immediately. Many veterinarians will turn the vaporizer directly to 5% (8% sevoflurane). This method is often used to induce fractious animals, because they are anesthetized sooner, and it also delivers high doses to animals that hold their breath. This helps expedite the process of moving a patient from stage 1 anesthesia to stage 3 anesthesia, skipping through stage 2 anesthesia, where animals tend to struggle. The potential disadvantage of this technique is that the animal can become deeply anesthetized and, if not monitored closely, can become apneic (stop breathing) and die. In the incremental approach, the inhalant anesthetic is delivered in increments to ensure a smooth procedure. The animal is started at 2%–3% (4%–5% sevoflurane) and the level increased or decreased based on the animal's status. The potential disadvantage of this technique is that induction can take a long time when the patient holds its breath and it is more likely to struggle as it moves to stage 3 anesthesia. Maintenance levels for isoflurane and sevoflurane are between 1.5% and 3.0% and 3.0% and 5.0%, respectively, but will vary from patient to patient. Anesthetic recovery for animals placed under general anesthesia (alone) is typically within 10–20 minutes after discontinuation of the gas.

Monitoring of the reptile or amphibian during an anesthetic or surgical procedure is often performed by the veterinary technician. The respiratory rate can usually be monitored by direct visualization of the body wall in snakes and lizards, whereas the gular area and "pumping" action of the legs are used to monitor respiration in chelonians.

Auscultation of the heart is very difficult in reptiles. Placement of the stethoscope bell directly on the scales results in an irritating friction-generated sound. Esophageal stethoscopes can be used; however, most reptile and amphibian patients are too small to accommodate these large tubes. Crystal ultrasonic Dopplers simplify monitoring the heart rate by producing a sound that verifies cardiac function. Pulse oximeters have gained in popularity in veterinary hospitals and provide not only the heart rate but also arterial oxygen saturation. ECGs can also be used.

There are a number of different probes that can be purchased with these systems. For mammals, C-clip probes are often used, but for reptiles these probes have limited usefulness because the signal cannot penetrate the colored scales. The cloacal probes appear to work best for reptiles. Although these devices can simplify the role of the veterinary technician, placement and repositioning might be required during the procedure.

The mucous membrane color and hydration status should also be monitored on a reptile or an amphibian during a surgical procedure. Amphibians should be kept moist throughout the procedure to prevent desiccation. If there is concern that an animal might experience significant blood loss during a procedure, it should be given fluids (e.g., IV or IO) or a blood transfusion.

Reptiles should be provided with heat during a surgical procedure. Water-circulating heat pads provide good results and are unlikely to cause thermal burns. When working with these heating elements, it is important to recognize that a reptile's sharp claws could tear the heating pad, so protection (e.g., a towel) should be used. Reptiles are dependent on the environmental temperature to maintain their metabolism and ability to process anesthetics and recover from surgery. Maintaining a reptile at an inappropriate temperature will prolong the recovery, with full recovery times lasting 1–3 days in some cases.

Amphibians do not tolerate excessive heat. When performing a procedure on an amphibian, it should be done at an appropriate temperature for that animal, typically 74°–78°F for tropical species and 68°–74°F for temperate species. Setting the ambient room temperature to an appropriate level is preferred over using heat lamps or heating pads, which can overheat the animal and promote desiccation.

Reptiles and amphibians have very unusual respiratory systems. The lungs of a reptile or amphibian are much simpler than those of mammals or birds, and reptiles and amphibians lack a true diaphragm. These anatomical features are important to consider when anesthetizing and maintaining a reptile or amphibian on inhalant anesthetics. Reptiles and amphibians normally breathe by movement of their body wall (intercostal muscles), limbs, and viscera; amphibians can also respire through their skin. When reptiles or amphibians are under general anesthesia, they might not be capable of breathing on their own and must be ventilated using positive pressure. Typically, 4–5 breaths a minute will be satisfactory. When a reptile or amphibian is ventilated, it is important to use a pressure of less than 12 cm of water to prevent their simple saclike lungs from rupturing.[11] The veterinary technician plays a vital role in the surgery and is often responsible for managing a number of tasks, including presurgical preparation of surgical supplies, preparing an aseptic surgical site, assistance during the surgical procedure, and anesthetic monitoring.

Preparing the surgical suite for a reptile or amphibian patient should follow the basic techniques used for preparing the suite for mammalian patients. The surgical packs should be sterilized by the same methods (e.g., autoclaved, gas) used to prepare surgical equipment for domestic species.

Selection of the appropriate suture material will reduce the possibility of incision dehiscence and poor healing. The absorbable synthetic sutures can be used for ligation and suture placement internally, and nylon sutures can be used to close skin incisions. Chromic catgut and stainless steel should not be used in reptiles or amphibians. In reptiles, the skin is considered the primary closing layer because it is unlikely to tear, whereas in mammals the linea alba is the primary closing layer. Skin sutures should remain in a reptile or amphibian patient for 4–6 weeks. This prolonged healing time is associated with the slower metabolism common to ectotherms.

The veterinary technician serves a primary role in monitoring asepsis during the surgical procedure. The surgical suite can become very busy, and it is important that the technician ensure that no individual compromises the sterility of the procedure. Preparation of the surgical site should follow standard protocol, wiping from the center of the surgical site in a circular motion until a desired area has been sterilized. Preparing the skin of reptiles can be difficult because of the scales, but attempts should be made to remove heavy debris. The skin of an amphibian is very thin, so minimal pressure should be applied when preparing the site. The surgical site should be prepared with a nonirritating solution, such as dilute chlorhexidine or betadine, followed by isotonic sterile saline. **Alcohol should never be used to disinfect a surgical site on a reptile or amphibian, because it creates an evaporative surface that can lead to significant body heat loss.**

During a surgical procedure, the veterinary technician is often expected to manage hemostasis. Hemostasis is essential in the reptile or amphibian patient because any excess loss of blood could prove to be life-threatening. In most cases, simply applying direct pressure using a sponge is sufficient. Do not wipe or smear the blood vessel, because this might cause an irritation or further damage the blood vessel. If direct pressure (30–120 seconds) is insufficient to stop the hemorrhage, the veterinary surgeon will consider other techniques such as suture or radiosurgery (Ellman International, Oceanside, NY).

Incision irrigation and lavage are other important functions that the veterinary technician performs when assisting the veterinarian during the surgical procedure. The irrigating or lavage fluid should be isotonic (e.g., normal saline) and prewarmed to the animal's body temperature (37°C is sufficient) to prevent cold stress. Cold stress can rapidly result in a cascade of physiologic changes that can alter the animal's response to

the anesthesia. Incisions should be irrigated liberally to improve the veterinary surgeon's view of the surgical site. When performing a lavage in the coelomic cavity of the reptile or amphibian, it is important to remember that it lacks a diaphragm and that excess irrigation fluid can place pressure on the animal's lung(s), making it difficult to breathe. To prevent this problem, lavage limited amounts of fluid at a time, removing any excess with sterile gauze or suction. Be careful when using suction because tissues can be damaged if they are pulled into the suction tube.

After the surgical procedure is completed, the animal should be moved to a clean, warm, quiet area to recover. Remove the animal from the anesthetic machine and allow it to recover on room air. Reptiles are stimulated to breathe when their blood oxygen levels decrease to a threshold; maintaining them on oxygen will only prolong the recovery.[13] The animal should not be extubated until it has started to swallow. Animals that have had a coeliotomy or fracture repair should not be provided with climbing branches until the veterinary surgeon feels that the animal is not in danger of wound dehiscence.

HEALTH MAINTENANCE AND DISEASE

The majority of the diseases encountered in pet reptile and amphibian medicine are directly related to inappropriate husbandry and are discussed below. Animals maintained under inappropriate temperatures, provided inadequate diets, or held under less than optimal housing conditions are at an increased risk of developing disease.

Husbandry-Related Problems
Thermal Burns

Reptiles will often seek heat to maintain their core body temperature. If an animal is placed in

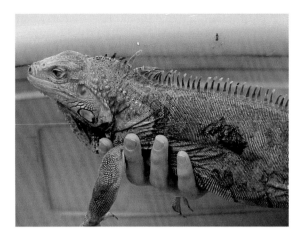

Figure 2.19 *Thermal burn in a green iguana.*

an enclosure that has an exposed lightbulb, heating pad, or heat rock as its only source of heat, the animal might remain on the device and develop severe life-threatening burns (Figure 2.19). These cases should be considered emergencies and treated appropriately. In severe burn cases, an animal can lose significant amounts of fluids through the burn sites and should be provided supplemental fluids. The wound should be assessed for severity. Deep contaminated wounds have a guarded prognosis. Prior to initiating wound management, the veterinary technician should collect a bacteriological sample and submit it for a culture and antimicrobial sensitivity to identify potential pathogenic organisms and an appropriate antibiotic.

Wound management should follow standard mammalian protocols. The wound should be irrigated with an isotonic saline solution and a nonirritating cleansing solution, such as chlorhexidine. Topical antimicrobials may be applied to prevent wound contamination. Topical creams or ointments should be applied in a thin coat over the wound, because excessive application can result in anaerobic conditions. Silvadene cream is an excellent antimicrobial cream that can be applied to thermal injuries.

Application of a wet-to-dry bandage can be used to reduce wound contamination and encourage wound healing. The bandage should be changed daily until the wound begins to "dry," and then as needed until the granulation tissue is considered adequate. It is important to remember that bandages that cover the body wall should not be too restrictive in order not to impede respiration. Animals with severe burns should be placed on antimicrobials. Enrofloxacin (5–10 mg/kg by mouth once daily) or trimethoprim-sulfa (15 mg/kg PO SID) provides excellent coverage and can be initiated while an antimicrobial sensitivity is pending.

Prey Bites

Reptiles and amphibians hunt food only when they are hungry. Most owners offer their reptiles and amphibians live foods, assuming that the pet will eat, or at least kill, the food item. Unfortunately, this is not always the case. Many prey items, including rodents and insects, will "attack" the predator if left unattended. A number of reports have cited large snakes that died from wounds inflicted by a mouse or rat. Even common crickets have been observed to "feed" on juvenile lizards. A prey bite should always be managed as a contaminated wound (see thermal burns). Owners should be educated about the dangers of feeding live prey and directed to observe their pet during feedings. All mammalian prey items (e.g., rats and mice) should be humanely euthanized before being fed to reptiles.

Dysecdysis

Reptiles shed the outer epidermal layer of their skin as they grow. In juvenile animals, shedding (ecdysis) occurs regularly and slows as the animal matures. Shedding of the skin is a routine and necessary behavior that all reptiles experience;

however, patterns of shedding differ among species. Chelonians and lizards routinely shed their skin in pieces, whereas snakes shed their skin in one entire piece. Most of the problems associated with shedding (dysecdysis) are reported in snakes, although dysecdysis can occur in all reptiles. Causes of dysecdysis in reptiles have been associated with low environmental humidity and temperature, ectoparasites, traumatic wounds, systemic disease, mishandling, and the lack of an adequate surface to assist with shedding.

Treatment for dysecdysis should include correcting any environmental and medical problems and soaking the animal in a shallow, warm (82°–84°F) water bath. The depth of the water bath should not exceed half the height of the animal. Never use a human water receptacle (e.g., bathtub or sink) to soak a reptile because of the potential for introducing zoonotic pathogens (e.g., *Salmonella* spp.). After soaking, a soft cotton towel can be used to gently wipe the animal down and remove any excess shed. Do not pull at skin that is not ready to come off because you could damage the underlying skin. Owners should be made aware of the importance of checking the spectacles or eye caps to make sure that they are removed after every shed. Retained spectacles can develop into subspectacular abscesses, which can lead to the loss of the eye if not managed appropriately.

Nutritional Diseases

Secondary Nutritional Hyperparathyroidism

The most common nutritional disease reported in reptiles is secondary nutritional hyperparathyroidism (SNHP). SNHP may occur as a result of a calcium-deficient diet, phosphorus-rich diet, or vitamin D deficiency. In this disease process, the parathyroid glands are activated and release parathormone, which mobilizes calcium from the skeleton for the animal to meet its daily needs. A thorough history will often guide a veterinarian in the diagnosis of this disease. Animals suffering from SNHP are often young, fast-growing animals or reproductively active adult females maintained at an inappropriate ETR (which reduces metabolism) and/or offered a calcium-deficient diet, excessive phosphorus diet, or not exposed to ultraviolet B wavelength light (which aids in synthesis of vitamin D).

On physical examination, the animal often has muscle tremors and fasciculations, "swollen" mandibles and long bones (fibrous osteodystrophy), and might suffer from seizures. Clinical diagnosis is made from a thorough history, physical examination, and radiographs. These animals should be considered critical care cases, and therapy should be initiated immediately. Medical management includes supplemental calcium and vitamin D therapy, fluids to rehydrate animals, enteral support to maintain energy demands, and treatment of secondary problems, such as splinting pathologic fractures.

Hypovitaminosis A

Chelonians offered inappropriate diets often develop hypovitaminosis A. Animals presenting with hypovitaminosis A are often young, fast-growing animals or long-term wild caught specimens maintained at inappropriate temperatures and offered a restricted, vitamin A–deficient diet. On physical examination, the animals will often have unilateral or bilateral blepharoedema (swelling of the eyelids), a nasal and ocular discharge, diarrhea, pneumonia, aural abscesses, and hyperkeratosis. Vitamin A deficiency leads to changes in the epithelial lining of the respiratory tract, oral cavity, skin, and urinary tract. The resulting squamous metaplasia reduces the tight junctions formed by the cells and allows for opportunistic pathogens to invade.[14] Diagnosis is often made from the history, physical examination, and response to treatment. Animals with respiratory disease should have a culture and sensitivity performed to evaluate appropriate antimicrobial therapy to manage opportunistic infections. Animals considered to have hypovitaminosis A should be administered vitamin A parenterally (500–1,500 IU/kg every 10 days for 1–4 treatments);[15] however, oversupplementation of vitamin A can lead to iatrogenic hypervitaminosis A. Hypervitaminosis A leads to skin sloughing and can be life-threatening.

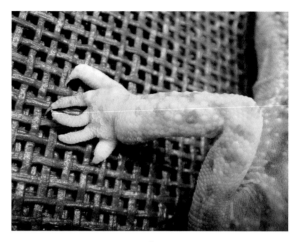

Figure 2.20 *Severe articular gout in a gecko.*

Gout

Gout results from the deposition of monosodium urate crystals into the viscera (visceral gout) or joints (articular gout) (Figure 2.20) as a result of the body synthesizing too much uric acid (e.g., high-protein diets), dehydration, or renal impairment. Animals presenting with gout are often adult and may be herbivores, omnivores, or carnivores. Generally, these animals are reported to be in good health, but become acutely depressed and lethargic. A review of husbandry practices will often reveal that these animals have been offered an inappropriate diet or not provided sufficient access to a water source. On physical examination, these animals are clinically dehydrated, have poor muscling condition, and are in overall poor condition. A thorough history, physical examination, plasma chemistry profile, and radiographs will help establish a diagnosis. Reptiles and amphibians with gout often have hyperuricemia; however, animals with gout can have normal plasma uric acid levels. If the kidneys are impaired as a result of the monosodium urate crystallization, the calcium-to-phosphorus levels will most likely be inverse (<1:1). Radiographs of a reptile with gout might reveal radiopaque lesions in joints or viscera. The goal of treatment for a reptile or amphibian with gout is to correct the original dietary (e.g., reduce dietary purine-based proteins, offer correct diet) and environmental (e.g., provide ad libitum access to water; do not restrict water) problems, reduce uric acid production in the body (allopurinol, 20 mg/kg by mouth once daily), and increase urate excretion (probenecid, 250 mg/kg, by mouth once daily).[16] The prognosis for these cases is guarded.

Infectious Diseases

Reptiles and amphibians are susceptible to a number of infectious agents, including viruses, bacteria, and fungi. The majority of cases presented to veterinary hospitals are directly related to inappropriate management. When a reptile or amphibian is maintained at low environmental temperatures, its immune function is reduced and it is prone to opportunistic infections. Another source of infectious diseases for reptile and amphibian collections is inadequate quarantine. Newly acquired animals should be segregated from other reptiles or amphibians to ensure that they are not shedding infectious agents that might contaminate a collection. The quarantine period for a reptile or amphibian should be a minimum of 60–90 days.[17]

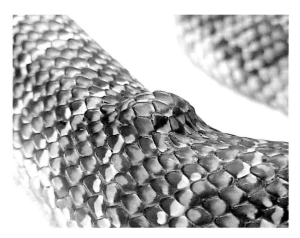

Figure 2.21 *A well-defined caseous abscess on the dorsum of a snake.*

Abscesses

Abscesses are a common finding in animals that are managed under inappropriate conditions. Abscesses are often the result of an infectious origin (e.g., bacterial infection), foreign body, or parasite. Abscesses in reptiles and amphibians can be found anywhere on the body and are commonly located on the toes and tail and in the oral cavity. Abscesses are often firm, well-circumscribed lesions (Figure 2.21). Diagnosis of an abscess is often made from the history, physical examination, and the results of an aspirate or biopsy of the mass. Reptile and amphibian abscesses are typically caseous or "cheesy" in nature, rather than liquefactive as in mammals. This difference is related to the reduced enzymatic firepower that reptile cells possess in relation to higher vertebrates.

Successful management of an abscess in a reptile or amphibian requires incision and curettage. Simply initiating systemic antibiotic therapy will be insufficient, because the inciting cause, or nidus, if bacterial, is often located in the center of the abscess and will be unaffected by any drugs. A local anesthetic line, or ring block using lidocaine,

should be performed prior to making the incision. A microbiological sample should be collected for culture and sensitivity once the incision is made. Caseous abscesses can generally be scooped out of the incision. The open wound should then be irrigated with a nonirritating disinfectant, such as diluted chlorhexidine. A single localized abscess can often be managed by irrigating it and applying a topical antimicrobial ointment. Generalized abscesses require systemic treatment and a systemic antibiotic, based on the sensitivity findings. The abscess should be managed as an open wound and allowed to heal by secondary intention.

Mycoplasmosis

Mycoplasmosis is a bacterial infection that has been associated with severe disease in chelonians. Affected animals might present with nasal and ocular discharge, conjunctivitis, palpebral edema, and pneumonia. Mycoplasmosis has also been identified in squamates and crocodilians. There are several diagnostic tests available to confirm mycoplasmosis in reptiles, including culture, an ELISA (*enzyme-linked immunosorbent assay*), and a PCR (*polymerase chain reaction*) assay. Microbiologic culture can be used to confirm an infection, but it is difficult and time-consuming to isolate this bacteria. Currently, parallel testing using both the ELISA and PCR assays provides the highest degree of sensitivity. Treatment may be attempted using tetracyclines and fluoroquinolones. Mycoplasmosis has been associated with declines in native tortoise populations in the United States, and treatment of wild specimens is not recommended.

Viruses

As diagnostic techniques to identify viruses improve, more and more of these pathogens are being associated with disease in reptiles and amphibians. The viruses that have received the most attention in pet reptile and amphibian medicine are paramyxovirus, retrovirus, herpesvirus, and ranavirus.

Paramyxoviruses are primarily associated with viperid snakes, although they have also been identified in nonviperid snakes.[18,19] This virus is typically spread from contact with respiratory secretions. Affected animals display clinical signs associated with respiratory disease, such as nasal and oral discharge, open-mouth breathing, increased lung sounds, and possible neurologic signs, including tremors and seizures. Diagnosis can be made antemortem from a blood test or postmortem from a histologic diagnosis.[20] Mixed results have been found among different laboratories using the antemortem serologic test for paramyxovirus, so caution should be used when interpreting the results.[21] There is no effective treatment for this virus.

Inclusion body disease primarily affects snakes in the family Boidae (e.g., boas and pythons). Historically, this virus was attributed to a retrovirus, although this has not been confirmed. The method of transmission of this disease is unknown, but it appears contagious and it is suspected that snake mites (*Ophionyssus natricis*) play a role in its dissemination. Affected boa constrictors present with chronic regurgitation, but might develop neurologic signs, including loss of righting reflex, tremors, and disorientation, as the disease progresses. Affected pythons develop severe neurologic signs, similar to those described for the boas, that progressively worsen. Animals typically succumb to this disease as a result of secondary infections and starvation. Diagnosis can be made antemortem from surgical biopsies and seeing inclusions in the cytoplasm of lymphocytes on a blood smear, and postmortem from histopathologic examination. There is no effec-

tive treatment for this disease. Affected animals should be euthanized to prevent the spread of the disease to other snakes.

Bearded dragon adenovirus was first reported in Australia in the early 1980s. The virus was not characterized in the United States until more than a decade later. Since that time, the virus has spread through the bearded dragon population in the United States and should be considered endemic. Transmission of the virus is primarily by the direct route (fecal-oral), although vertical transmission might also be possible. Affected animals might present with anorexia, weight loss, limb paresis, diarrhea, and opisthotonus. Concurrent dependovirus and coccidial infections have also been observed in neonatal bearded dragons.[22] Biopsies of the liver, stomach, esophagus, and kidney may be collected to confirm diagnosis (antemortem). On histopathology, basophilic intranuclear inclusion bodies are strongly suggestive of adenoviral infection. Antemortem diagnosis can also be made using PCR (fecal shedding). There is no effective treatment for adenoviral infections, although supportive care (e.g., fluids, enteral nutrition, antibiotics) can be useful in stemming the secondary effects of the disease.

The incidence of herpesvirus infections in chelonians has been on the rise since originally being isolated from sea turtles in 1975. Herpesvirus infections have been identified in freshwater, marine, and terrestrial species of chelonians. Transmission of the herpesvirus is believed to be via the horizontal route, although it has been suggested that a vertical route of transmission is also possible. Affected animals might present with rhinitis, conjunctivitis, necrotizing stomatitis, glossitis, enteritis, pneumonia, and neurological disease. Molecular diagnostics, electron microscopy, and viral isolation have been used to diagnose herpes infections in chelonians. Affected animals should be given appropriate supportive care (e.g., fluids, enteral nutrition, and antibiotics) to control clinical signs. Acyclovir has been used with some success by reducing viral replication. However, there is no effective treatment for this virus. Affected animals should not be released into the wild, to prevent translocation of the virus to naïve chelonians.

Ranaviruses are members of the family Iridoviridae. These viruses have historically been an important pathogen in amphibians, more specifically anurans. In recent years, they have been found to cross over into other classes of animals, including reptiles and fish. They have been found in both wild and captive chelonians (e.g., box turtles). Clinical signs in affected animals might include anorexia, depression, upper and lower respiratory tract disease, cervical cellulitis, and death. This virus will likely become more prevalent in both wild and captive populations over time as natural habitats of turtles are further encroached upon by humans and animals, and as turtles are brought into captivity without appropriate quarantine methods.

Fungi

Fungi are being diagnosed more frequently in captive reptile and amphibian cases. The apparent increased prevalence can be attributed to better diagnostic testing and a greater awareness of these pathogens among veterinarians. Although most cases are associated with opportunistic infections, there has been a rise in cases attributed to obligate fungal pathogens in both reptiles and amphibains.

The *Chrysosporium* anamorph of *Nanniziopsis vriesii* has been found to infect snakes, lizards, and chelonians. Bearded dragons appear to be very susceptible. Often called "the yellow fungus" in these lizards, this fungal pathogen can be fatal

to animals. Affected animals typically present with yellow crusts that can be found anywhere on their body. The crusts can progress into pyogranulomatous inflammation. Diagnosis can be made from biopsy samples submitted for histopathology and culture. Treatment needs to be aggressive and should include both topical (chlorhexidine and miconazole cream) and systemic (itraconazole, 5 mg/kg by mouth once daily) treatment.

Chytrid fungi are a problem in both captive and wild populations of amphibians. This fungus has been attributed to worldwide population declines in amphibians. Affected animals lose their ability to regulate their fluid balance, because the pathogen has a predilection for the keratinized tissues associated with their ventral abdominal patch, and become susceptible to other opportunistic infections. Diagnosis can be made from histopathology and culture. A PCR assay is also available. Topical and systemic antifungals should be used to treat affected animals.

Parasites

Cryptosporidium serpentis is considered a "plague" of captive snake collections. This apicomplexan parasite has been associated with both high morbidity and mortality in captive collections. Affected snakes commonly regurgitate their meals, have a midbody swelling, and are dehydrated. A variety of methods can be used to diagnose cryptosporidiosis in snakes. Acid-fast cytology of a regurgitated meal or fecal sample is often diagnostic; however, multiple samples might be needed to confirm the presence of the parasite, because they can be transiently shed. Because there is currently no effective treatment, affected animals should be culled. *Cryptosporidium saurophilum* is a more recently diagnosed species associated with lizards. Whereas *C. serpentis* is associated with the stomach, *C. saurophilum* is associated with the intestine. Currently,

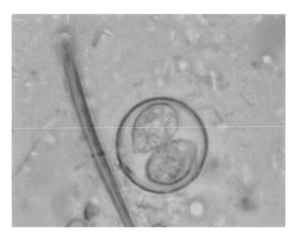

Figure 2.22 *Coccidiosis in a bearded dragon. This particular organism is* Isospora amphiboluri.

no consistent treatment is available for *C. saurophilum* or *C. serpentis.*

Coccidiosis is a major cause of morbidity and mortality in reptiles. A species of special concern, *Isospora amphiboluri*, is found in bearded dragons (Figure 2.22). These endoparasites are especially problematic in neonatal dragons, often resulting in stunting, diarrhea, and death. Whereas most coccidial infections in higher vertebrates are self-limiting, these infections often persist in bearded dragon colonies, because animals are held in high densities and autoinfection is common in vivaria that are not cleaned regularly. Historically, eliminating coccidia from bearded dragons was difficult because most of the therapeutics used to eliminate the parasites were coccidiostatic (i.e., suppresses but does not kill coccidia). Ponazuril (30 mg/kg by mouth once, with a second treatment 48 hours later) is coccidiocidal (i.e., kills coccidia) and has excellent therapeutic value against *I. amphiboluri*. Quarantine and environmental disinfection/sanitation should also be done to eliminate coccidia from dragon colonies.

Microsporidians are obligate intracellular parasites. The life cycle of these parasites includes both merogenic and sporogenic phases. These parasites are common in lower vertebrates (e.g., fish), but have also been implicated as a concern in humans with acquired immunodeficiency virus. Bearded dragons infected with these parasites can present with a clinical picture similar to that of as adenovirus or coccidiosis. Affected dragons are anorexic, unthrifty, cachectic, and may die acutely. Diagnosis is generally made postmortem. Hepatic and renal necrosis is common, although other organ systems (e.g., intestine and gonads) might also be affected. There is no effective treatment. To limit the likelihood of introducing this parasite into a collection, herpetoculturists should acquire animals only from reputable breeders and quarantine any new arrivals for a minimum of 60–90 days.

ZOONOTIC DISEASES

The veterinarian and veterinary technician serve vital roles in educating their support staff and clients about the potential diseases that their patients (reptiles and amphibians) might spread to humans (zoonoses). Many zoonotic diseases can be prevented by practicing strict hygiene and using common sense. Exotic pets should not be recommended for households with infants and young children, immunocompromised individuals, or the elderly, because the immune systems in these groups of individuals are often naïve or inefficient at protecting them against most pathogens.

The most notorious reptile zoonosis is *Salmonella* spp., a Gram-negative rod that is a facultative anaerobe (can live in the absence of oxygen). There are more than 2,435 serotypes of *Salmonella* spp.[23] All *Salmonella* spp. should be considered pathogenic to humans.

In the early 1970s, there were more than 280,000 human cases of salmonellosis in the

United States attributed to reptiles (turtles).[24] Attempts to certify the animals (turtles) as *Salmonella*-free in the United States failed because the animals were found to be latent shedders of the organism (i.e., they could test negative one week and positive weeks or months later). In 1975, the United States Food and Drug Administration put an inter- and intrastate shipping ban on turtles with a carapace under 4", effectively halting the sale of turtles in the United States. The ban on turtles proved to be successful as follow-up research indicated a 77% decrease in turtle-associated salmonellosis.[25]

In the late 1980s and through the 1990s, reptile-associated salmonellosis again received national attention. Many of the cases during this period included infants, with one infant dying. These cases differed from the turtle-associated salmonellosis cases because the infants did not have direct contact with the reptile in their household. Owners should be warned of these potential hazards and should practice strict hygiene, including hand washing after handling their pet or cleaning its environment, removing fecal wastes and cleaning the reptile's/amphibian's habitat with an appropriate disinfectant, and wearing gloves during the procedure. They should also not handle the animals near human food preparation sites or wash receptacles (e.g., sinks and bathtubs) and should not allow the animal to roam free within a human domicile.

There are other species of bacteria (Gram-positive and Gram-negative) that have been isolated from both clinically healthy and diseased reptiles that can cause disease in humans, including *Aeromonas* spp., *Campylobacter* spp., *Citrobacter* spp., *Edwardsiella* spp., *Escherichia coli*, *Klebsiella* spp., *Mycobacterium* spp., *Pasteurella* spp., *Proteus* spp., *Staphylococcus* spp., and *Streptococcus* spp. The population at risk is similar to that defined for *Salmonella* spp. and includes infants, immunocompromised individuals, and the elderly—although clinically healthy adults can also develop infections under certain circumstances. Humans can be exposed to these pathogens through wound contamination (e.g., scratch or bite wounds), water exposure, or fecal-oral exposure. Adhering to strict hygiene practices, such as hand washing, wearing protective gloves when cleaning reptile/amphibian enclosures, and not handling or allowing the animals near human food preparation sites should prevent disease.

SELF-STUDY QUESTIONS

1. Why is an environmental temperature range important for reptiles? Describe different methods for providing a temperature gradient for reptiles.

2. Why is ultraviolet B radiation (UVB) important for reptiles? What recommendations would you make to clients to ensure their pet reptile is provided with an appropriate source of UVB?

3. Describe the three different types of feeding strategies used by reptiles. Why is it a challenge to meet the needs of these animals in captivity?

4. What are the recommended techniques to restrain a snake, chelonian, and lizard?

5. How is the hydration status of a reptile evaluated?

6. Describe the proper methods of performing a physical examination on a lizard, snake, and chelonian.

7. How do you determine the sex of a snake, lizard, and chelonian?

8. How much blood can be safely collected from a reptilian patient?

9. Describe blood collection techniques used for reptilian patients.

10. How can you minimize the likelihood of "smudgeocytes" in a reptile blood smear?

11. How are erythrocytes and leukocytes different between reptiles and mammals?

12. What types of anesthetics can be used for reptiles and amphibians?

13. How do you assess depth of anesthesia in amphibians and reptiles?

14. Name three common nutritional diseases reported in captive reptiles.

15. What are the different routes for replenishing fluids in a reptile patient?

16. What are common infectious disease presentations in reptiles? Why are viral infections on the rise?

17. Which zoonotic disease in reptiles has been associated with high morbidity in humans?

REFERENCES

1. Acierno M, Mitchell MA, Roundtree M, and Zachariah T. Evaluating the effect of ultraviolet B radiation on 1,25 hydroxyvitamin D levels in red-eared sliders (*Trachemys scripta elegans*). *American Journal Veterinary Research* 2006;67:2046–49.
2. Acierno M, Mitchell MA, Roundtree M, Zachariah T, Kirchgessner M, and Sanchez-Migallon Guzman D. Effects of ultraviolet radiation on plasma 25-hydroxyvitamin D concentrations in corn snakes (*Elaphe guttata guttata*). *American Journal Veterinary Research* 2009;67:294–97.
3. Frye FL, and Boyer TH. Captive Reptile Husbandry. In: Frye, FL, ed. *Reptile care*. Neptune City, NJ: Tropical Fish Hobbyists Publications, Inc.; 1991:23–26.
4. Allen ME, Oftedal OT, and Ullrey ED. Effect of dietary calcium concentration on mineral composition in fox geckos (*Hemidactylus garnoti*) and Cuban tree frogs (*Osteopilus septentrionalis*). *Journal of Zoo and Wildlife Medicine* 1993;24:118.
5. Donoghue S, and Langenberg J. Nutrition. In: Mader, DR, ed. *Reptile medicine and surgery*. Philadelphia: WB Saunders; 1996:148–74.
6. Boyer TH. Metabolic bone disease. In: Mader, DR, ed. *Reptile medicine and surgery*. Philadelphia: WB Saunders; 1996:385–92.
7. Jacobsen ER. Blood collection techniques in reptiles: Laboratory investigations. In: Fowler, ME, ed. *Zoo and wild animal medicine: Current therapy 3*. Philadelphia: WB Saunders; 1993:144–52.

8. Myers D, Mitchell MA, Fleming G, et al. Determining the value of bovine albumin as a blood cell stabilizer for pancake tortoises (*Malacochersus tornieri*) blood smears. *Journal of Herpetological Medicine and Surgery* 2009;18.

9. Wright KM. Amphibian husbandry and medicine. In: Mader DR, ed. *Reptile medicine and surgery*. Philadelphia: WB Saunders; 1996:436–59.

10. Lane TJ, and Mader DR. Parasitology. In: Mader DR, ed. *Reptile medicine and surgery*. Philadelphia: WB Saunders; 1996:185–203.

11. Bennett RA. Anesthesia. In: Mader DR, ed. *Reptile medicine and surgery*. Philadelphia: WB Saunders; 1996:241–47.

12. Divers SJ. The use of propofol in reptile anesthesia. Proceedings of the Association of Reptile and Amphibian Veterinarians, 1996:57–59.

13. Diethelm G, and Mader DR. The effect of FlO_2 on post anesthetic recovery times in the green iguana. Proceedings of the Association of Reptile and Amphibian Veterinarians, 1999:169–70.

14. Frye FL. Nutritional disorders in reptiles. In: Hoff GL, Frye FL, and Jacobson ER, eds. *Diseases of amphibians and reptiles*. New York: Plenum Press; 1984:640–42.

15. Fowler ME. Comparison of respiratory infection and hypovitaminosis A in a desert tortoise. In: Montali RJ, and Migaki G., eds. *Comparative pathology of zoo animals*. Washington, DC: Smithsonian Institute; 1980:93–97.

16. Mader DR. Gout. In: Mader DR, ed. *Reptile medicine and surgery*. Philadelphia: WB Saunders; 1996:374–79.

17. Lloyd ML, and Flanagan JP. Recent developments in ophidian paramyxovirus research and recommendations on control. South Padre Island, Texas. Proceedings of the American Association of Zoo Veterinarians, 1990:151–56.

18. Ahne W, Neubert WJ, and Thomson I. Reptilian viruses: Isolation of myxovirus-like particles from the snake *Elaphe oxycephala*. *Journal of American Veterinary Medicine* 1987;34:607.

19. Jacobsen ER, Gaskin JM, Simpson C, et al. Paramyxo-like virus infection in a rock rattlesnake. *Journal of American Veterinary Medicine* 1980; 177(9):796.

20. Schumacher J. Viral diseases. In: Mader DR, ed. *Reptile medicine and surgery*. Philadelphia: WB Saunders; 1996:224–34.

21. Allender MC, Mitchell MA, Dreslik MJ, et al. Measuring agreement and discord among hemagglutination inhibition assays against different ophidian paramyxovirus strains in Eastern massasauga (*Sistrurus catenatus catenatus*). *Journal Zoo Wildlife Medicine* 2008;29:358–61.

22. Kim DY, Mitchell MA, and Bauer R. An outbreak of adenoviral infection in inland bearded dragons (*Pogona vitticeps*) coinfected with dependovirus and coccidial protozoa (*Isospora* sp.). *Journal Veterinary Diagnostic Investigation* 2002;14:332–34.

23. Popoff MY, and Leminor L. Antigenic formulas of the *Salmonella* Serovars, 7th revision. World Health Organization Collaborating Center for Reference Research on *Salmonella*, Pasteur Institute, Paris, France, 1997.

24. Lamm SH, Taylor A, Gangarosa EJ, et al. Turtle-associated salmonellosis I: An estimation of the magnitude of the problem in the United States, 1970–1971. *American Journal of Epidemiology* 1972; 95(6):511–17.

25. Cohen ML, Potter M, Pollard et al. Turtle-associated salmonellosis in the United States. Effect of public health action, 1970–1976. *Journal of the American Veterinary Medical Association* 1980; 12(243):1247–49.

26. Jacobson ER. Use of chemotherapeutics in reptile medicine. In: Jacobson ER, and Kollias GV, eds. *Exotic animals.* New York: Churchill Livingston; 1988:35–48.

27. Jacobson ER. Antimicrobial drug use in reptiles. In: Prescott JF, and Baggot JD, eds. *Antimicrobial therapy in veterinary medicine.* Ames: Iowa State University Press; 1993:543–52.

28. Allen DG, Pringle JK, and Smith D. *Handbook of veterinary drugs.* Philadelphia: JB Lippincott; 1993:534–67.

29. Klingenberg RJ. Therapeutics. In: Mader DR, ed. *Reptile medicine and surgery.* Philadelphia: WB Saunders; 1996:299–321.

30. Jacobson ER. Snakes *Veterinary Clinics of North America Small Animal Practice* 1993;23:1179–1212.

CHAPTER 3

Ferrets

INTRODUCTION

The ferret, *Mustela putorius furo*, belongs to the order Carnivora and the family Mustelidae. These animals initially became popular as pets in the United States during the 1970s. Over the next two decades their numbers increased significantly, with estimates of more than 7 million ferrets being kept as pets in 1990.[1] More recent surveys conducted by the American Veterinary Medical Association suggest that their popularity has continued to rise into the new century, with a 6.5% increase in pet ferret numbers being reported between 2001 and 2007 (http://www.avma.org/reference/market stats/ownership.asp). The ferret has endeared itself to humans because of its "spunky" disposition and small stature. The ferret has also become quite popular in urban domiciles (e.g., apartments) that might be too small to house dogs or cats.

Domestication of the ferret is not recent; it has been recorded that ferrets were used for hunting more than 2,000 years ago.[2] The ferret was originally introduced into the United States more than 300 years ago.[3] In other parts of the world, such as England, the ferret serves in a working role as a hunter of rabbits and rodents. Male ferrets are called hobs, females, jills, and their young, kits. Sexing ferrets is straightforward; males have a prepuce on their ventral abdomen, similar to dogs, and females have a vulva ventral to their anus. The ferret is also used extensively in research.

Although the domestic ferret continues to gain in popularity in the United States, it cannot legally be kept as a pet in all states. The ferret has developed an unfortunate reputation in certain areas as dangerous around children or a threat to native wildlife. In California, a 1933 law regulating the importation of mustelids is responsible for the current prohibition on pet ferrets in California. Local ordinances in certain "ferret-legal" states might also prohibit ferrets as pets, so it is important to research the laws in your state and local

Table 3.1 **Ferret Basic Information**

BODY WEIGHT	
Adult Male (Hob)	
Intact	1.0–2.0 kg[3]
Neutered	0.7–1.1 kg
Adult Female (Jill)	
Intact	0.5–1.0 kg[3]
Neutered	0.5–0.7 kg
Birth Weight (Kit)	8–10 grams[3]
TEMPERATURE, PULSE, AND RESPIRATION	
Rectal Body Temperature	100°–103°F
Normal Heart Rate	170–230 beats/minute
Normal Respiratory Rate	25–40 breaths/minute
REPRODUCTIVE CYCLE	
Sexual Maturity	4–8 months of age[3]
Gestation	41–42 days[3]
Estrous Cycle	Induced ovulator
Weaning Age	6–8 weeks
Life Span	4–9 years average, up to 11–12 years

municipality to protect yourself and your clients. In many states, the wildlife and fisheries department regulates permits for domestic ferrets; it should be contacted regarding official regulations.

Success in working with the ferret, as with all exotic species, requires veterinary technicians to develop a basic knowledge of the anatomy and physiology of the animal (Table 3.1), so that they can perform a thorough physical examination, administer medical therapy, and answer an owner's questions about his or her pet.

Anatomy and Physiology

The technician should become familiar with those anatomical characteristics in the ferret that differ from other domestic mammals. The ferret has a long, tubular body that enables it to maneuver through burrows when hunting prey. It has sharp, nonretractable claws, which it uses to dig and burrow, and ferret owners are often scratched by their pets while playing with them. Ferret owners might request to have their pet declawed; however, the procedure would be very painful and should never be performed.

The majority of ferrets offered for sale in pet shops are de-scented and neutered. These procedures are commonly done to minimize the odor associated with these animals. Although the overwhelming majority of ferrets presented to veterinary hospitals will have had these procedures done at the commercial breeders, there remain some private breeders who will sell their animals intact. Removing the scent glands (anal glands) and neutering/spaying a ferret are similar to the procedures described for dogs and cats, respectively. Neutered animals might weigh significantly less than their intact counterparts (Table 3.1). Ferrets can lose a significant amount of weight during the summer months, only to gain the weight back in the winter. Indoor domestic ferrets can experience a 10%–30% weight change, whereas an outdoor intact animal can fluctuate by as much as 40% of its body weight.[3]

More than 30 hair coat color variations are recognized in the domestic ferret. The most common colors, sable and albino, are naturally occurring patterns, whereas many of the other variations are the result of selective breeding (Figures 3.1 and 3.2). Ferrets undergo routine spring and fall seasonal molts, similar to domestic dogs. Ferrets have very thick skin and a technician might find it difficult to inject vaccinations or subcutaneous fluids between the shoulders. This thick skin over the nape of the neck is a site where ferrets bite during reproduction and territorial fighting.

The ferret has a pair of anal glands that produce a musky odor. Commercial breeding farms de-scent and neuter kits prior to shipping them

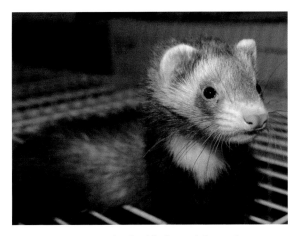

Figure 3.1 *A standard sable ferret. This is the most common color produced in captivity.*

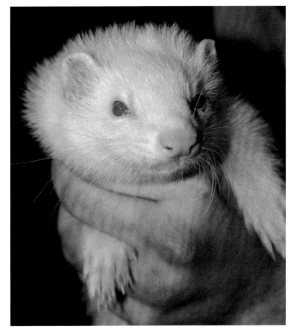

Figure 3.2 *An albino ferret. Note the general loss of pigment throughout the hair coat and irises.*

to pet stores, whereas private breeders will often leave that option to the new owner.

Female ferrets are induced ovulators and must be bred by a male to stimulate ovulation. A female that is not bred or spayed could develop a life-threatening estrogen-induced anemia. Male ferrets have a *j*-shaped os penis. Because of the shape of their os penis, calculi (mineral deposits) can sometimes become obstructive. Male ferrets also have a prostate. This accessory sexual organ was originally not considered to be present in ferrets until cases of prostatomegaly became apparent with adrenal gland disease.

Ferrets are true carnivores and have a relatively short gastrointestinal tract, which makes them capable of processing a meal within 3–4 hours. This is important to consider when performing a gastrointestinal radiographic contrast series.

HUSBANDRY

Environmental Concerns
Ferrets may be maintained indoors or outdoors. They are primarily maintained indoors in the United States, whereas they are often maintained outdoors in Europe. Ferrets kept outdoors should be protected from extremes of heat and cold. During the summer months, animals should be provided shelter and fresh water and should be removed from direct sun. Ferrets do not tolerate temperatures over 88°–90°F. In the winter, animals should be provided a shelter with straw or hay. When the temperature drops below freezing (32°F), ferrets should be brought into a warm shelter.

Ferrets should be given a well-ventilated, spacious enclosure. Glass fish tanks are not suitable for ferrets because they do not allow for adequate ventilation. Animals maintained in glass enclosures often develop respiratory problems. Galvanized metal cages or wood-frame cages are routinely used to house ferrets. Galvanized metal is composed of zinc and could expose those animals that lick and chew the bars to heavy metal toxicity. Reports of heavy metal toxicity in ferrets are rare, but should be considered in animals that display neurologic signs, vomiting, diarrhea, or hematochezia.

The enclosure should be large enough to provide the animal an area to sleep, eat, exercise, and have a latrine. Ferrets urinate and defecate in corners and can be trained to use a litter box. Owners should be advised that they might need to place a litter box in multiple corners to ensure their pet will use it. Litter pans should have low sides to allow an animal easy access. Fecal and urine material should be removed from the litter pan daily. Clients should be taught what to watch for when evaluating fecal and urine output in ferrets. Because several gastrointestinal diseases are associated with changes in fecal appearance and consistency (e.g., coronavirus infection: green, mucoid diarrhea; gastric ulcers: melena), the client's ability to describe fecal changes can be important to the veterinary personnel working on a diagnosis. Also, because cystic calculi and prostatomegaly are found in captive ferrets, historical information regarding the production of urine and whether a ferret is straining to urinate are important pieces of information to guide veterinary personnel toward a diagnosis.

Ferrets naturally tend to burrow and hide when they sleep, and it's important to tell clients to provide their pet with a sleeping shelter. A number of commercial ferret hammocks or slings can be purchased, although most old towels or shirts work fine. Owners should be advised to observe their pet closely to ensure that it does not attempt to ingest any of the material. Cardboard box shelter can be provided to animals that are at risk with the cloth material.

Ferrets should remain in their cage and only be allowed to roam free in a home under close supervision. These animals are capable of fitting into small crevices between furniture and ventilation systems and are notorious for getting into trouble. The ingestion of foreign material is the most common problem reported in unsupervised ferrets.

Commercial ferret harnesses can be used to walk an animal indoors or outdoors.

Nutrition

As mentioned, ferrets are true carnivores, as evidenced by their relatively short gastrointestinal tract. The gastrointestinal transit time of the ferret is rapid (3–4 hours), so food quality is important to ensure maximal nutritional benefit. The diet of a ferret should consist primarily of high-quality protein and fat. The exact nutritional requirements for the ferret have not been established, although it is generally accepted that adult altered animals require 30%–40% protein and 18%–20% fat.[5] Breeding animals and young, fast-growing kits require significantly more protein (minimum 35%) and fat (minimum 25%). Although readily accepted by ferrets, carbohydrates (e.g., sweets) should be minimized in the animal's diet. Carbohydrates, especially simple sugars, can also prove problematic in ferrets with insulinoma. Feeding simple sugars can exacerbate the disease by increasing insulin levels and further decreasing glucose levels. The provision of simple sugars (e.g., Karo syrup) to a ferret with an insulinoma should be reserved for emergency cases (e.g., animal is severely depressed, seizures). The short gastrointestinal tract of the ferret is not dependent on dietary fiber, as is the case with herbivores. Most commercial ferret diets contain minimal quantities of fiber.

A number of commercial diets can provide a ferret with adequate nutrition. In recent years, commercial ferret diets have been offered for sale at retail pet stores. Ferret owners should be encouraged to read the labels of commercial diets to ensure that the appropriate levels of protein and fat are offered, based on the animal's age and reproductive status. Commercial feline growth diets are also routinely recommended for ferrets.

Again, the ingredient list should be evaluated and recommendations made based on the animal's needs. The list of ingredients should start with poultry products rather than vegetable (corn) products. Canine diets should never be recommended for ferrets, because they do not provide adequate protein or fat and contain significant amounts of carbohydrates. A ferret can be offered food ad lib. Ferret diets can be supplemented with lean meats such as chicken or beef, or meat-based (onion salt–free) baby foods.

Ferrets should be offered fresh, clean water daily. Water can be offered in heavy ceramic water bowls or hanging sipper bottles. The bowl should be placed in a corner where it is unlikely the ferret will tip it over. Water sipper bottles should be placed in an area of the cage that is readily accessible to the animal. Water-soluble vitamins are not necessary for ferrets that are fed a good-quality commercial ferret or feline growth diet.

Transport

Owners should know that ferrets should be transported in a carrier when they visit the veterinarian. If these animals are allowed free roam in a car during transport, they could get into a particular area that makes them difficult to retrieve, or they could ingest foreign material (e.g., coins) lying on the floor of the automobile. Ferrets should also be maintained in a transport carrier while they are in the waiting room to prevent contact with other animals or a dog or cat attack. Tell owners that they can reduce their ferret's stress during transport by placing a towel in the carrier to provide the animal a place to burrow and hide.

Grooming

Ferrets naturally have a musky odor, which is especially evident in intact animals during the breeding season. Ferrets do not require regular bathing; however, they may be bathed once a month, if desired. The most appropriate shampoo is one that is pH balanced, such as a commercial ferret or kitten shampoo. Excessive bathing might lead to the development of dry, pruritic skin.

In the wild, ferrets use their sharp nails to dig; however, in captivity the need for this activity is reduced, so regular nail trimming is recommended to avoid painful scratches when interacting with owners. Ferret nails can be trimmed in the same fashion as described for dogs and cats. If the nail is cut short and the animal bleeds, an appropriate styptic powder can be applied. On occasion, veterinary personnel are asked about the possibility of declawing a ferret. Ferret nails are nonretractable, like dog nails. Therefore, an onchiectomy should never be performed on this species.

Ferrets can develop significant dental tartar over time. To prevent potential dental problems, the animal's teeth should be brushed regularly. Commercially available toothbrushes and toothpaste available for use in dogs and cats can also be used to clean ferret teeth. Ferrets with dental tartar should be scheduled for a scaling (tartar removal) to minimize the risk of long-term gingival and dental disease. These types of procedures, as with dogs and cats, require general anesthesia.

HISTORY

A thorough history is essential to making an appropriate diagnosis for any exotic animal case, because many of the problems identified in exotic animals are directly related to inappropriate husbandry. A veterinary technician should first collect the signalment, including age, sex, and color variety. Knowledge of the animal's age and sex can be useful when developing a differential diagnosis list. For example, an adult intact female ferret with a history of weakness and lethargy might be suffering from an estrogen-induced anemia, whereas an adult male or female kit would be very unlikely to develop the same problem. Knowledge of the color variety is also important because differences in physiologic parameters, such as hematology, can vary (see Tables 3.2 and 3.3).

After the technician defines the signalment, he or she should focus on collecting background information, including where the animal was acquired, length of time owned, if the owner has other pets, if he or she recently acquired another ferret, the interaction between the owner and the pet, and the animal's vaccination history (canine distemper virus and rabies) and heartworm prevention status. This information should provide the technician with an initial understanding of the client's knowledge of the pet ferret.

The next set of questions should focus on how the animal is managed at home (husbandry),

including whether the animal is housed indoors or outdoors, if it has supervised or unsupervised run of the house, cage size and material, cage location in the house, whether ferrets are housed singly or together, substrate used in the cage, how often the cage is cleaned and the type of disinfectant used, whether a litter pan is used, the brand of cat litter, and the types of cage furniture (e.g., ferret hammock) and toys. Questions about the animal's nutrition are also important and should include type of food (e.g., ferret or cat), brand, amount fed, frequency, supplements, water source, and how often the food and water are changed.

Finally, questions should focus on the animal's current health status and should include past medical history, current presenting problem, and duration of the complaint. Although it is natural to want to focus on the problem at hand, a great deal of information could be overlooked if the

Table 3.2 **Ferret Hematological Reference Ranges[4,6]**

DETERMINATION	ALBINO		FITCH	
	Male	Female	Male	Female
PCV (%)	55 (44–61)	49 (42–55)	43 (36–50)	48 (47–51)
RBC (10^6/µl)	10.2 (7.3–12.2)	8.1 (6.8–9.8)	n/a	n/a
Hemoglobin (g/dl)	17.8 (16.3–18.2)	16.2 (14.8–17.4)	14.3 (12.0–16.3)	15.9 (15.2–17.4)
Leukocytes (10^3/µl)	9.7 (4.4–19.1)	10.5 (4.0–18.2)	11.3 (7.7–15.4)	5.9 (2.5–8.6)
Neutrophils (%)	57 (11–82)	59.5 (43–84)	40.1 (24–78)	31.1 (12–41)
Bands (%)	n/a	n/a	0.9 (0–2.2)	1.7 (0–4.2)
Lymphocytes (%)	35.6 (12–54)	33.4 (12–50)	49.7 (28–69)	58 (25–95)
Eosinophils (%)	2.4 (0–7)	2.6 (0–5)	2.3 (0–7)	3.6 (1–9)
Monocytes (%)	4.4 (0–9)	4.4 (2–8)	6.6 (3.4–8.2)	4.5 (1.7–6.3)
Basophils (%)	0.1 (0–2)	0.2 (0–1)	0.7 (0–2.7)	0.8 (0–2.9)
Platelets (10^3/µl)	453 (297–730)	545 (310–910)	n/a	n/a
Reticuloytes (%)	4.0 (1–12)	5.3 (2–14)	n/a	n/a

Table 3.3 **Ferret Serum Biochemistry Reference Ranges**[4,6,7]

DETERMINATION	ALBINO	FITCH
Glucose (mg/dl)	136 (94–207)	101 (63–134)
Blood urea nitrogen (mg/dl)	22 (10–45)	28 (12–43)
Creatinine (mg/dl)	0.6 (0.4–0.9)	0.4 (0.2–0.6)
Total bilirubin (mg/dl)	<1.0	n/a
Cholesterol (mg/dl)	165 (64–296)	n/a
Calcium (mg/dl)	9.2 (8.0–11.8)	9.3 (8.6–10.5)
Phosphorus (mg/dl)	5.9 (4.0–9.1)	6.5 (5.6–8.7)
Alkaline phosphatase (IU/L)	23 (9–84)	53 (30–120)
Alanine aminotransferase (IU/L)	n/a	170 (82–289)
Aspartate aminotransferase (IU/L)	65 (28–120)	n/a
Sodium (mmol/L)	148 (137–162)	152 (146–160)
Chloride (mmol/L)	116 (106–125)	115 (102–121)
Potassium (mmol/L)	5.9 (4.5–7.7)	4.9 (4.3–5.3)
Total protein (g/dl)	6.0 (5.1–7.4)	5.9 (5.3–7.2)
Albumin (g/dl)	3.2 (2.6–3.8)	3.7 (3.3–4.1)
Globulin (g/dl)	n/a	1.8 (1.3–2.1)

technician fails to collect the historical information in a thorough and systematic way.

RESTRAINT

Employing the appropriate technique when restraining a ferret is essential to the protection of the veterinarian, the technician, and the animal. Ferrets can be safely restrained by scruffing—a technique commonly used by the jill to move her kits. Scruffing is accomplished by grasping the skin over the dorsal cervical area (nape) with the index finger and thumb (Figures 3.3A and 3.3B). Once the animal is scruffed, it will often relax and offer little resistance. The handler's second hand should be placed along the spine to protect it from injury. Do not hold the rear legs or allow the animal to place them on the table, because this often stimulates the animal to struggle. Ferrets will often yawn while being scruffed, which will facilitate examination of the oral cavity.

Adult pet ferrets rarely bite, but might if they are in pain. A ferret will often make a hissing sound to warn of their dissatisfaction prior to attempting to bite. Animals that are too difficult to handle can be sedated using anesthetics. Kits, on the other hand, are naturally very playful (and teething) and are likely to bite. Fortunately, their bite is similar to a puppy or kitten bite and rarely breaks the skin of the handler. Moribund and cooperative animals can simply be restrained on the examination table; however, any invasive procedure (e.g., vaccination, rectal temperature, injection) will require scruffing.

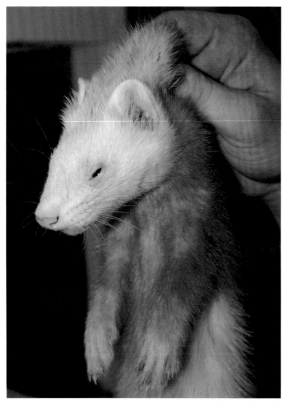

Figure 3.3A *Grasping the nape of a ferret is an excellent way to gently restrain these animals.*

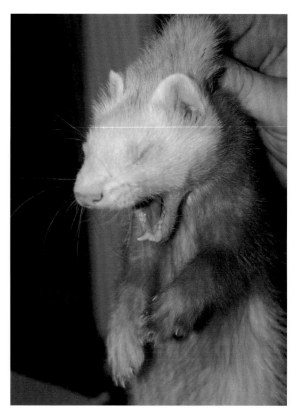

Figure 3.3B *Most ferrets will yawn when scruffed, which allows veterinary personnel to examine the oral cavity.*

PHYSICAL EXAMINATION

Ferrets are stoic animals and might not display overt clinical signs until late in the course of a disease; therefore, the veterinarian will perform a thorough physical examination on every animal presented to the veterinary hospital. Proper restraint is essential for a veterinarian to perform a thorough physical examination, so it is important for a veterinary technician to be on hand to assist in the procedure. Physical examination of the ferret follows the standard protocol recommended for domestic species.

The ferret should be observed from a distance to assess those functions, such as locomotion, behavior, and respiration, that could be altered by restraint. The ferret should be mobile, aware of its surroundings, and its breathing pattern consistent and not labored. Ferrets are naturally nasal breathers, so open mouth breathing is an indication of a problem. Coughing, sneezing, and nasal discharge also should be considered abnormal findings. A ferret presenting with dyspnea should immediately be placed in an oxygen cage or provided oxygen via a face mask.

When removed from the carrier, the animal should be bright, alert, and responsive. If the ferret is limp or nonresponsive, this behavior should be considered abnormal and managed as an emergency. A thorough physical examination can always be delayed while stabilizing the patient.

The animal's eyes should be clear and free of discharge. A fluorescein stain should be performed on any animal in which a corneal ulcer is suspected. In some cases the corneal ulcer will be readily apparent because of gross changes to the corneal surface, whereas in other cases it might be more subtle and present in the form of increased blinking or just holding an eye closed because it is painful. Ferret pupils have a small oval shape and horizontal position. It can be difficult to perform a fundus examination in a ferret without using mydriatics drugs (e.g., atropine).

The nares should be clear and free of any crusting or discharge. Ferret ears can have a dark, ceruminous wax buildup. If an excessive amount of wax is identified, a cotton-tipped applicator should be dipped in mineral oil and a sample of the wax collected and tested for ear mites (*Otodectes cynotis*). The majority of ferrets presenting to veterinary hospitals in the United States will have two small ink tattoos in their right ear (Figure 3.4), which were originally used to identify ferrets raised by Marshall Farms (North Rose, NY), the largest captive producer of ferrets in the United States. Other ferret producers have begun using this method to mark their animals, too. The tattoos indicate that the animal has been spayed/ neutered and de-scented (anal glands removed).

The oral cavity should be thoroughly evaluated. The teeth should be free of obvious dental caries or fractures. The amount of dental tartar should be recorded, and animals with moderate to severe dental tartar should be scheduled for a dental scaling. The mucous membranes should be moist and pink. The capillary refill time should be less than 2 seconds. The veterinarian will assess hydration status by evaluating the mucous membrane quality and capillary refill time, packed cell volume, skin elasticity, and retrobulbar fat. A ferret with a decreased capillary refill time (>2 seconds) and

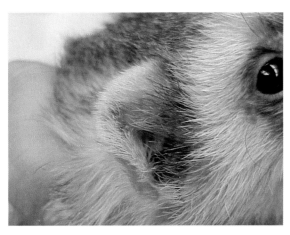

Figure 3.4 *Ferrets tattooed with two ink dots in the right ear were most likely raised at Marshall Farms. The two tattoos indicate that the ferret was spayed/ neutered and de-scented.*

delayed skin elasticity should be considered 5% dehydrated. When an animal also presents with sunken eyes, resulting from the loss of fluid from the retrobulbar fat, the animal should be considered at least 8%–10% dehydrated.

The length and condition of a ferret's hair coat can vary with the season, with the hair coat being much thinner in the summer than during the winter. Seasonal tail alopecia is also a common finding reported in ferrets during the late summer and early fall. Animals that develop symmetrical alopecia or thinning of the skin might have an endocrinopathy (e.g., adrenal gland disease) (Figure 3.5).

The veterinarian will thoroughly evaluate the skin for defects such as tumors; mast cell tumors are an especially common finding in ferrets. The ferret has peripheral lymph nodes similar to those of the cat and dog, including the submandibular, cervical, prescapular, axillary, abdominal, inguinal, and popliteal lymph nodes. Examination of the lymph nodes is especially important in ferrets that can develop lymphoma. Normal lymph nodes are not typically palpated in a ferret. When

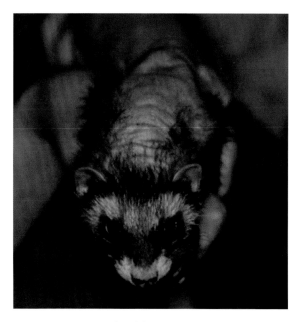

Figure 3.5 *Generalized hair loss (alopecia) is one of the most common clinical signs associated with adrenal gland disease. The skin in these animals also appears thin compared with that of unaffected animals.*

a lymph node can be palpated, the veterinarian will order a fine needle aspirate and cytologic evaluation of the sample. Obese animals might appear to have a lymphadenopathy when, in reality, the nodes palpate larger than normal because of excessive fat accumulation.

Abdominal palpation is much more rewarding in ferrets than in other mammals. The veterinarian will palpate the spleen by grasping the left side of the abdomen with the index finger and thumb. Splenomegaly is a common finding in mature ferrets, so the organ is often easy to identify. There are a number of different reasons that splenomegaly occurs in ferrets, including extramedullary hematopoiesis, neoplasia, and trauma. Palpating the surface of the spleen can provide some insight into the underlying cause of disease, because neoplastic conditions often affect the surface texture of the spleen (e.g., make it more "lumpy").

The stomach is located medial to the spleen and typically palpates as a large empty tubular structure unless the ferret has eaten a recent meal or has a gastric foreign body. The veterinarian will slide his or her fingers more medially to find the left kidney. It should have a uniform texture and be approximately 2–2.5 cm. The right kidney can be palpated by switching to the right side of the abdomen. The right kidney is located cranial to the left kidney and is often located under the last ribs. It should have a texture and size similar to the left kidney. Medial and slightly cranial to the kidneys lie the adrenal glands. These structures can be palpable in ferrets with adrenomegaly associated with adrenal gland disease. The urinary bladder should be palpable in the caudal abdomen if urine is present. A large firm prostate may be palpable caudal and dorsal to the urinary bladder in male ferrets with prostate/adrenal gland disease. Unless there is an intestinal foreign body, ileus, or significant ingesta in the intestines, the intestines are not typically palpable. Likewise, unless there is significant pathology to the liver (e.g., hepatomegaly), this organ is not typically palpated on a routine physical examination.

A veterinarian will usually also perform a neurological examination during a routine physical examination, especially in animals with a history of weakness, paresis, or paralysis. The limbs of the animal will be thoroughly palpated to rule out fractures. The range of motion and reflexes associated with the shoulder, elbow, carpus, pelvis, stifle, hock, and digits will be evaluated and any crepitus or problems recorded. Animals showing deficits associated with the cranial nerves (e.g., drooping eyelids, facial paralysis, hypersalivation) will also be given a thorough evaluation.

The veterinarian will evaluate the anus, ensuring that the perianal region is free of fecal staining. The vulva of the neutered jill should be small (<2 mm) and free of discharge or staining. Jills that are intact or have adrenal disease might develop an enlarged and turgid vulva (Figure 3.6). Often these animals will have a purulent vulvar discharge. The penis of the hob might be difficult to extract from the prepuce in an animal that is awake. If there is a history of stranguria, hematuria, or anuria, the animal should be sedated to thoroughly examine the penis.

Auscultation of the heart and lungs is an important component of the physical examination. In most mammals, the heart is located at the point of the elbow, whereas in the ferret the heart is located in the mid-thoracic region between ribs 6 and 8. Placement of the stethoscope bell housing in the appropriate location is vital to evaluating the heart. The ferret heartbeat is much more rapid than that of domestic mammals, and a sinus arrhythmia is a common finding.

Checking the rectal temperature of a ferret can be a real challenge. A digital thermometer is preferred over a glass thermometer, because of the risk of breakage and injury to the animal. The ferret's normal body temperature should be between

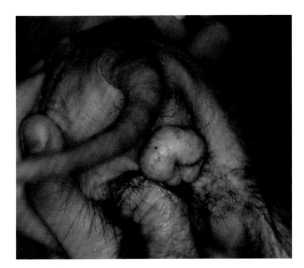

Figure 3.6 *Female ferrets with adrenal gland disease can develop significantly enlarged vulvas.*

100° and 103°F. Animals that struggle during the examination could have a falsely elevated body temperature.

After the examination is completed, the technician should record abnormal findings, and a problem list with differential diagnoses should be established. Based on the top differential diagnoses, diagnostic tests are prioritized to confirm a diagnosis or to determine the severity of the disease.

DIAGNOSTIC SAMPLING

Blood Collection

Obtaining a blood sample from a ferret might prove challenging at first, but with experience the procedure will become routine. Ferrets that are not effectively immobilized using simple restraint should be anesthetized. The advent of inhalant anesthetics in veterinary medicine has simplified this procedure, allowing for rapid induction and recovery. The site chosen for venipuncture will depend primarily on the volume of sample required and the technician's skill level. Most clinical laboratories can perform complete blood counts and serum chemistry analysis on 1–2 ml of blood, significantly reducing the volume of blood required for testing. In certain cases, such as a blood transfusion, the technician might need to collect a larger volume of blood. The blood volume of a ferret has been estimated to be between 5% and 6% of the animal's body weight, and up to 10% of the animal's blood volume (5–6 ml/kg of body weight) can be safely collected at one time.[4]

A number of different venipuncture sites have been described to collect blood samples from the ferret. The volume that can be collected and the quality of the sample might vary from site to site. In general, the cranial vena cava and jugular vein are the preferred sites for sample collection, because large volumes of blood can be collected from them relatively easily. Other sites include the cephalic and saphenous veins and the tail artery. The cephalic vein should be reserved for intravenous catheterization and used for venipuncture only as a last resort. Some have recommended clipping a nail to collect a blood sample, but this should not be performed because it is painful and yields lymph-diluted samples.

To collect a sample from the cranial vena cava, place the animal in dorsal recumbency. A total of three people will be required to collect the sample if the animal is not anesthetized: two handlers and one sample collector. One handler should grasp the head and stretch it forward with one hand, while using his or her second hand to pull the front legs back. The second handler should restrain the animal's rear legs. The technician should anesthetize an animal that struggles during restraint before performing the procedure. The landmarks for the venipuncture site are the manubrium and first right rib. The site should be aseptically prepared, using an appropriate antiseptic to prevent the introduction of bacterial contaminants into the thorax. A 25-gauge needle fastened to a 3 ml syringe should be used to collect the sample (Figure 3.7). The needle should be inserted at a 45° angle to the body at the juncture of the manubrium and first right rib and directed toward the right rear leg. The cranial vena cava can also be approached by inserting the needle at the junction of the manubrium and left first rib and directing it toward the right rear leg; however, many veterinarians prefer the former technique, because it doesn't require passage of the needle through mediastinal tissues. The level of the cranial vena cava can vary from animal to animal; however, most samples can be collected by inserting the 5/8", 25-gauge needle to approxi-

mately half its depth. Apply negative pressure to the syringe once the needle has entered the thorax until blood fills the syringe. In cases where a large volume of blood is required, such as for a transfusion, a 25-gauge butterfly catheter can be attached to a 12 or 20 ml syringe to facilitate collection.

The jugular vein should also be considered when large volumes of blood are required. There are two restraint techniques that can be used to prepare an animal for jugular venipuncture. The first technique is similar to that described for cats, where the animal's front legs are held over the edge of the table and the neck is stretched up. The second technique is performed on an animal in dorsal recumbency and restrained using the same technique described for the cranial vena cava technique.

Animals that are difficult to manually restrain should be anesthetized. The jugular vein of the ferret courses in a more lateral direction than that in dogs and cats. Shaving the hair over the ventral cervical area can facilitate visualization of the vein; however, the ferret jugular vein is often surrounded by fat and difficult to see. The site should be aseptically prepared using an appro-

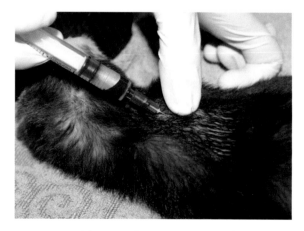

Figure 3.7 *The cranial vena cava is a preferred site for collecting blood from a ferret.*

priate antiseptic. A 22-, 23-, or 25-gauge needle fastened to a 3 ml syringe can be used to collect the blood sample.

The trachea is located on the ventral midline of the cervical region and can be used as a landmark. Apply gentle pressure with your thumb at the thoracic inlet to increase visibility and resistance in the vein. A slight bend (20° angle) in the needle can be made to improve access to the vein. The skin in the cervical region is more difficult to penetrate than in other regions of the body; therefore, be prepared to exert additional force. In those cases where the jugular vein is not visible, a "blind-stick" will be necessary. Inserting the needle just cranial to the thoracic inlet provides the greatest success for collecting a jugular blood sample. By using this site, the technician can gain access to the vessel as it leaves the thorax and before it makes a lateral deviation in the neck. Do not be overly aggressive when searching for the jugular, because there are other vital tissues in the cervical area that could be damaged.

The cephalic and saphenous veins can be used to collect small volumes of blood (<0.5 ml), but should be reserved to use as intravenous catheter sites when an animal presents for any disease condition that might require fluid therapy. The cephalic vein is located over the antebrachium, as in dogs, although the vein courses more laterally in the ferret. The lateral saphenous vein can be located at the level of the hock and courses diagonally in an anterior to posterior fashion (Figure 3.8). Shaving the hair over the venipuncture sites will facilitate visibility. The site should be aseptically prepared using an appropriate antiseptic. The ferret should be restrained using the same techniques used to restrain a cat when collecting a blood sample from the cephalic or saphenous vein. A 25- or 26-gauge needle fastened to a 1 or 3 ml syringe can be used to collect the sample.

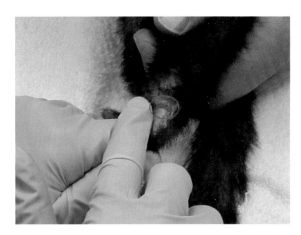

Figure 3.8 *The lateral saphenous vein is an excellent site for collecting small to moderate volumes of blood from a ferret.*

Again, a slight bend (20° angle) in the needle might simplify the approach to the vessel.

Blood samples can also be collected from the tail artery, although this technique is rarely used. The tail artery is located 2–3 mm deep to the midline of the ventral tail. The animal should be restrained by scruffing and pulling the legs caudally. The site should be aseptically prepared using an appropriate antiseptic. A 22-gauge needle fastened to a 3 or 6 ml syringe can be used. The needle should be inserted into the ventral midline of the tail and negative pressure applied until blood is observed filling the syringe. Because this is an artery, direct digital pressure should be applied to the site for a minimum of 2 minutes after withdrawing the needle.

Observed reference ranges for the ferret complete blood count (CBC) and serum chemistry panel are listed in Tables 3.2 and 3.3, respectively. These values represent observed reference ranges and should not be considered complete.

Bone Marrow Aspiration

Ferrets might develop several diseases that can lead to a suppression of the progenitor cells of the bone marrow, including estrogen-induced anemia, neoplasia, and adrenal gland disease. Animals with a nonregenerative anemia, thrombocytopenia, leukopenia, or pancytopenia are good candidates for this diagnostic procedure.

There are a number of sites that can be used to collect a bone marrow sample (humeral, femur, iliac crest); however, the proximal femur and proximal tibia are the most frequently used sites because of accessibility. Ferrets undergoing a bone marrow aspiration should be given general anesthesia. For the proximal femur bone marrow aspirate, place the ferret into lateral recumbency and shave the fur over the proximal femur. The site should be aseptically prepared using an appropriate antiseptic, and the procedure should be performed using sterile techniques. The veterinarian will make an incision, using a #15 scalpel blade, over the greater trochanter of the femur. A 20- or 22-gauge 1–1.5" spinal needle can be inserted into the femur to collect the sample. A 6 ml syringe can be fastened to the spinal needle to aspirate the sample. For the proximal tibia, the same restraint, site preparation technique, and equipment can be used. The landmark for the tibia is the tibial plateau. The needle can be inserted in a slight posterior direction so that it will slip into the medullary cavity of the tibia.

Splenic Aspirate

Splenomegaly is a common finding in adult ferrets. A splenic aspirate is a relatively noninvasive technique compared with biopsy, and can be used to collect a sample for cytology. It is important for clients to understand, however, that this technique can lead to seeding the abdomen with cancerous cells. Animals that are fractious should be anesthetized to prevent splenic laceration. The ferret should be restrained in right lateral recumbency, and the left side of the body wall in the area of the spleen should be shaved and aseptically prepared. This procedure will introduce a needle into the abdomen, so it is vital that sterile techniques be followed closely.

The spleen can be immobilized by grasping it through the skin and holding it between the thumb and index finger. A 22- to 25-gauge needle fastened to a 3 ml syringe can be used to collect the sample. The needle should be inserted into the spleen and negative pressure applied by rapidly pulling the plunger back several times. The needle should be removed from the spleen and the sample prepared for cytology. Remember that the sample is in the needle, and pulling back on the plunger, once the needle is removed from the spleen, can result in the sample being pulled into the syringe and lost. Always remove the needle from the syringe, then pull air into the syringe, refasten the needle, and spray the sample onto microscope slides. Different types of stains can be used to evaluate the slides (e.g., Diff Quik, Gram stain), so it is important to ascertain which stains the laboratory or pathologist reading the cytology prefers.

Urine Collection and Interpretation

The collection of uncontaminated urine is essential to evaluating the true status of a sample. Free-catch urine samples are often contaminated with bacteria and can be misinterpreted by the novice. Fortunately, cystocentesis can be performed relatively easily on an unanesthetized ferret. The animal should be placed in dorsal recumbency and the ventral abdomen aseptically prepared. The urinary bladder is located cranial to the pelvis and should be identified prior to attempting this procedure. If the bladder cannot be palpated, it is best to delay the procedure until sufficient urine accumulates within the bladder. Using your index finger and thumb, gently grasp the abdomen in the area of the bladder and move your hand in a cranial to caudal motion. The urinary bladder should palpate like a water-filled balloon. A 25-gauge needle fastened to a 3 or 6 ml syringe can be used to collect the sample. Isolate the bladder between your index finger and thumb and insert the needle perpendicular to the body wall. Maintain a steady hand and prevent excessive movement of the needle within the abdomen.

Urinary catheterization can also be used to collect a urine sample, but this procedure is difficult in ferrets and requires anesthesia. In the female, the urethral opening is located approximately 1 cm cranial to the clitoral fossa.[8] A vaginal speculum can be used to visualize the urethral opening and introduce an appropriate-sized catheter (e.g., 3.5 French). This procedure is best performed with the ferret in sternal recumbency with the caudal half of the body elevated (e.g., place a rolled towel under the abdomen). In the male, the penis must be gently exteriorized from the prepuce. An appropriate-sized catheter (e.g., 3.5 French) can be introduced into the urethra and sutured to the skin to maintain urethral patency. This procedure is best performed with the ferret in dorsal recumbency. Identifying the tip of the urethra can be difficult in hobs, especially if there is pathology associated with this structure. Some veterinarians have used a technique whereby sterile water or saline is infused through the tip of the catheter while searching for the urethra to facilitate the dilation of the urethral tip.

Ferret urine should be yellow and have little turbidity (Table 3.4). These animals are true carnivores and should have a urine pH between 6.5 and 7.5.[9] Animals with alkaline urine might be predisposed to calculi formation. There should be no blood or bacteria from a sample collected via cystocentesis or catheterization.

Radiology

Radiographs serve as an important diagnostic tool in ferret medicine. Standard safety protocols should be employed when radiographing ferrets. Ferrets should be anesthetized to ensure that quality radiographs are taken. Isoflurane is the anesthetic of choice. A ferret radiographic technique chart should be established based on the capabilities of a facility's radiographic machine. A high-capacity radiographic unit capable of producing 300-milliampere exposures at times of at least 1/60th of a second is recommended. The kilovoltage peak (kVp) settings should be adjustable by increments of 2 to provide finite detail. A thorough understanding of ferret anatomy is essential to radiographic interpretation.

Table 3.4 **Urinalysis Results in the Ferret**[6]

DETERMINATION	MALE	FEMALE
Color	Yellow	Yellow
Turbidity	Minimal	Minimal
Volume (ml/24 h)	26 (8–48)	28 (8–140)
Sodium (mmol/24 h)	1.9 (0.4–6.7)	1.5 (0.2–5.6)
Potassium (mmol/24 h)	2.9 (1.0–9.6)	2.1 (0.9–5.4)
pH	6.5–7.5	6.5–7.5
Protein (mg/dl)	7.0–33.0	0–32.0

Parasitology

External Parasites

Ear mites (*Otodectes cynotis*) are a common finding in ferrets, especially kits. Animals with ear mites will often present with a thick, brown discharge in the ear. Owners often complain that the animal shakes and scratches at its ears. A cotton-tipped applicator dipped in mineral oil can be used to collect a sample from the ear for diagnosis. The sample should be placed onto a glass slide and evaluated under light microscopy.

Fleas that parasitize dogs and cats can also prey on ferrets. Ferrets with a flea infestation will often present with a history of pruritis and tail base alopecia. On close examination of the animal, the fleas or their feces ("flea-dirt") will be obvious. Kits or severely compromised adult animals can become severely anemic if they have a heavy flea burden. In these cases, a minute blood sample (<0.1 ml) can be collected and a packed cell volume determined. Animals with a packed cell volume less than 15% might require a blood transfusion. Flea eradication is similar to that performed for cats, and the owner should be made aware of the importance of treating both the animal and the environment.

Ferrets maintained outdoors might be susceptible to fly-strike, especially if they have a skin laceration. Animals maintained outdoors should be monitored closely for any injuries and the animal given shelter and protection against flies. Animals that develop a maggot infestation should have the site shaved, maggots removed, and a topical antiseptic cream applied to protect the injury site.

Internal Parasites

Gastrointestinal parasitism is uncommon in ferrets. Ferrets allowed to play outdoors are more likely to develop a patent parasite infection than animals maintained indoors. A fecal sample should be submitted for a saline direct smear and a fecal float for kits at the time of their initial examination and for adult animals on an annual basis.

Ferrets are susceptible to *Dirofilaria immitis*, and animals in heartworm-endemic areas should be tested and given a heartworm preventive. Diagnosis of heartworm disease in ferrets can be difficult. The two most commonly used diagnostic tests in veterinary clinical practice are the Knott's test and the enzyme-linked immunosorbent assays (ELISA). The Knott's test is used to diagnose circulating microfilaria, and the ELISA test is used to diagnose circulating antigens produced by gravid female worms. Sensitivity of these tests is often lower in ferrets than in canids, because adult worm burdens are low (e.g., 1 worm) or occult (e.g., same sex) in ferrets. With the limitations of the currently available heartworm tests, echocardiography might provide a more definitive and consistent approach to heartworm disease diagnosis in the ferret.

VACCINATIONS

Canine distemper virus (CDV) is associated with high mortality in affected ferrets. Ferret owners should be made aware of the risks of this disease and the likelihood of exposure, even to indoor animals. Vaccination is the best protection against infection. The preferred vaccine against CDV in ferrets is the Purevax ferret distemper vaccine (Merial Inc., Athens, GA). This vaccine is a canarypox-derived vaccine and appears to have fewer side effects than canine combination or ferret-cell origin vaccines. The vaccine should be administered subcutaneously in the area between the shoulder blades or over one of the rear legs. The site of the injection should be recorded in case a reaction is noted. The standard CDV vaccine protocol for a kit should include a vaccine at 6 weeks, 10 weeks, and 14 weeks. A booster vaccine should be administered annually to adult animals. Ferrets >12 weeks of age with an unknown vaccine history should be given 2 vaccinations 3 weeks apart to stimulate an appropriate humoral response.

Ferrets are susceptible to rabies and should be vaccinated against this devastating disease. There is one USDA-approved vaccine (Imrab 3, Rhone-Merieux Inc., Athens, GA) for use in ferrets. The rabies vaccine should be administered to a kit at ≥12 weeks of age and a booster administered annually. The vaccine can be administered subcutaneously or intramuscularly, and administration should align with local rabies ordinances. Again, the vaccination site should be recorded in case vaccine reactions are noted later. Vaccinated ferrets are currently protected under the same statutes as dogs and cats, whereas an unvaccinated ferret should be managed as a wild animal under circumstances of questionable rabies exposure. Ferret owners should be made aware that, by law, unvaccinated ferrets that bite a human are supposed to be treated like a wild animal, which could include euthanasia for rabies testing.

Postvaccination hypersensitivity reactions are not an uncommon occurrence in ferrets. These hypersensitivity reactions have been reported following single vaccinations, especially with some of the former ferret distemper vaccines (Fervac-D, United Vaccine, Madison, WI), and vaccinations combining a distemper vaccine and rabies vaccine. Ferrets that experience a hypersensitivity reaction might develop gastrointestinal signs, including vomiting and diarrhea, become dyspneic, or develop other systemic signs (e.g., depression, lethargy, and erythematous skin).

Treatment of a ferret experiencing a vaccine reaction should follow the standard protocol for mammals and include diphenhydramine hydro-chloride at 0.5–2.0 mg/kg, IM or IV.[4] When the postvaccination reaction becomes life-threatening (e.g., severe dyspnea from inflammation in the airway), a potent steroid (e.g., prednisone or dexamethasone) and oxygen should be given. Animals that have had a previous vaccine reaction should be premedicated with oral diphenhydramine hydro-chloride 15 minutes prior to the vaccination. As a matter of protocol in some veterinary practices, all ferrets are premedicated with diphenhydramine hydrochloride prior to being vaccinated. In addition, it has been recommended that only one vaccine per visit be given to ferrets to limit the occurrence of vaccine reactions. In cases when the veterinarian or client is concerned about the severity of a vaccine reaction in a ferret, alternatives to vaccination, such as monitoring antibody titers, can be done.

THERAPEUTICS

There are no approved therapeutics for the ferret in the United States. Current recommendations should follow those described for cats. The same routes of administration apply, including *per os* (PO), subcutaneous (SC), intramuscular (IM), intraosseus (IO), and intravenous (IV). Animals that are critical require routes of administration that provide rapid drug delivery, such as IM, IO, or IV, whereas less critical animals can be given therapeutics PO or SC. Intravenous injections should be administered through an IV catheter to limit the likelihood of perivascular contamination. The preferred site for IV catheterization is the cephalic vein (Figure 3.9); however, if it is not possible to catheterize this vein, the lateral saphenous vein or jugular vein can also be used to provide IV access. Intraosseus injections can be given into the femur or tibia. It should be noted that catheter placement into the tibia is more direct than into the femur. Intramuscular injections are routinely

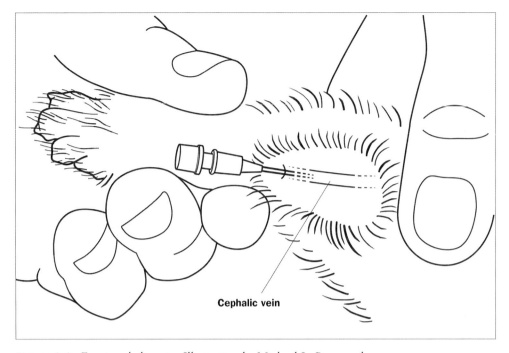

Cephalic vein

Figure 3.9 *Ferret cephalic vein. Illustration by Michael L. Broussard.*

administered into the epaxial muscles along the spine or in the muscle bellies (e.g., quadriceps or hamstring: semimembranosus, semitendinosus, biceps femoris) of the rear limbs.

The muscle masses of the ferret limb are relatively small in comparison with those of other mammals; therefore, the volume of the injection should be limited. It is very difficult to orally administer tablets or capsules to a ferret. Fortunately, there are a number of commercial pharmacies that can compound oral therapeutics into flavored liquids to simplify delivery of the drug.

Fluid administration protocols for ferrets should follow those described for dogs and cats. The fluid maintenance rate for ferrets is 80–100 ml/kg/day. It is important to recognize that fluid replacement in a ferret, or in any vertebrate for that matter, should include both the daily maintenance needs of the patient and a correction for its deficit (% dehydrated). The daily maintenance

rate is especially important to consider in patients that are not eating or drinking. Animals that are mildly dehydrated (<5%) can be administered fluids PO or SC, whereas an indwelling IV or IO catheter should be placed in any animal that is greater than 5% dehydrated.

Intraperitoneal delivery of fluids can also be considered for more critical cases where IO or IV access might not be possible. Fluids should not be administered orally to any animal with gastrointestinal disease. Giving fluids to a patient with delayed gastrointestinal emptying or diarrhea could exacerbate these disease conditions. Subcutaneous fluids can be administered in the SC space between the shoulder blades or along the lateral body wall. The cephalic and lateral saphenous veins are routine sites for catheter placement.

The jugular vein can also be used if the other vessels become unavailable. Ferrets that are alert and responsive will require sedation for this procedure, which can be accomplished by masking the animal with isoflurane anesthesia. A moribund animal will not require sedation. The animal should be placed in sternal recumbency for cephalic catheter placement, although the animal may be placed into lateral recumbency for lateral saphenous catheterization. One individual will need to "hold off" the vessel by grasping the animal at the elbow for the cephalic vein and above the hock for the lateral saphenous vein. IV catheters often become damaged when they are inserted through tough skin. To avoid this problem, make a puncture in the skin lateral to the vessel using a 22-gauge needle. A heparinized 22- to 24-gauge catheter can be introduced into the skin puncture and threaded into the vessel. An injection port should be fastened to the catheter, and the device can be secured to the animal's leg using tissue glue and appropriate bandage material.

Placement of a tongue depressor splint can reduce the likelihood of catheter failure. To do this, place a tongue depressor on the posterior aspect of the forelimb. Measure the distance from the toes to the elbow. Cut the tongue depressor to fit this distance. Trim the cut end to minimize the potential for splinters. Secure the tongue depressor to the limb with tape, and then incorporate it into the bandage.

Ferrets that are very active and chew at the catheter might require an Elizabethan collar, which is commercially available or can be fashioned from exposed radiographic film. The catheter should be flushed regularly (e.g., q4h) with 0.9% heparinized saline. The animal should be observed regularly to ensure the catheter remains patent and the animal does not become entangled in its fluid line.

Blood transfusions might be required in animals with severe anemias (PCV <15%). Because ferrets lack distinct blood groups, they can be used as universal donors. Blood can be collected from an anesthetized blood donor from either the jugular vein or anterior cranial vena cava, using a 23-gauge butterfly catheter fastened to a 6 or 12 ml syringe. The syringe should be preloaded with an anticoagulant (e.g., acid-citrate dextrose) at a ratio of 1 ml of anticoagulant to 6 ml of blood.[10] The blood should be administered to the recipient animal via a syringe pump or slow bolus through a cephalic or jugular catheter. The animal should be observed for any reactions to the transfusion. The volume of blood that can be collected from the donor and the volume required by the recipient can be determined using the formulae described in small animal medicine.

Table 3.5 **Injectable Analgesic and Anesthetic Dosages for the Ferret[11]**

DRUG	DOSE	COMMENTS
Ketamine	10–20 mg/kg IM 30–60 mg/kg IM	Tranquilization Anesthesia
Ketamine and Acepromazine	20–25 mg/kg (K) IM 0.2–0.35 mg/kg (A) SC, IM	Anesthesia
Ketamine and Diazepam	10–20 mg/kg (K) IM 1–2 mg/kg (D) IM	Anesthesia
Ketamine and Xylazine	10–25 mg/kg (K) IM 1–2 mg/kg (X) IM	Anesthesia Avoid in sick animals
Butorphanol	0.1–0.5 mg/kg IM q12h	Analgesia
Buprenorphine	0.01–0.03 mg/kg SC, IM q12h	Analgesia

SURGICAL AND ANESTHETIC ASSISTANCE

A variety of anesthetic agents can be used for ferrets (see Table 3.5), although the inhalant anesthetics are by far the most commonly used. Injectable anesthetics can be used to preanesthetize the animal or in situations where an inhalant anesthetic is not available. For procedures that will induce pain, an appropriate analgesic protocol should be established. Ferrets, like other mustelids, are very responsive to opioids (e.g., butorphanol, 0.05–0.3 mg/kg intramuscular).

Ferrets should be fasted for a minimum of 4 hours prior to an anesthetic procedure, although special precautions should be taken (e.g., IV dextrose) for an animal susceptible to a hypoglycemic episode (e.g., ferret with insulinoma). A water source can be left with the ferret up to the time of the procedure. Ferrets should be maintained on a water-recirculating heating pad during any anesthetic procedure and recovered in a warmed environment to prevent hypothermia.

For short procedures, such as venipuncture or radiography, inhalant anesthetics can be used to facilitate sample collection. Ferrets can be "masked down" using an appropriately sized mask, or placed into an induction chamber and anesthetized (Figure 3.10). Inducing anesthesia via face mask at 5% isoflurane or 8% sevoflurane expedites the process of getting the animal through the sedation phase, which is the time they struggle. Once the ferret has lost its righting reflex, it can be maintained at 1%–2% isoflurane or 2%–3% sevoflurane. Anesthetized ferrets should be intubated to gain control over their respiration. Ferrets can be intubated using a 2.0 to 4.0 mm OD endotracheal tube, depending on their size. A laryngoscope can be used to visualize the airway. The animal should be monitored closely during the procedure using appropriate equipment (e.g., Doppler, pulse oximeter, and EKG).

Surgical preparation of the ferret should follow the same protocols described for dogs and cats. The surgical site should be shaved, using a standard grooming clipper at a slow, cautious speed to prevent clipper burn and tearing of the skin. The shaved area should be uniform and provide the surgeon ample room to perform the surgery without the risk of contamination (Figure 3.11). The surgical site should be aseptically prepared, using a surgical

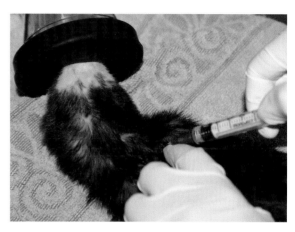

Figure 3.10. *Ferrets can be "masked down" with isoflurane or sevoflurane.*

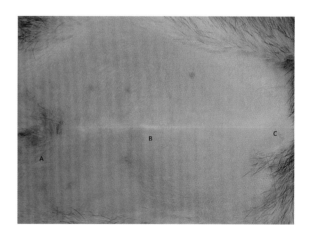

Figure 3.11 *It is important to create an appropriately sized sterile field for a surgical procedure; the size of the field will vary depending on the procedure. The surgical approach for a ferret with insulinoma and adrenal gland disease should include the area between the manubrium of the sternum and cranial pelvis.*

scrub and warmed sterile saline. Avoid using alcohol to prepare the surgical site because it can result in significant heat loss. The surgical site should be covered with a sterile drape until the surgeon begins. The surgical instruments used to perform surgery on dogs and cats can also be used for ferrets.

HEALTH MAINTENANCE AND DISEASE

Gastrointestinal Diseases

See "Emerging Diseases," below, for information on other common gastrointestinal diseases.

Ingestion of Foreign Bodies

The curious nature of the ferret, in combination with its voracious appetite, is likely the reason why it ingests foreign material. Ferrets should always be monitored closely when they are outside of a cage. Kits are notorious for ingesting foreign material, including metal, paper, and plastic, whereas adults are more likely to develop trichobezoars. Taking time to ask the client about the different types of material a ferret might be exposed to in its environment can be helpful when pursuing these cases, especially if the material is not radiopaque (e.g., plastic). Affected ferrets might exhibit lethargy, inappetence, vomiting, or diarrhea. The degree to which they express certain clinical signs will vary based on the location and extent of the obstruction (e.g., partial vs. complete). The veterinarian will thoroughly evaluate ferrets suspected of ingesting a foreign body by performing a physical examination and surveying radiographs. In some cases, the foreign material and secondary gas accumulation (e.g., ileus) will be palpable. A contrast series might be necessary if the suspected foreign material is not evident on survey radiographs. Surgical correction is necessary to remove the foreign material. The veterinary technician should stabilize the surgical candidate prior to the procedure. The techniques used to remove a gastric foreign body (e.g., endoscopy, gastrotomy) or small-intestine foreign body (enterotomy) should follow protocols described for domestic species.[12,13]

Gastric Ulcers

Gastric ulcers are often reported in ferrets that experience chronic stress. A number of different etiologies have been associated with gastric ulcers in the ferret, including primary gastritis, neoplasia, infection (e.g., *Helicobacter mustelae*), foreign body ingestion, and inappropriate drug use (e.g., corticosteroids). Ferrets that present with gastric ulcers are often inappetent, vomiting, and have melena or diarrhea. Many of these animals also grind their teeth and hypersalivate, symptoms that appear to be associated with upper gastrointestinal pain. Diagnosis of gastric ulcers should follow standard protocol. A complete blood count and serum chemistry panel should be performed to evaluate the animal's general health. Animals with chronic gastric ulcers could be anemic. Survey radiographs can be beneficial in identifying potential causes of the gastric ulcer. Endoscopy can be used to visualize the ulcers and collect biopsies for culture and histopathology. This technique is preferred when attempting to determine if an animal has *H. mustelae*. Ferrets should fast for at least 3 hours before the technician performs radiographs or endoscopy to ensure no food remains in the stomach. Treatment for gastric ulcers depends on the etiology. In cases when a biopsy is not possible, empirical therapy is initiated that includes antibiotics (metronidazole and amoxicillin), an H_2 antagonist, and a gut protectant such as sucralfate.

Respiratory Diseases

Ferrets are susceptible to many of the same respiratory infections that are common to dogs and cats. Animals that develop clinical signs associated with respiratory disease, such as coughing, sneezing, and dyspnea, should undergo diagnostic testing in accordance with those described in other species.

Ferrets are susceptible to canine distemper virus, with mortalities approaching 100%. This virus replicates in the respiratory tract of the ferret, and affected animals develop a chronic cough.[14] Anorexia, lethargy, and pyrexia are also common findings, especially early in the development of clinical signs. Ferrets with canine distemper can also develop symptoms associated with the skin (e.g., crusting under the chin and hyperkeratosis of the footpads) (Figure 3.12), eyes (e.g., blindness), and the central nervous system (e.g., incoordination). Diagnosis is typically achieved in animals with clinical disease by submitting fecal samples for polymerase chain reaction testing. Treatment is unrewarding, and affected animals should be humanely euthanized. Prevention can be achieved through routine vaccination (see "Vaccinations").

Ferrets are susceptible to the human influenza virus, as well as the highly pathogenic avian influenza virus (H5N1) and swine (H1N1) influenza virus. The human influenza virus primarily affects the upper respiratory system of ferrets, and clinically ill animals might exhibit signs of sneezing, coughing, difficulty smelling (nasal discharge and not using olfaction as they normally would), inappetence, and lethargy. Humans can infect their pets and vice versa. Diagnosing this viral infection in ferrets is not commonly done; instead, affected animals are provided supportive care (e.g., fluid therapy, enteral support, antibiotics against secondary bacterial infections), and a presumed diagnosis comes through a response to therapy. Affected animals should also be kept away from infants, the elderly, and those individuals with reduced immune function. The H5N1 (avian) and H1N1 (swine) influenza viruses can also cause severe systemic disease in ferrets, ultimately leading to their death.

Neoplasia

Neoplasia is a common finding in ferrets and can affect any age group.[15] The most common neoplastic diseases reported in ferrets are adrenal gland neoplasia, insulinoma, and lymphoma. Adrenal gland disease seems to be by far the most common disease presentation for adult ferrets, with insulinoma being the second most common presentation among adult animals. There are a number of potential etiologies for the high incidence of neoplasia in ferrets, including genetics, early-age spay/neutering, diet, photoperiod, and infectious agents; to date, no specific cause has been identified.

Adrenal gland disease is most commonly diagnosed in adult ferrets (>3 years of age). Currently, there is no documented sex predilection associated with the disease. Ferrets affected with adrenal gland disease often present with focal or generalized alopecia, pruritis, thinning of the skin, and weight loss. A majority of the animals remain active with

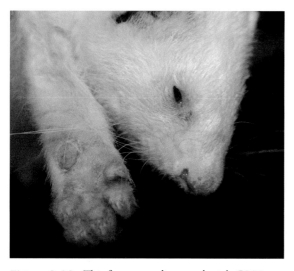

Figure 3.12 *This ferret was diagnosed with CDV. Note the severe hyperkeratosis of the footpads.*

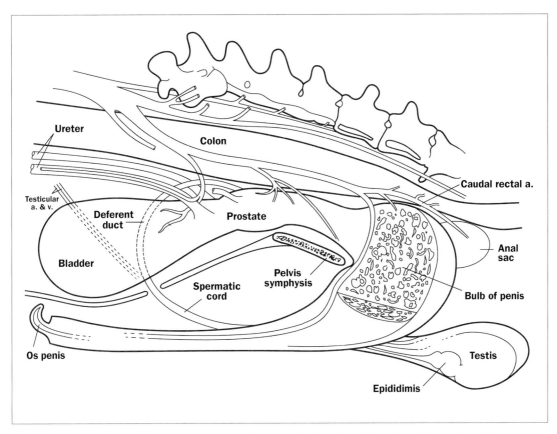

Figure 3.13 *The ferret prostate, when enlarged, can easily be palpated. Hobs with an enlarged prostate often present for stranguria. Illustration by Michael L. Broussard.*

the disease. Hobs that are affected with adrenal gland disease can develop secondary prostatic disease, which can affect their ability to urinate (Figure 3.13). In severe cases, hobs can present for stranguria; clients might complain that the ferret acts as if it wants to urinate, but can't. These animals will often vocalize as they strain because of the pain associated with their inability to evacuate their bladder. Because ferret adrenal gland disease is associated with increased production of sex hormones, hobs might also display sexual aggression (e.g., aggression toward or attempts to mount other ferrets). Jills with adrenal gland disease often develop a swollen vulva, and sexual behaviors (e.g., standing for coitus) might also be

noted in them. In both genders a pancytopenia might develop. To diagnose adrenal gland disease, a series of diagnostic tests should be performed, including a complete blood count, chemistry panel, radiographs, ultrasound, and measurement of steroid hormone concentrations. Current recommendations for treatment of adrenal gland disease focus on surgical intervention as the best chance for eliminating the cancer, although some successful medical therapies (e.g., leuprolide acetate) have been reported. Adrenal gland neoplasia is most commonly identified in the left adrenal gland, but can occur in both glands. It is not uncommon to perform a unilateral adrenalectomy (Figure 3.14) only to have the contralateral gland

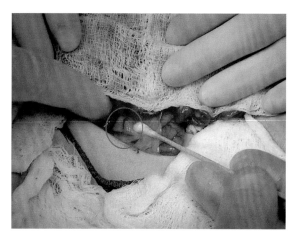

Figure 3.14 *An enlarged left adrenal gland at surgery. This tumorous gland was removed and submitted for histopathology. Final diagnosis: adenoma.*

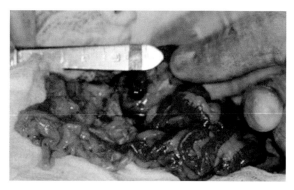

Figure 3.15 *Insulinoma in a ferret. Note the nodular appearance of these tumors.*

be affected later. Biopsy/histopathology of the affected gland(s) should be performed. Adrenal gland hyperplasia, adenoma, and adenocarcinoma are the most common histopathologic diagnoses associated with adrenal gland disease in ferrets. The medical management of adrenal gland disease with leuprolide acetate is not curative, but will alleviate clinical signs. Clients opting to pursue medical management should be informed that the treatment is lifelong and that it will not eliminate the cancer, thus a lapse in therapy will result in the return of clinical signs.

Insulinomas are another common tumor found in adult ferrets and are often identified concurrently in ferrets with adrenal gland disease. These beta-cell tumors can coalesce to form gross nodules within the pancreas (Figure 3.15). Affected animals often present with a glassy-eyed appearance, hind leg or general weakness, hypersalivation (accompanied by pawing at the mouth), or seizures. Blood work, including a fasting blood glucose, insulin level, complete blood count, and chemistry panel, should be performed to confirm the diagnosis. If an animal is suspected of being hypoglycemic, a fast is

unnecessary. Survey radiographs and ultrasounds rarely prove to be diagnostic, but can be useful in identifying concurrent problems such as adrenal gland disease. Current recommendations for treatment are focused on surgical intervention, although medical therapies have been reported with some success. Performing a nodulectomy does not guarantee remission of the neoplasia. In cases where the neoplasia recurs, medical management using prednisone and diazoxide might be considered. Some ferrets have lived up to 3 years postdiagnosis through medical management alone.

Lymphoma is the most common tumor in young ferrets.[15] Affected animals can be clinically normal or might present with weakness, lethargy, generalized lymphadenopathy, splenomegaly, or dyspnea. Diagnosis of lymphoma should include a complete blood count, chemistry panel, radiographs, ultrasound, and biopsy of affected tissues. Treatment can be difficult and remission is likely. Most ferrets diagnosed with lymphoma rarely live for more than a year even with treatment. There are a number of different chemotherapeutic protocols that can be used to treat an affected animal. The treatment protocol should be based on the animal's condition and the owner's comfort level.

Cardiovascular Diseases

Dilated and hypertrophic cardiomyopathies have been reported in ferrets. Affected animals often present with many of the same clinical signs reported in dogs and cats, including weakness, lethargy, dyspnea, exercise intolerance, and hind leg weakness. A full cardiac diagnostic series should be performed to assess the animal's condition and should include a complete blood count, serum chemistry profile, radiograph(s), echocardiograph, and EKG. Medical management of the heart condition will vary depending upon the animal's general physical condition upon presentation and the extent of the disease.

Dirofilaria immitis, the parasite associated with heartworm disease in dogs and cats, can cause severe disease in ferrets. The majority of the cases reported in ferrets are from the southeastern United States, where mosquitoes can be active year-round; however, this disease can occur in ferrets anywhere it is found in dogs and cats. Being housed indoors is protective, but does not ensure an animal will not become infected. Heartworm infestations in ferrets are typically at a lower worm burden (1–4 worms) than those in dogs, but the pathology is more severe because of the small size of the ferret heart. Affected animals often present with lethargy, depression, weakness, rear leg paresis, and exercise intolerance. Unfortunately, by the time most affected animals present, the disease is severe. Confirmation of heartworm disease can be made in ferrets using a Knott's test (although a rare occurrence, ferrets can have patent infections with microfilaria), ELISA heartworm tests, radiographs, and ultrasound. Ultrasound is often the test of choice, because it allows the veterinarian to see the parasites within the heart. Treatment is difficult because of the potential for thromboembolic disease. Because of the severity of this disease,

prevention is key. Ferrets can be placed on the same preventives used for dogs and cats (adjusted for weight).

Reproductive Diseases

Ferrets are induced ovulators and an intact jill that is not bred can develop a life-threatening, estrogen-induced anemia. Affected animals will have a history of being intact and not bred, and will have a swollen vulva, pale mucous membranes, and a history of weakness and lethargy. A blood sample can be collected to assess the erythron and leukon. In most cases, a pancytopenia will develop. Prevention is key, and any female ferret not being used for breeding should have an ovariohysterectomy performed. Animals that are intended as breeders and affected with the disease should be induced to ovulate and provided appropriate supportive care, including fluid therapy and a blood transfusion, if necessary.

Urogenital Diseases

Ferrets can develop urolithiasis if they are maintained on a low-quality cat or dog food. Magnesium ammonium phosphate is the most common urolith identified in the ferret.[16] Cystitis might also be identified in animals with urolithiasis and should be managed accordingly. A thorough diagnostic screening should be performed on affected animals and should include a complete blood count, chemistry panel, radiograph(s), urinalysis, and urine culture. Affected animals often have alkaline urine as a result of a predominance of plant-based proteins in their diet, whereas an animal offered a high-quality, meat-based diet will have an acidic urine (normal). In males a blockage of the urethra should be considered an emergency, and immediate steps should be taken to remove the offending calculi. In severe cases, surgical removal of the uroliths might be required.

Renal cysts are an incidental finding often reported at necropsy.[17] A specific etiology for renal cysts has not been determined. On occasion, renal cysts will be identified on routine examination, survey radiographs, or ultrasound. A thorough diagnostic workup, including an analysis of blood and urine, should be performed to determine if the animal has any renal compromise as a result of the renal cysts.

Bacterial Diseases

Ferrets are susceptible to opportunistic Gram-positive and Gram-negative pathogens. Kits and geriatric animals are typically more susceptible to bacterial pathogens than a healthy adult animal. Animals being maintained on immunosuppressive doses of corticosteroids (e.g., high doses of prednisone for insulinoma treatment) are also more susceptible to opportunistic infections. Sample collection should follow standard sterile techniques. A commercial sterile culturette and transport media can be used to collect samples and protect them from desiccation during transport to a diagnostic laboratory. Standard microbial techniques can be employed to isolate a potential pathogen. Most opportunistic infections are associated with aerobic infections; however, in certain abscesses facultative or obligate anaerobic organisms should be considered. *Helicobacter mustelae* are Gram-negative rods that are routinely cultured from gastric ulcers. Most bacterial infections are associated with pneumonia, urinary cystitis, dermatitis, and diarrhea. A number of pathogens have been isolated from these different organ systems, including *Streptococcus zooepidemicus* and *S. pneumoniae*, *E. coli*, *Klebsiella* spp., *Pseudomonas* spp., and *Bordetella* spp. Fungal infections in ferrets are rare. In cases where a fungal infection is suspected, the techniques used to collect and process samples employed in other domestic species may be followed.

Emerging Diseases

There are several recent diseases that appear to be emerging in captive ferrets. Unfortunately, there is much we do not know about these diseases, so it is important to record and share these findings with others. By disseminating new knowledge we will be able to further elucidate the epidemiology of these diseases and establish preventive methods to minimize their dissemination into captive populations and design effective treatments.

Ferret enteric coronavirus has been associated with epizootic catarrhal enteritis, a severe disease in ferrets characterized by severe dehydration, a green-mucoid diarrhea, and death. The disease tends to be introduced into established ferret households by newly introduced kits that are carriers. A variant of this virus appears to be associated with a feline infectious peritonitis (FIP)–like disease in ferrets (ferret infectious peritonitis).[18] The systemic disease in ferrets is characterized by widespread dissemination of the virus; two of the more interesting findings are generalized nodules throughout the abdomen and abdominal masses (palpable on examination). Currently there is no effective treatment for this disease; however, some veterinarians are using some of the treatments used for cats with FIP.

Disseminated immunopathic myositis is a disease that tends to affect young ferrets (kits to young adults).[18] This disease is characterized by a fatal, inflammatory condition of the muscles. The most common findings in affected ferrets are a high fever (105°–108°F; 40.5°–42.2°C), anorexia, and an inability to move. The etiology of this syndrome is not known, and currently there is no effective treatment.

Mycoplasmosis is a disease that is well-known in chelonians, birds, and rats. Recently, this disease has also been reported in ferrets.[18] Affected animals display typical signs for this pathogen, including conjunctivitis, sneezing, wheezing, and coughing.[18] In more severe cases the pathogen can move from the upper to the lower respiratory tract. A novel *Mycoplasma* spp. has been identified in affected animals.[18] Treatment for this disease should include antimicrobials with good specificity against *Mycoplasma* spp. and supportive care.

Other diseases that appear to be emerging in ferrets remain classified based on clinical presentation or diagnostic testing and require additional research, including oral ulceration syndrome, acute hemorrhagic syndrome, and aplastic anemia/bone marrow hypoplasia syndrome.[18]

SELF-STUDY QUESTIONS

1. What are the terms used to define a male, female, and juvenile ferret?

2. What type of enclosure is appropriate for ferrets?

3. What type of diet should a ferret be provided?

4. What are some common grooming concerns for captive ferrets?

5. Describe how to properly restrain a ferret.

6. Describe how to examine a ferret.

7. What are some common venipuncture sites in a ferret? How much blood can you collect from a ferret?

8. What are some common ectoparasites found on ferrets?

9. Which vaccinations are considered essential in ferrets?

10. What are the different routes for replenishing fluids in a ferret patient?

11. What preanesthetic recommendations would you make to a client to minimize complications with an anesthetic event?

12. What are two common gastrointestinal diseases of captive ferrets?

13. What are the common presenting signs of a ferret with adrenal gland disease?

14. What are the common presenting signs of a ferret with insulinoma?

15. Which parasite of dogs is also found in ferrets? How can you diagnose it?

16. Name three emerging diseases in ferrets.

REFERENCES

1. Rupprecht CE, Gilbert J, Pitts R, et al. Evaluation of an inactivated rabies virus vaccine in domestic ferrets. *Journal of the American Veterinary Medical Association* 1990;193:1614–16.
2. Fox JG. Taxonomy, history and use. In: Fox JG, ed. *Biology and diseases of the ferret.* Philadelphia: Lea and Febiger; 1988:3–13.

3. Brown SA. Basic anatomy, physiology and husbandry. In: Hillyer EV, and Quesenberry KE, eds. *Ferrets, rabbits and rodents: Clinical medicine and surgery.* Philadelphia: WB Saunders; 1997:3–13.
4. Fox JG. Normal clinical and biological parameters. In: Fox JG, ed. *Biology and diseases of the ferret.* Philadelphia: Lea and Febiger; 1988:159–73.
5. Bell J. Ferret nutrition and diseases associated with inadequate nutrition. Proceedings of the North American Veterinary Conference, Orlando, FL, 1993:719–20.
6. Thorton PC, Wright PA, Sacra PJ, et al. The ferret, *Mustela putorius furo*, as a new species in toxicology. *Lab Animals* 1979;13:119–24.
7. Kawasaki TA. Laboratory parameters in disease states in ferrets. Proceedings of the North American Veterinary Conference, 1992:663–67.
8. Quesenberry KE. Basic approach to veterinary care. In: Hillyer EV, and Quesenberry KE, eds. *Ferrets, rabbits and rodents: Clinical medicine and surgery.* Philadelphia: WB Saunders; 1997:14–25.
9. Williams CSF. *Practice guide to laboratory animals.* St. Louis, MO: CV Mosby; 1976:66.
10. Hoefer, HL. Transfusions in exotic species. In: Hohenhaus AE, ed. *Transfusion medicine.* Philadelphia: JB Lippincott; 1992:625–35.
11. Brown SA. Ferret drug dosages. In: Bauck L, Boyer TH, Brown SA, et al., eds. *Exotic animal formulary.* Lakewood, CO: American Animal Hospital Association; 1995:5–11.
12. Orsher RJ, and Rosin E. Small intestine. In: Slatter D, ed. *Textbook of small animal surgery.* Philadelphia: WB Saunders; 1997:593–612.
13. Van Sluys FJ. Gastric foreign bodies. In: Slatter D, ed. *Textbook of small animal surgery.* Philadelphia: WB Saunders; 1997:568–71.
14. Pearson RC, and Gorham JR. Viral disease models. In: Fox JG, ed. *Biology and diseases of the ferret.* Philadelphia: Lea and Febiger; 1988:305–14.
15. Brown SA. Neoplasia. In: Hillyer EV, and Quesenberry KE, eds. *Ferrets, rabbits and rodents: Clinical medicine and surgery.* Philadelphia: WB Saunders; 1997:99–114.
16. Hillyer EV. Urogenital diseases. In: Hillyer EV, and Quesenberry KE, eds. *Ferrets, rabbits and rodents: Clinical medicine and surgery.* Philadelphia: WB Saunders; 1997:44–52.
17. Fox JG. Systemic diseases. In: Fox JG, ed. *Biology and diseases of the ferret.* Philadelphia: Lea and Febiger; 1988:255–73.
18. Johnson-Delaney K. Emerging ferret diseases. *Journal of Exotic Pet Medicine* 2010;20:1–4.

FURTHER READING

Fox JG. Anesthesia and surgery. In: Fox JG, ed. *Biology and diseases of the ferret.* Philadelphia: Lea and Febiger; 1988:289–30.
Heard DJ. Principles and techniques of anesthesia and analgesia for exotic practice. *Vet Clinic of North Am/Small Animal Practice* 1993;23:1301–27.
Hillyer EV, and Brown SA. Ferrets. In: Birchard SJ, and Sherding RG, eds. *Saunders manual of small animal practice.* Philadelphia: WB Saunders; 1994:1317–44.

Rabbits

CHAPTER 4

INTRODUCTION

One of the most common misconceptions regarding rabbits is that they belong to the order Rodentia, which includes mice, rats, and guinea pigs. Rabbits belong to the order of animals called Lagomorpha, which also includes hares and pikas. Rabbits differ from mice, rats, and guinea pigs because they have a second pair of underdeveloped smaller peg teeth directly behind the primary incisors, which rodents do not have. This classification difference is important to point out in the beginning of this chapter, because rabbit husbandry and health concerns are very different from those of rodents. Many rabbits are obtained through impulse purchases during the spring and Easter season. Often these impulse purchases do not include education on proper husbandry, nutrition, or health maintenance. It is hoped that new rabbit owners will schedule an appointment with a veterinarian for a routine health examination and, most importantly, receive an education during the visit on the requirements for maintaining a healthy, happy pet. Frequently, an owner will ask questions regarding the basic physiologic values of their new pet rabbit. It is important for the technician to know the normal physiologic values not only to answer owners' questions, but also to assess the patients' health status upon presentation to the clinic and to administer medical therapy (Table 4.1).

Anatomy and Physiology

The technician needs to become familiar with a few areas of rabbit-specific anatomy. It might seem that rabbits are very docile animals. Although rabbits can be very gentle, they are territorial and will mark and viciously defend their territory. The chin glands, anal glands, and inguinal glands are used to mark territory and young. Males mark most often, followed by dominants of both sexes over subordinates.[1] The scrotal sacs are cranial and lateral to

Table 4.1 **Rabbit Basic Information**[1]

GENERAL CATEGORY	CLASSIFICATION	PHYSIOLOGIC PARAMETERS
Body Weight	Adult Male (Buck)	2–5 kg
	Adult Female (Doe)	2–6 kg
	Birth Weight (Bunny)	30–80 g
Temperature, Pulse, and Respiration	Rectal Body Temperature	101.3°–104°F
	Normal Heart Rate	180–250 beats/minute
	Normal Respiratory Rate	30–60 breaths/minute
Amounts of Food and Water	Daily Food Consumption	50 g/kg
	Daily Water Consumption	50–150 ml/kg
	Daily Urine Excretion	10–35 ml/kg
Age at Onset of Puberty and Breeding Life	Sexual Maturity, Male	22–52 weeks
	Sexual Maturity, Female	22–52 weeks
	Breeding Life, Male	60–72 months
	Breeding Life, Female	24–36 months
Female Reproductive Cycle	Estrous Cycle	Induced ovulation
	Estrus Duration	Prolonged
	Ovulation Rate	6–10 eggs
	Pseudopregnancy	16–17 days
	Gestation Length	30–33 days
	Litter Size	4–12 bunnies

the urethral opening, which in many cases is near or over the anus. The penis can be pushed out of the urethral opening by applying gentle pressure to the base of the prepuce.

The female might have a large "dewlap" or fold of skin under her chin. During nesting, the female sometimes removes hair from the dewlap as a source of soft nest material. The external genitalia are cranial to the anus, and the urogenital orifice is located between the folds of skin at this site. The ears make up a large percentage of the rabbit's body. At no time should the animal be picked up by the ears. Regarding other parts of the rabbit's body, they have footpads like cats, dogs, and rodents. Their feet are covered with fur that provides protection to the plantar surface of the foot. In the "Rex" breed this fur is absent, which predisposes these animals to sore hocks. This fur has developed to protect the feet in the rabbit's natural habitat, not in wire-bottomed cages. Large, obese rabbits can develop sores on the ventral surface of their hocks, because that part of the leg is in contact with the cage surface when they are resting.

Owners and rabbit handlers must be cautious of the sharp claws, especially the claws on the rear legs. When struggling, a rabbit will kick forward with the rear legs and scratch, sometimes severely, an unprepared holder. Declawing rabbits is not recommended. The underlying tissue support and footpads are not present to aid and protect the foot when healing. Sharp claws should be trimmed to blunt the sharp points, or the plastic rubberized Soft-Paws can be used (Figure 4.1).

HUSBANDRY

Environmental Concerns

Pet rabbits are very sensitive to heat. When educating a rabbit owner, emphasis must be placed on their pet's intolerance to heat. It would be most appropriate to give owners this information in the spring, when many of these pets are purchased. They have a well-developed hair coat that protects them against cold weather, but they quickly overheat when environmental temperatures are high. When a rabbit is housed outside in a nonair-conditioned house or apartment or in a car (when traveling), the owner must implement precautions to prevent hyperthermia. The rabbit should not be maintained in outdoor temperatures over 90°F or humidity over 90%. Common housing precautions against heat stress include providing a shaded enclosure (roof or natural setting), placing 2-liter soda bottles filled with frozen water in the cage, keeping the rabbit in an air-conditioned room during the summer months, and providing a fan for an animal housed outside. During the winter months, when humans need extra clothing, pet owners might erroneously assume that extra measures are needed to keep their pet rabbits warm. If a plywood "house" is placed in the animal's enclosure and lined with hay, this should protect the animal in temperatures down to 32°F (Figures 4.2A, 4.2B, and 4.2C).

Rabbit owners will house their pets either primarily inside or primarily outside. Animals that are housed inside can be allowed to roam outside in the grass within a fenced enclosure. No exposure to other animals such as dogs or cats is recommended because of the unpredictable

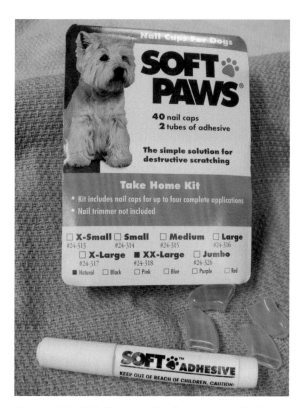

Figure 4.1 *Soft-Paws can be placed on a rabbit's claws to diminish its ability to scratch its owner.*

nature of a natural hunter when a prey animal (the rabbit) is observed. If rabbits are allowed to roam the house, plants and electrical cords need to be removed or made inaccessible. These animals can maneuver behind furniture and "dig" under rugs; hiding cords under rugs does not prevent the rabbit from gnawing on them. The recommendation for allowing pet rabbits to roam free within a given area includes making it impossible for the rabbit to escape, and observing the animal while it is out of the cage. A special wire enclosure or grazing ark can be made with wire sides and top for use outside. The open bottom of the special enclosure allows the animal to graze protected and unattended. Because the grazing ark is mobile, the owner can move the enclosure to fresh grass as needed.

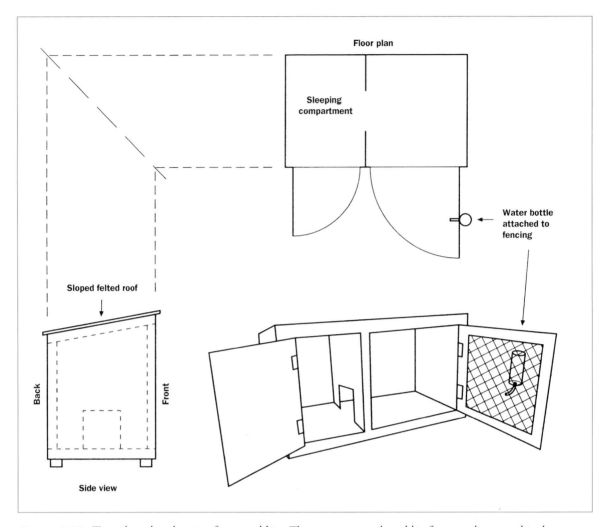

Figure 4.2A *Typical outdoor housing for pet rabbits. The cage protects the rabbit from predators and inclement weather. Illustration by Michael L. Broussard.*

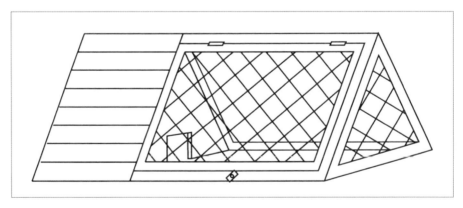

Figure 4.2B *Morant pen. This outdoor hutch allows the rabbit access to the sun and grass while providing shelter in the event of a storm. Illustration by Michael L. Broussard.*

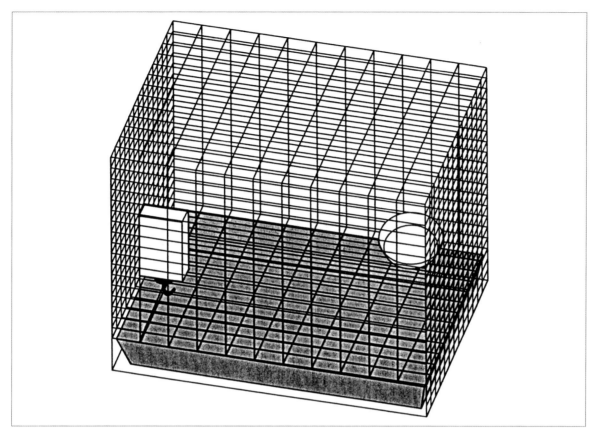

Figure 4.2C *Indoor rabbit housing. This pop-up style rabbit hutch has a place for food and water. Illustration by Michael L. Broussard.*

A rabbit can be house-trained to use a litter tray as soon as it is brought into a house. If the rabbit will be housed in a cage and allowed to free-roam, it is best for the animal to use a litter box that has been placed in its cage. Close the cage and allow the rabbit to develop a sense of location for its latrine. Once the latrine area has been established, place a litter box in that location again, allowing the rabbit to use the litter box a number of times before opening the cage door. When the cage door is finally opened, the rabbit should go back to the cage to defecate and urinate in the litter box. If the rabbit is free-roaming within the house, the owner will have to determine where the rabbit's latrine is and place the litter box in that location. The rabbit will dictate where the litter box is placed in the house. It is preferable to have a rabbit cage to put the rabbit in at night and establish the latrine location within that enclosure. The tray should have low sides and be filled with a preferable substrate (recycled paper substrate, hay, straw), and, when first acquired, the new pet should be placed in the tray every few minutes.[1] Litter training is possible with most rabbits, but owners should be informed that these animals are very territorial, and adult bucks might mark different areas of the house with strong-smelling feces to identify their territory.

These animals are prey species in their natural setting and propagate readily. Pet rabbits should not be housed together after they reach sexual maturity, because of their strong territorial nature.

It is not uncommon for two males housed together to viciously fight when they reach sexual maturity. Fighting can even occur when a male and a female are housed together, with the female fighting the male rabbit in her territory. If a breeder asks about breeding without causing fighting, tell the client to always bring the female rabbit into the male's enclosure for the act of breeding, and then return the doe to her cage.

Commercial cages are available to house rabbits indoors. These relatively small cages are excellent for the dwarf and mini breeds, but lack the exercise space needed for the larger breeds. If owners prefer to build the rabbit cage, inform them that two functional spaces are needed: one space for resting and sleeping, and the other for exercise. As mentioned earlier, rabbits are susceptible to foot/leg problems (sore hocks) if they are large and are housed in a wire-bottom cage. The cage bottom must have a solid surface in part of the area, and the other section (which is usually wire) should be covered with a layer of substrate—either hay or large pine shavings. The sides of the cage must be made of wire to allow for ventilation. The top can be made of wire, but if the cage is to be kept outdoors, the area in which the rabbit sleeps needs to be covered with plywood or corrugated fiberglass roofing material to protect against precipitation. Owners should be encouraged to clean the cage every one to two days.

Because rabbits are natural prey species, owners should be informed that living with dogs and cats is a potential danger. At no time should rabbits be allowed to commingle with dogs or cats, and they should be allowed out of their cage only under supervision. Rabbits and birds can live in the same house without any problem, but rabbits should not be housed with guinea pigs. Without any ill effects to themselves, rabbits can carry and transmit *Bordetella bronchiseptica*, a disease that is deadly to guinea pigs.[1] Fly-strike is a common sequel for rabbits in outdoor environments that develop open wounds. There have been rare reports of rabbits that are housed outside being exposed to and becoming infected with rabies.[2]

Nutrition

Rabbits normally feed in the early morning and in the evening. Pet owners should be made aware that rabbits also eat their feces to reinoculate their digestive system with good bacteria. The process of eating feces is called coprophagy, and this usually occurs 3–8 hours after eating.[3] These soft and sweet-smelling feces, or cecotropes, are often produced in the early hours of the morning. The cecotropes contain high levels of vitamins B and K and have twice the protein and half the fiber of regular hard feces.[4]

Rabbits should be fed free-choice timothy or grass hay and a regulated grass-based pelleted diet (Figures 4.3 and 4.4). These pellets can be purchased with protein contents that range from 10%–12% to 22%–24%. Pellets containing 16% protein are the most commonly fed. Recommend that your clients offer pellets with a fiber content of more than 16% to guard against anorexia and diarrhea. A higher fiber content helps reduce the onset of obesity, which is common in pet rabbits. Free-choice feeding of pellets also encourages obesity; therefore, sedentary pet rabbits should be fed $1/8$ to $1/2$ cup per day, depending on their size.[4] The exceptions to this rule are lactating does and growing young, which need as much food as they will eat. Tell the pet owner to wait 5 days after birth and then start increasing the amount of pellets by 150 grams, or 5 ounces, per day.[4] If there are no pellets left in the food container over the next 5-day period, they should add 150 grams more food. They should reduce the amount of pellets in the diet only when some of the pellets remain the next morning.

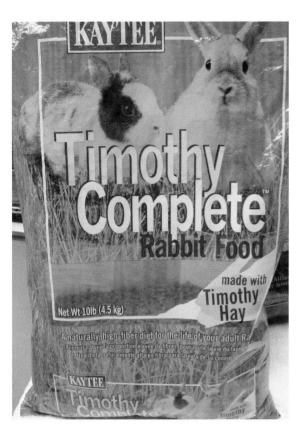

Figure 4.3 *A timothy grass–based pelleted diet is recommended for pet rabbits.*

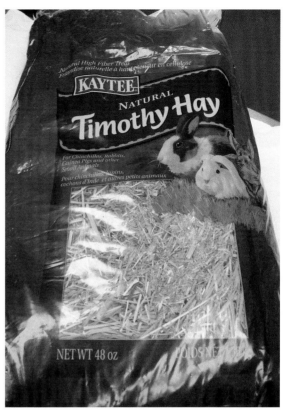

Figure 4.4 *Grass hay is recommended to maintain the overall health of a rabbit.*

At weaning, it is recommended that the doe be removed from the cage to reduce the stress of a new environment on the young. There has been an emphasis on the importance of fiber in a rabbit's diet to prevent obesity, diarrhea, and hairballs. Timothy hay is recommended as the best source of rabbit fiber and is universally available along with other grass hays (e.g., orchard grass, prairie grass). Overall, the best daily diet for pet rabbits is a measured timothy grass–based pellet with free-choice grass hay and a treat of dark green leafy vegetables.[4] To increase or improve hay consumption, tell clients to introduce a variety of grass hays to young rabbits and offer at least half a body size in volume per day. Often more hay is eaten when placed in the litter box (remove soiled hay), when pelleted food is hidden in the hay, or when the hay is lightly misted with water.[5]

Water is extremely important, and access to clean tap water needs to be provided. Rabbits easily learn to drink from inverted water bottles that have a stainless steel tube extending down into the cage (Figure 4.5). These water containers are commonly sold as Lix-it bottles. Rabbits, like most animals, drink from water bowls, but their low profile often contaminates the water bowl with food and feces. Drinking from the water bowl will also moisten the dewlap on large females, predisposing them to bacterial and fungal dermatitis. The water bottle must be kept clean and full of fresh water at all times.

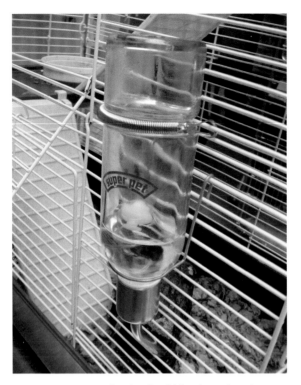

Figure 4.5 *Water bottles should be cleaned and re-filled on a regular basis.*

Transport

A plastic pet carrier filled with a recycled paper product substrate is recommended to transport rabbits to a veterinary clinic. In many cases a rabbit patient should be removed from and placed back in the carrier by removing the top of the carrier. When lifting the patient out of the carrier the rear leg must always be supported. Never place a rabbit headfirst into a cage or pet carrier; always put the animal in tail first. Rabbits will kick out with their rear legs and cause serious spinal damage; therefore, proper handling and supporting the rear legs at all times will reduce unintended injuries.

Grooming

Rabbits have powerful rear legs and sharp claws. Claw trimming is an important procedure in pet rabbits to reduce owner injury. Traditional dog nail trimmers can be used on rabbit claws. In many rabbit patients the vascular "quick" can be observed through the clear claw. With the rabbit well restrained the claw is clipped below the level of the blood line. If the claw is cut too close and bleeding occurs, a silver nitrate hemostatic stick can be used to apply the chemical cautery agent. Plastic nail caps that are applied with tissue glue can also be used to prevent owner injury caused by sharp claws. Rabbits should never be declawed because they have a different foot anatomy than a cat. If a rabbit is declawed, permanent foot injury will result from which most will not recover.

HISTORY

Veterinary technicians must obtain a thorough history of the patient before an educational recommendation can be given or a proper physical exam performed. The name, breed, sex, and age of the animal to be examined are the first questions to ask when taking a patient's history. As noted in Table 4.1, there is quite a difference in the physiologic parameters when comparing sex and rabbit breed. As with most species, smaller breeds of rabbits will mature faster than larger breeds. Common breeds of large pet rabbits are Angora, Lop-Eared, and New Zealand White; common small breeds are Mini Lop-Eared and Netherlands Dwarf (Figures 4.6A and 4.6B).

The next group of questions centers on general background information, such as length of time owned, where the animal was acquired, how often the animal is handled, and character of the fecal material. After getting answers to these preliminary questions, the veterinary technician should start to have a basic understanding of the owner's knowledge of rabbits and care provided. Husbandry questions should follow, including

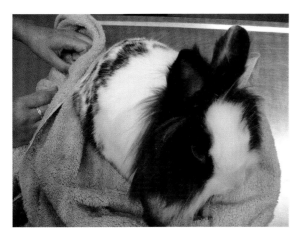

Figure 4.6A *Many different rabbit breeds are maintained as companion animals. This is a lion-headed rabbit.*

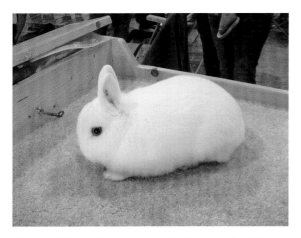

Figure 4.6B *This is an example of a dwarf rabbit.*

its life expectancy. One area of questioning that must not be overlooked is the status of other pets or animals in the house. Housing other pets with rabbits exposes them all to disease and injury. Finally, the technician should obtain information about past health problems and the reason the patient is presenting.

Many larger-breed rabbits can weigh up to 6 kilograms. The smaller breeds seem to be the most popular companion animals. Many unwanted older rabbits are large-breed animals that were sold as bunnies, either unknowingly or unscrupulously, as a dwarf breed. The owner who brings in a rabbit that he or she believes is a dwarf breed when it is not should be informed of this.

RESTRAINT

It is very difficult to restrain most rabbit patients. These small mammals have very strong muscles in their rear legs and jump quickly, with force. If not maintained in a proper position, a patient can jump out of the technician's arms onto the floor. An unexpected fall of this magnitude often creates an injury that was not present at the beginning of the appointment. To prevent this tragic scenario, there are certain guidelines to follow when holding a rabbit for examination, transport, and placement in or removal from a cage.

Ears are not handles. Although rabbit ears are usually large and appear to be an excellent piece of anatomy to grasp, do not succumb to this illusion. The ears are delicate, and when they are pulled, a rabbit will use its powerful rear legs to escape. When a rabbit kicks its rear legs and its body is unsupported, spinal trauma or fracture can occur, which can cause temporary or even permanent paralysis. Always support the body by placing a hand on the rear of the animal during transport

indoor/outdoor roaming habits, cage location, type and size of caging, cage substrate, frequency of cage cleaning, and type of disinfectant (if any) used when cleaning the cage. Some of the most important questions a technician should ask a rabbit owner are the type of food and water that are offered and how much and how often the bowls are cleaned and refilled. The rabbit's gastrointestinal system is very sensitive, and rabbits are susceptible to obesity; therefore, educating clients in husbandry will help a pet rabbit reach or examination (Figure 4.7). When removing the patient from a cage or pet carrier, grab the scruff with one hand, placing the other hand under its tail, supporting the rear legs. Place the animal on an examination table that is covered with a towel, which provides a nonslip surface. This towel can then be wrapped around the animal's body, forming a "bunny burrito" and preventing leg movement (Figure 4.8). While it is in a bunny burrito, the animal's head and tail can be examined and oral medications can be administered. The towel must be removed to perform a full-body examination and auscultation. If the animal is to be transported, place its head in the crook of one elbow, with the arm supporting the body of the rabbit and the hand of that arm over the rump. The opposite hand should grab the scruff (Figure 4.9). When placing a patient into a cage or carrier, always back the animal into the enclosure. If rabbits are placed headfirst into an enclosure, they might jump out of a handler's grasp into the cage, possibly injuring themselves or the handler.

PHYSICAL EXAMINATION

The rabbit physical examination should always take place on a properly restrained animal. This is easier said than done on many rabbit patients, but veterinary technicians should heed this advice to prevent tragedies from occurring. Observation of the animal in the carrier initiates a physical examination (Figure 4.10). Observe and note the animal's attitude, posture, and physical activity (if any) in the record. Closely examine the hair coat and skin next, looking for hair loss, skin lesions, and ectoparasites. Rabbits are susceptible to respiratory disease, ear mites, and ocular trauma. You must consider these disease problems during an external physical examination of the eyes, nose, and ears.

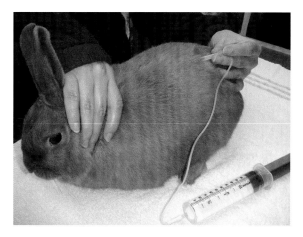

Figure 4.7 *A rabbit's rear should be supported to prevent the patient from kicking and injuring its back.*

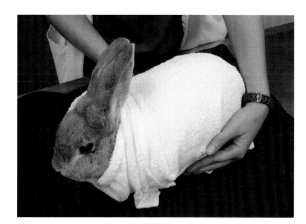

Figure 4.8 *A "bunny burrito" can be used to restrain rabbit patients.*

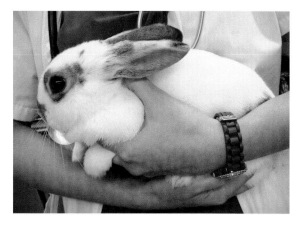

Figure 4.9 *When carrying a rabbit, support the rear legs and apply a firm grip to the dorsal cervical area.*

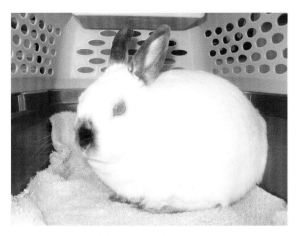

Figure 4.10 *Rabbits should be transported to and from the veterinary clinic in a plastic pet carrier. Always back a rabbit into a cage or carrier.*

One major problem rabbits often present with is malocclusion of the incisors or molars. Rabbit patients generally do not like people looking in their mouths, especially if they have dental problems. Proper restraint is emphasized for the oral examination. You can manipulate the lips with a tongue depressor, which will allow you to observe the front teeth. Rabbit patients have been known to bite an unsuspecting veterinarian or technician during this procedure, so use caution. An easy way to examine the molars in the back of a rabbit's small mouth is to use an otoscope with an appropriate-sized head. This is about the only way to simplify a difficult operation.

Hydration status of the animal can be checked during the oral examination through mucous membrane capillary refill time or packed cell volume percentage, or corneal moisture. Palpation of the body and extremities is necessary to look for possible fractures and lymph node or organ enlargement. The examination should be completed with a neurologic assessment, auscultation of the heart and respiratory system, and examination of the external reproductive structures and anus.

After you complete the examination, record any abnormal findings and establish a list of differential diagnoses. Finally, prioritize diagnostic tests to confirm a diagnosis or to determine the severity of the disease.

DIAGNOSTIC SAMPLING

Blood Collection

Rabbits can be difficult patients from which to obtain blood for diagnostic testing. Covering a rabbit's eyes might help reduce movement of the patient and the stress associated with restraint. In many older textbooks, the larger rabbit species were used to show how to collect blood from the marginal ear vein or central ear artery (Figure 4.11A and 4.11B). In larger rabbit species, these sites are effective for obtaining blood at volumes necessary for diagnostic tests, but this is not the case with smaller, popular companion rabbit species. Although the marginal ear vein and central ear artery might be considered as sites of blood collection in small rabbit breeds, they are often too small to collect any significant amount of blood. The ear vein and artery have a tendency to develop thrombi, leading to vascular ischemia, which ultimately causes necrosis of the affected area on the dorsal surface of the ear. For this reason, only experienced phlebotomists should collect blood from these areas.

Other recommended venipuncture sites are the jugular vein (site of choice for smaller rabbit breeds) (Figures 4.12A and 4.12B), the cephalic vein (Figure 4.12C), and the lateral saphenous vein (Figure 4.12D). The jugular and lateral saphenous veins are the blood collection sites of choice for most rabbit patients. Because rabbit fur is dense and difficult to shave and the skin is easily ripped by the blade of a clipper, it is preferable to pluck the hair over the vein rather than shave it, after

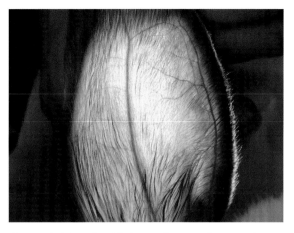

Figure 4.11A *A rabbit's ear, showing the central artery and marginal ear vein.*

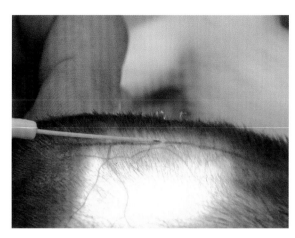

Figure 4.11B *Collecting blood from the marginal ear vein.*

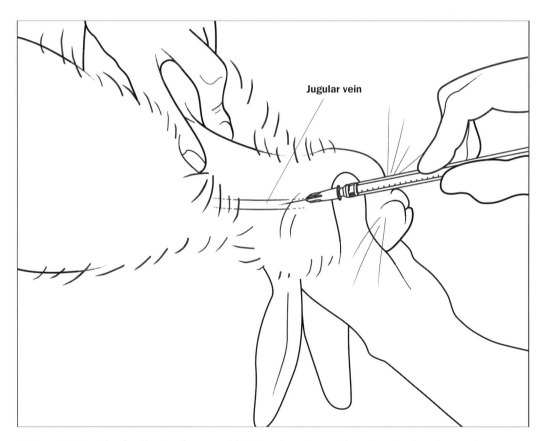

Figure 4.12A *Blood collection from a rabbit's jugular vein, with patient in dorsal recumbency. Illustration by Michael L. Broussard.*

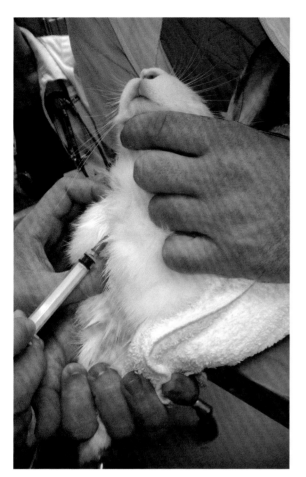

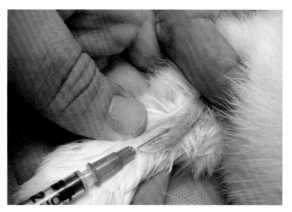

Figure 4.12C *Collecting blood from the cephalic vein of a rabbit.*

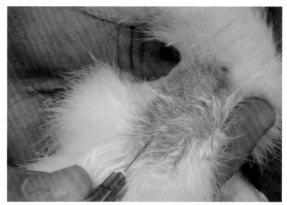

Figure 4.12B *Blood collection from a rabbit's jugular vein, with patient in ventral recumbency.*

Figure 4.12D *Collecting blood from the saphenous vein of a rabbit.*

which an alcohol wipe can be used to help identify the collection site. The vein should be clamped with two fingers proximal to the venipuncture area to increase vascular pressure and dilate the vessel. A small-gauge (25-, 26-, or 27-gauge) needle is used to penetrate the vein from which blood is being collected. If blood collection is slow owing to vessel size, using a heparinized needle will help prevent blood clotting in the syringe. To avoid collapse of the vein or artery caused by excess pressure during collection with a syringe or vacutainer tube, insert a needle without a syringe

attached into the vessel and allow the blood to drip from the needle into an open blood tube.[6]

The cephalic vein is accessible, more so in larger breeds than in smaller breeds, because of the short antebrachial length and small vein size in the diminutive rabbits. This is also true of the saphenous vein, which courses across the lateral aspect of the tibia. Again, always pluck the hair over the collection site instead of shaving to prevent clipper trauma to the skin.

As stated, the site of choice for blood collection in most rabbit species of varying sizes is the jugular vein, but ear veins can also be used, and they can be used for intravenous catheter placement.

Although some rabbit patients do not need to be sedated for blood samples to be obtained, it might be easier to give the patient a small amount of sedation to reduce stress and possible injury to the patient or veterinary personnel. Isoflurane inhalation anesthesia (induction 5%, then maintain at 1.5%–2% with a 1.5 L flow rate of oxygen) administered through a face mask is probably the easiest, quickest, and safest method to sedate a rabbit for venipuncture and other diagnostic collection techniques (Figure 4.13). When collecting any diagnostic sample from a rabbit patient that is fractious, always consider sedation to prevent injury to the patient. The neck should be carefully shaved from the mid-cervical to the caudal cervical area on the ventral, ventrolateral aspect of the body.

To collect the blood, the rabbit should be placed in dorsal recumbency with its head over the edge of the table and its feet held in a caudal position. Take care not to overextend the neck in this position, or respiratory compromise might occur. Even the smallest rabbit breeds have a large

Table 4.2 **Rabbit Complete Blood Count Reference Ranges**[6,7,8]

CELL TYPES	NORMAL RANGE
Erythrocytes	5.1–7.9 x 10^6/µl
Hematocrit	36 48%
Hemoglobin	10.0–15.5 mg/dl
Leukocytes	5.2–12.5 x 10^3/µl
Neutrophils	20–74%
Lymphocytes	30–85%
Eosinophils	0–4%
Monocytes	1–4%
Basophils	2–7%
Platelets	122–795 x 10^3/µl
Serum Protein	5.4–7.5 g/dl
Albumin	2.7–4.6 g/dl
Globulin	1.5–2.8 g/dl

enough blood volume to safely collect enough to obtain diagnostic results. Rabbit blood volume has been recorded to be between 57 and 78 ml/kg.[7] Reference ranges for complete blood counts and serum chemistry panels are listed in Tables 4.2 and 4.3, respectively.[6,8,9]

Bone Marrow Aspiration

Recommended sites for collecting bone marrow in rabbits include the femur, humerus, pelvis, and proximal tibia. The technician should follow the same precollection protocol when obtaining a bone marrow aspirate in a rabbit as with any other small animal. The patient must be anesthetized for this procedure.

Collection of Cerebrospinal Fluid

This is not a very common diagnostic procedure performed on pet rabbits, but it could be helpful in diagnosing listeriosis if the cerebrospinal fluid (CSF) is cultured.[7] CSF samples should be either submitted quickly or refrigerated to prevent cellular degradation, which occurs rapidly at room

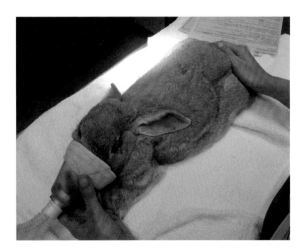

Figure 4.13 *Rabbits can be induced and maintained for short procedures using a face mask.*

Table 4.3 Rabbit Serum Biochemistry Reference Ranges[6,7,8]

ANALYTES	NORMAL RANGE
Serum Glucose	75–150 mg/dl
Blood Urea Nitrogen	17.0–23.5 mg/dl
Creatinine	0.8–1.8 mg/dl
Total Bilirubin	0.25–0.74 mg/dl
Serum Lipids	280–350 mg/dl
Phospholipids	75–113 mg/dl
Triglycerides	124–156 mg/dl
Cholesterol	35–53 mg/dl
Serum Calcium	5.6–12.5 mg/dl
Serum Phosphate	4.0–6.2 mg/dl
Alkaline Phosphatase	4–16 U/L
Alanine Aminotransferase (ALT)	48–80 U/L
Aspartate Aminotransferase (AST)	14–113 U/L
Lactate Dehydrogenase	34–129 U/L

temperature. The correct position for this procedure is to place the rabbit in lateral recumbency with its head flexed to the ventral chest wall. The area from the occipital protuberance to the level of the third cervical vertebra and laterally past the margin of the atlas needs to be prepped for the collection procedure.[6] This external skin preparation is similar to the methods used for CSF in canine patients. A 22-gauge, 1.5–3.5" spinal needle is recommended for this procedure in rabbits. A stylet is always recommended to prevent blockage of the needle in this very critical procedure. The spinal needle should enter the skin halfway between the cranial margins of the wings of the atlas and the occipital protuberance, slowly advancing toward the nose until penetration is felt through the dura and subarachnoid membranes.[7] The CSF should be allowed to drip into a plastic collection device, because leukocytes adhere to glass.[7] As with other companion animal species, the area being tested is surrounded by very vascular tissue, and blood contamination of the CSF sample commonly occurs; therefore, the sample should be monitored for quality during collection.

Urine Collection Using Cystocentesis

A cystocentesis can be successfully accomplished on most rabbit patients without sedation or anesthesia. Rabbits can be hypnotized while in dorsal recumbency, which is the position of choice for cystocentesis collection. The patient's scruff and rear limbs need to be restrained to prevent any sudden movements while the needle is in the bladder collecting urine. A 22-gauge needle attached to a 10 ml syringe is the recommended collection combination for cystocentesis. The bladder should be palpated cranial to the pelvis along the ventral midline of the body prior to placing the needle in the abdomen.[7] Cystocentesis preparation for rabbits is similar to that for dogs and cats. It is imperative that all precautions be considered to prevent an iatrogenic bladder infection.

Midazolam, 0.5–2 mg/kg intramuscularly, will provide excellent sedation for catheterization of the urethra in male and female rabbits.[10] The male is collected with a well-lubricated 9 French catheter.[7] The patient is best positioned in a sitting posture to extend the penis and access the urethra. The female's urethral orifice is located on the floor of the vagina and is best catheterized with the patient in sternal recumbency.[7]

Normal rabbit urine ranges in color from orange to brown. The urine color corresponds to diet, concentration of crystals, and urinary tract health. Normal rabbit urine is cloudy, containing many ammonium magnesium phosphate, calcium carbonate monohydrate, and anhydrous calcium carbonate crystals. The veterinary technician should understand that this finding is different from that in any other companion animal, but it is a normal finding. Table 4.4 lists the normal parameters of a rabbit urinalysis.[10]

Table 4.4 Rabbit Normal Urinalysis Values

URINARY PARAMETERS	NORMAL RESULTS
Urine Volume	
Large	20–350 ml/kg/day
Average	130 ml/kg/day
Specific Gravity	1.003–1.036
Average pH	8.2
Crystals Present	Ammonium Magnesium Phosphate, Calcium Carbonate Monohydrate, Calcium Anhydrous Carbonate
Casts, Epithelial Cells, or Bacteria	Absent to rare
Leukocytes or Erythrocytes Present	Occasional
Albumin Present	Occasional in young rabbits

Microbiology

Rabbits are predisposed to *Pasteurella multocida* infections that usually present as respiratory disease. P. *multocida* infections are so common in rabbits that they are often called "snuffles," because of the nasal and ocular discharge associated with the disease. To culture the organism for isolation, introduce a mini-tipped culturette into the deep nasal sinuses to the level of the medial canthus of the eye.[7] If the rabbit is too fractious, sedation is recommended. Abscesses that may or may not be caused by P. *multocida*, *Staphylococcus aureus*, *Pseudomonas aeruginosa*, *Proteus* spp., or *Bacteroides* spp. have to be cultured on the interior wall of the lesion, because most rabbit abscesses are sterile in the center. All other culture procedures used to collect fungal and bacterial organisms in rabbit patients are similar to those employed on dogs and cats.

Radiology

Many rabbit case presentations require radiographic evaluation, including fractures, malocclusion, inter-

nal abscesses, and reproductive, gastrointestinal, and respiratory diseases. It is recommended that rabbits be sedated or maintained under general anesthesia for the radiographic procedure. This prevents injury and stress to the patient and usually prevents poor radiographic images owing to patient movement. Most importantly, it reduces the chance of human skeletons (hands and fingers) showing up in the film. Isoflurane is the general anesthesia of choice for rapid induction and recovery.

Other Diagnostic Imaging Modalities

Rabbits can be imaged using ultrasound (US), computed tomography (CT), and magnetic resonance imaging (MRI). These advanced imaging modalities allow greater interpretation of disease conditions within the skull and body cavity. Ultrasound imaging is useful for determining and evaluating reproductive tract disorders (e.g., uterine adenocarcinoma). Preparation of the patient for US, CT, and MRI is similar to that described for obtaining traditional radiographic images. In some cases in which the patient is compliant, US examinations can take place using light sedation and proper restraint.

Parasitology

External Parasites

The advent of new ectoparasitic medications allows the use of one product to effectively treat or prevent many different parasites that infest rabbits. One example of these new products is imidacloprid and moxidectin topical solution (Advantage Multi for cats 9 weeks of age and older, 5.1–9 lbs; Bayer HealthCare LLC, Animal Health Division, Shawnee Mission, KS) used at a dose of one 0.4 ml tube, placing the contents on the skin between the scapulas, once a month. This solution will treat or prevent fleas, *Psoroptes cuniculi, Cheyletiella parasitivorax, Listrophorus gibbus,* and *Trichostron-gylus* spp.

Psoroptes cuniculi, or the rabbit ear mite, is a very common finding in pet rabbits (Figures 4.14A and 4.14B). The animal usually presents with thick crust originating from the base of the external ear canal extending up to, and sometimes out of, the ventral aspect of the pinna. Identification of the mite can be made through a direct examination of the ear crust or observation of the mites within the ear canal, using an otoscope. Treat with ivermec-

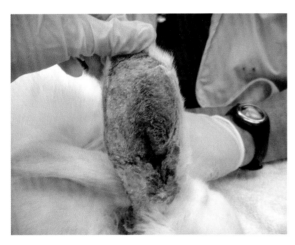

Figure 4.14A *Typical ear presentation of a rabbit with* Psoroptes cuniculi.

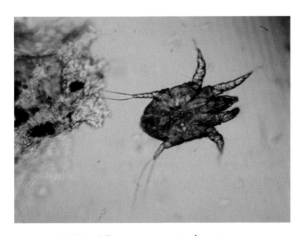

Figure 4.14B *A* Psoroptes cuniculi *mite.*

tin (Ivomec, Merck AgVet Division, Rahway, NJ) at 0.4 mg/kg SC once every two weeks for three treatments, or once and repeated in 18 days.[11] The crusts should not be cleaned, because the underlying tissue is very irritated. After the mites have been killed and healing takes place, the crust usually sloughs in one piece. Topical treatment of the infestation is not necessary if ivermectin is being used, but it might help as adjunct therapy to expedite the healing process. The use of fipronil is contraindicated in rabbits. Do not use it, because it has been associated with neurologic disease and death in these animals.

Cheyletiella parasitivorax is commonly called walking dandruff, or the rabbit fur mite. This ectoparasite can also infect humans and other companion animals. *C. parasitivorax* is rather large, and the dandruff and debris that are collected from a suspect case can be examined under a microscope by picking up the material on a piece of scotch tape. This is commonly called the "Scotch Tape" test in dermatology. The life cycle of the rabbit fur mite is about 5 weeks, and avermectin is the treatment of choice. The pet's environment should also be treated with flea-control products to prevent reexposure. Other mites have been diagnosed in rabbits, including *Sarcoptes scabiei, Notoedres cati,* and *Demodex cuniculi,* but these are relatively uncommon findings.[11]

Fleas also feed on rabbits. As with other companion animals, signs of infestation include dried bloody flea feces ("flea dirt"), itching, and the appearance of fleas themselves. Treatment is similar to that for cats, and the owner must be reminded to treat the environment as well as the patient.[11]

Large maggot larvae and smaller fly larvae affect rabbits. The large maggot larvae from flies (*Cuterebra* spp.; Figure 4.15) are usually noted as a swelling in the ventral cervical, axillary, or inguinal area or the dorsal rear.[11] Maggots must

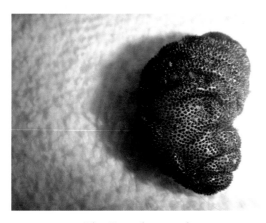

Figure 4.15 *This* Cuterebra *spp. larvae was removed from a rabbit patient.*

be surgically removed and surrounding tissues treated to prevent any secondary complications. Smaller fly larvae are attracted to moist, matted fur around the anogenital area. The patient that is suffering from maggot infestation needs to have its fur trimmed and skin treated. Cleaning and removal of maggots are best accomplished on a sedated patient.

Internal Parasites

The most common intestinal parasite class that affects rabbits is coccidia of the genus *Eimeria*. E. *stiedae*, which affects the liver, is very common in mismanaged rabbit breeding operations. All other rabbit coccidia affect the intestinal tract, with diarrhea being the most common clinical presentation. Coccidia (sulfamerazine; 100 mg/kg orally), protozoan parasites (metronidazole; 20 mg/kg, orally), nematode (fenbendazole; 10 mg/kg, orally, repeat in 14 days), and cestode (praziquantel; 5.10 mg/kg, subcutaneous, repeat in 10 days) parasites can be diagnosed through direct fecal examinations and fecal flotations. Once the parasite has been correctly identified, the appropriate medication should be prescribed.

THERAPEUTICS

Often rabbit patients do not present in a condition that would initially seem critical. After a thorough history and physical examination, the veterinarian might decide that the patient is in distress and the technician must be prepared to provide the necessary critical care. If injections need to be administered, subcutaneous sites of choice include the dorsal cervical region and lateral flank area; the intramuscular sites are the epaxial muscles that course along the caudal vertebral column or the cranial aspect of the quadriceps muscle group in the rear leg.[6]

Oral suspensions that have been flavored by a compounding pharmacy are the recommended method for administering oral medications. Other oral medication flavoring options are strawberry jam, a small piece of banana, and piña colada mix. Crushed tablets or pills can be mixed in a gel substance, for example Nutracal, and placed on the fur around the mouth. Rabbits, being fastidious groomers, will readily lick their fur clean and ingest the medication.

Lacrimal Duct Cannulation

It is not uncommon to have a rabbit patient present with epiphora and concurrent facial dermatitis associated with the moisture around the eye. The epiphora is often caused by an occluded nasolacrimal duct caused by collected debris or inflammation associated with an upper respiratory bacterial infection. The nasolacrimal duct should be flushed using a lacrimal cannula (straight or curved) or a small-gauge IV catheter with the needle removed. The ocular opening to the nasolacrimal duct is located behind the ventral lid margin near the medial canthus. The lid margin is retracted along with excess conjunctival tissue revealing the punctum. The cannula/catheter is gently inserted into the punctum, while sterile saline is gently flushed into the duct (Figure 4.16). Antibiotic solutions can be used to treat infections involving the nasolacrimal duct, and radiopaque dyes are used to determine if the duct is patent in cases where this is not evident.

Fluid Therapy

For rabbit patients the cephalic or lateral saphenous veins are recommended for indwelling catheter placement when providing fluid therapy. In dwarf breeds, 24- or 27-gauge catheters can be used, whereas in larger breeds (e.g., New Zealand white) a 22-gauge catheter is optimum. If an intravenous catheter cannot be placed because of a dehydrated or hypotensive condition, an intraosseous (IO) catheter is the best option.[12] The IO catheter of choice for rabbits is a 20-gauge, 1" spinal needle, which should be inserted into the greater trochanter of the femur, passed parallel to the long axis of the femur or into the tibial plateau and passed parallel to the long axis of the tibia.[12] The IO catheter should be maintained in place similar to the way an IV catheter would be maintained, but placement can be validated through radiographic imaging. Maintenance fluid requirements of 75–100 ml/kg/day have been published and should be provided in critically ill patients as a continuous infusion.[12] Colloidal fluids (e.g., hetastarch) should be provided for hypoproteinemic patients or when crystalloid (e.g., lactated Ringer's solution) is unable to increase blood pressure.[12] Subcutaneous fluid administration, 1–2 times daily at 50–100 ml/kg, can be provided if the rabbit is stable, and preferably, if the rabbit is drinking, oral fluids should be accessible.[12]

Critical Care Diet

Commercially produced, supportive liquid diets can provide nutrition to critically ill anorexic

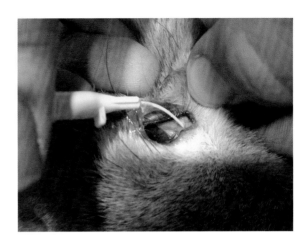

Figure 4.16 *Flushing a rabbit patient's nasal lacrimal duct.*

patients. It is recommend to feed 50 cc of mixed Critical Care for Herbivores (Oxbow Pet Products, Murdock, NE, and Lafeber Company, Cornell, IL) per kilogram of body weight divided between 4 and 6 feedings per day (Table 4.5).[13] To feed supportive liquid diets a "catheter tipped" 50 ml syringe is recommended. Once it is filled, a small amount (5–10 ml) is injected into the oral cavity through the side of the mouth. The patient should be allowed to swallow the liquid before it is given more. Usually a maximum of 20 ml of supportive diet is provided to the patient at each feeding.

If the rabbit patient cannot or will not accept the supportive diet through syringe feeding, a nasogastric tube can be put in place. The nasogastric tube can be used once (e.g., to remove air from the stomach or administer food or medication), or it can be maintained in place for a period of time (e.g., long-term food supplementation). Four to eight French tubes (it is recommended to use nasogastric tubes manufactured for rabbits) can be placed in both conscious and anesthetized animals. The tube should be premeasured to the level of the seventh rib and marked at the level of

Table 4.5 Recommended Amount to Feed 50 ml of Mixed Critical Care™ for Herbivores (Oxbow Pet Products, Murdock, NE) per Kilogram of Body Weight Divided Between 4 and 6 Feedings per Day[13]

WEIGHT OF RABBIT (Kg)	NUMBER OF FEEDINGS PER DAY			
	3	4	5	6
0.5	8 ml	6 ml	5 ml	4 ml
0.9	15 ml	11 ml	9 ml	8 ml
1.4	23 ml	17 ml	14 ml	11 ml
2.3	38 ml	28 ml	23 ml	19 ml
3.2	53 ml	40 ml	32 ml	27 ml

the nose. The tube should not be placed any further than the nasal marking on the tube. A local anesthetic agent is applied to the tube and inside the nasal opening into which the tube is being inserted. The latex catheter is then placed in the nares and pushed through the upper respiratory sinus into the esophagus and finally into the stomach. The place marked prior to tube insertion should be immediately outside the nasal opening when the procedure is finished. The tube can then be sutured to the top of the head, and an Elizabethan collar placed on the patient if it tries to disturb the sutured area (Figure 4.17).

SURGICAL AND ANESTHETIC ASSISTANCE

Once the decision has been made to perform a surgical procedure, certain equipment requirements must be met for proper surgical preparation. To aid in the intubation process, a short narrow laryngoscope and a rigid plastic catheter are needed. All other surgical equipment is similar to that used for small kittens and dogs. Medical skin staples allow for rapid closure in the thin elastic skin, and most rabbit patients are unable to remove them.

Preparation of the patient prior to surgery starts with food removal 2–4 hours before the

procedure. Presurgical antibiotic therapy is dependent on the procedure being performed and the patient's medical history. Intravenous or intraosseous catheters can be placed prior to surgery, and also in emergency situations, if fluid replacement or therapeutic agents need to be quickly assimilated. All veins that were mentioned as sites for venipuncture can be used for intravenous catheter placement, but the larger veins (e.g., cephalic and saphenous) are recommended.[6] Complications, such as venous thrombi and eventual skin sloughing of the affected area, make the ear vessels a poor choice for indwelling catheter placement. If

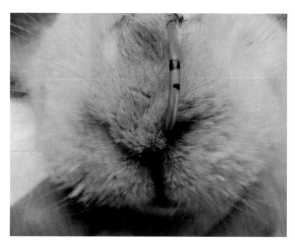

Figure 4.17 *Nasogastric tube in place to provide supplemental nutrition.*

an intravenous catheter cannot be placed because of vascular complications, an intraosseous catheter should be placed in the greater trochanter of the femur. Rabbit daily fluid requirements range between 50 and 100 ml/kg/day and can be replaced daily, divided into 2 equal amounts, or continuously provided through an infusion pump.[6] If the patient does not accept the catheter, a collar should be applied.

Preparation of the surgical area is important and difficult when clipping thick, fine rabbit fur. In addition, the skin is thin, elastic, and easily traumatized. The clipper blade should be held flat, close to the skin, and the fur clipped at a slow, cautious speed. Regular cleaning of the clipper blade during the preparation will improve the ability of the blade to cut the fine fur.

The surgical site should be prepped after clipping to reduce the heat loss in these small animals. General recommendations to reduce heat loss are listed in Table 4.6.[14]

When anesthetizing a rabbit, the biggest difficulty facing the technician is the intubation process. The mouth does not open widely, the distal portion of the tongue is muscular, the larynx is in the caudal oropharynx, and rabbits are predisposed to having laryngospasms.[14] Various methods of intubation can be used, other than the oral route, including nasotracheal and a blind technique, using an endotracheal tube attached to a standard stethescope.[15] The most successful and least traumatic method for intubating a rabbit is using a rigid endoscope and visualizing the tracheal opening (Figure 4.18). Most rabbit surgical procedures that require a short time period to complete might be accomplished by inducing the patient using indicated anesthetic agents and maintaining it via face mask on isoflurane inhalation anesthesia. Tables 4.7 and 4.8 list sedation and anesthetic agents.

Table 4.6 Rabbit Surgery Preparation

1. Warm the immediate environment with the use of circulating water blankets or heat lamps.

2. Clip the minimum amount of hair from the body surface at and around the surgical site.

3. Use warmed surgical scrub solution for surgical site preparation.

4. Avoid alcohol rinses for surgical preparation, substituting warmed saline.

5. Cover the exposed surface of the animal with a drape.

6. Minimize the duration of surgery and anesthesia.

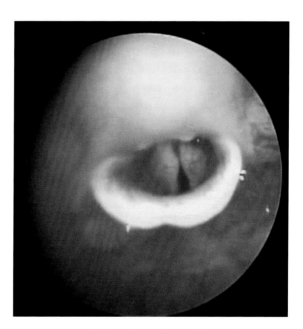

Figure 4.18 *Rabbit glottis observed through an endoscope prior to intubation.*

HEALTH MAINTENANCE AND DISEASE

Gastric Stasis or "Wool Block"

As discussed earlier in this chapter, rabbits are predisposed to hairballs when fed an improper diet. Because rabbits are unable to vomit or regurgitate stomach contents, hairballs have to be digested or passed through the intestinal tract. When hairballs

Table 4.7 **Rabbit Premedication, Sedation, and Chemical Restraint Agents**[10]

DRUG	DOSE	COMMENTS
Acepromazine	0.25–1.0 mg/kg IM or SC*	Good for preanesthetic use and for mild tranquilization
Diazepam	1–5 mg/kg IM or IV	Preanesthetic/tranquilizer
Fentanyl-Droperidol	0.13–0.22 ml/kg IM or SC	Excellent restraint, good analgesic qualities
Medetomidine	0.25 mg/kg IM	Sedatic Reversal agent: Atipamezole (0.001 mg/kg SC, IV, IP)
Midazolam	1–2 mg/kg IM, IV	Preanesthetic/tranquilizer
Xylazine	1–5 mg/kg IM or SC	Good sedation/analgesia Might produce respiratory depression and slow heart rate Reversal agent: Yohimbine (0.2 mg/kg IV)

*SC = subcutaneously, IM = intramuscularly, IV = intravenously

Table 4.8 **Rabbit Injectable Anesthetic Agents**[10]

DRUG	DOSE	COMMENTS
Diazepam/Ketamine	Diazepam (0.5 mg/kg) and Ketamine (10–20 mg/kg) IV	Good for sedation and adjunct to supplemental inhalation anesthesia
Medetomidine/Ketamine	0.35 mg/kg IM and 5 mg/kg IV	Anesthesia: Surgical depth approximately 19 minutes
Tiletamine-Zolazepam	5–25 mg/kg IM	Light sedation and general anesthesia High dose could cause severe depression, slow recovery, and possible nephrotoxicity
Xylazine/Ketamine	1. Xylazine (3–5 mg/kg) and Ketamine (20–40 mg/kg) IM	Good for some surgical procedures
	2. Xylazine (3mg/kg) and Ketamine (10 mg/kg) intranasal	Xylazine can cause respiratory depression and hypotension Intranasal administration good for short-term anesthesia

become too large, gastric motility is affected, and the animal becomes anorexic. Treatment includes antibiotics, cisapride (0.5 mg/kg SC q8.12h) to stimulate gastric motility, and syringe feeding the patient. A recommended recipe for syringe feeding is one cup rabbit pellets, one 8 oz. can Ensure, and one 8 oz. container fruit yogurt; blend and feed via syringe. If obese rabbits are not fed and subsequently develop a negative energy balance, hepatic lipidosis will occur.

Prevention of hairballs in rabbits is initiated through owner education on proper dietary requirements. Since the recommendation of grass diets, there appears to be a significant reduction in the number of rabbit patients presenting with trichobezoars.

Gastroenteritis

Antibiotics can cause a fatal gastrointestinal bacterial overgrowth if administered to rabbits. **Never use the following unless they are the absolute last resort for treatment: clindamycin, amoxicillin and derivatives, ampicillin, penicillin, cephalosporins, and erythromycin.** Always make sure that the drug being given is appropriate to use in rabbits. Treatment of gastroenteritis is similar to that for other pets; that is, maintaining hydration status, identification of the causative agent, and proper treatment. E. *coli, Clostridium piliforme, Salmonella* spp., and *Pseudomonas* spp. are common bacterial organisms that cause gastroenteritis.

Pasteurella Multocida "Snuffles"

This is the most common disease affecting pet rabbits. *Pasteurella multocida* can infect all major body systems (especially the respiratory system) and major organs, and it can cause subcutaneous abscesses. Another common presentation is a head tilt, which is often the result of an internal ear infection associated with *P. multocida*. This bacterium can survive within a rabbit host for years without causing any overt disease signs. During this period, shedding can take place, which can then infect any rabbit that comes into contact with the infected animal. Treatment has improved with Baytril enrofloxicin 5–20 mg/kg PO, once a day for up to 21 days. As with any antibiotic treatment administered to rabbits, during the treatment period owners should be advised to closely observe their pet's eating habits, stool, and general disposition. If there is any decrease in food consumed, change in fecal consistency, or depression, the antibiotic treatment should be stopped and the case reassessed. There is no guarantee that the treatment will cure the patient of the infection, but treatment is usually successful in reducing the disease signs associated with the infection. The bacterial organism is transmitted through direct contact, fomites, and sexual intercourse, but usually gains entry into the host through the nares or wounds. Culture of the respiratory system, through the nares, is usually the best way to confirm a diagnosis, but response to treatment of this pervasive disease precludes diagnostic testing. The best prevention of this disease is client education and the purchase of rabbits from reputable breeders who have a P. *multocida*–free herd.

Malocclusion

Overgrowth of the incisors or the cheek teeth is a problem often affecting pet rabbits (Figures 4.19A and 4.19B). Malocclusion of the teeth might present as the rabbit not being able to chew and hold food in its mouth or excessive drooling around the edges of the mouth. A complete oral examination is required for each patient. The incisors can be examined by using a tongue depressor and moving the lips to observe the teeth. In most cases of rabbit malocclusion, the upper incisors grow behind the bottom incisors. Genetics and traumatic injury appear to be the main sources of this disease.

The cheek teeth are best examined using an otoscope (Figure 4.20) or a small rigid endoscope (Figures 4.21A, 4.21B, and 4.21C). The teeth can be trimmed using small clippers and the cheek teeth floated, using a dental unit, small rabbit floats, or a Dremel tool with special rabbit tooth-trimming bits and specula for exposure in the small oral cavity (Figure 4.22). In the majority of cases, affected patients never "grow out" of this problem and have to be treated on a regular basis, about every 6 weeks. Removal of the overgrown teeth is not recommended, unless there is a complicating abscess at the base of the tooth. This is a very common problem in pet rabbits, and

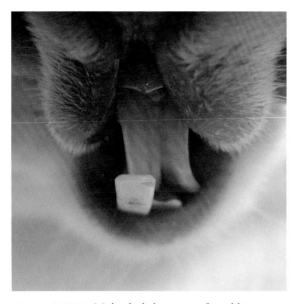

Figure 4.19A *Maloccluded incisors of a rabbit.*

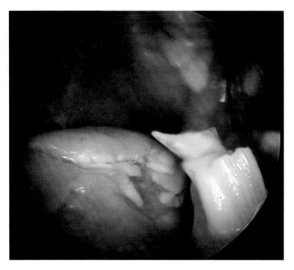

Figure 4.19B *Maloccluded molars of a rabbit, showing enamel projections and irritated lingual surface.*

further reading is recommended in more detailed texts.[16,17]

"Sore Hocks" or Ulcerative Pododermatitis

Ulcerative pododermatitis is an infection of the plantar surface of the hock. This condition is usually the result of poor husbandry practices by the

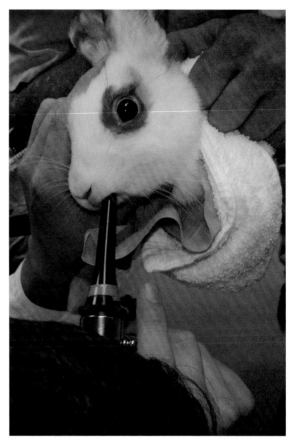

Figure 4.20 *Examination of a rabbit's teeth using an otoscope.*

owner. Once the hock area ulcerates because of improper flooring, secondary bacterial infections infiltrate the wound. This is a very difficult disease to treat, and owner understanding and compliance are essential for a successful outcome. The importance of proper husbandry practices should be stressed to clients. The environment needs to be cleaned, and the wounds must be cleaned and bandaged.

ZOONOTIC DISEASES

There are not many cases of diseases being transmitted from rabbits to their human caretakers. Although uncommon, such disease transmission

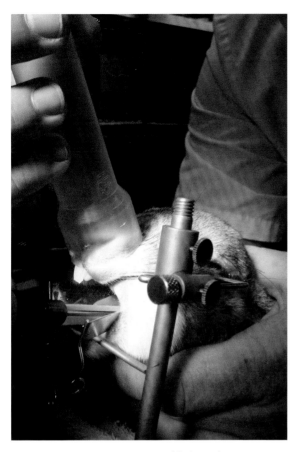

Figure 4.21A *Examining a rabbit's teeth using an endoscope.*

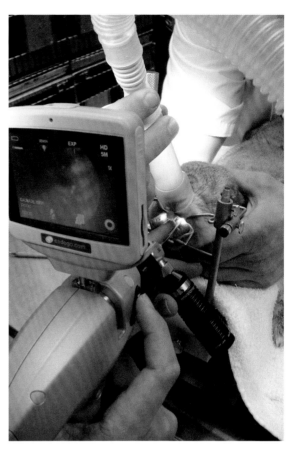

Figure 4.21B *Trimming a rabbit's teeth using a Dremel tool.*

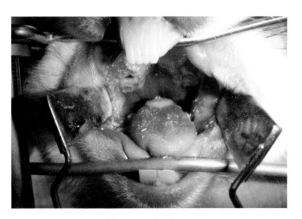

Figure 4.21C *Rabbit's teeth after trimming.*

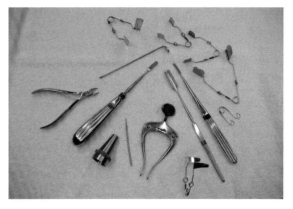

Figure 4.22 *Dental instruments for use with rabbits.*

can and does occur. Common bacterial pathogens that can be transferred include *Salmonella* spp., *Pasteurella multocida*, and bacteria through scratches or bites. Dermatophyte (ringworm) infections can cause dry, crusty lesions on rabbits that exhibit hair loss. The most common dermatophyte isolated in pet rabbits is *Trichophyton mentagrophytes*, which is extremely zoonotic to children and older adults.

SELF-STUDY QUESTIONS

1. How would you determine the sex of a rabbit?

2. What would you recommend to owners if they complain their rabbit is scratching them with its sharp claws?

3. Describe the proper husbandry and nutritional recommendations for rabbits.

4. How do you house-train a rabbit?

5. Describe how one properly restrains a rabbit for a physical examination. What are the possible consequences if the rabbit is not properly restrained?

6. Describe how to examine a rabbit.

7. What is the procedure for collecting blood from a rabbit? Bone marrow? Cerebrospinal fluid? Urine?

8. How should you sedate a rabbit for diagnostic sample collection?

9. What is "snuffles," and how is it treated?

10. Describe diagnostic imaging modalities used to examine rabbits. What are the advantages and disadvantages of each?

11. What are the common rabbit parasites and treatment options for each of them?

12. Describe the procedure for cannulating the lacrimal ducts of rabbits.

13. Describe fluid therapy administration in rabbits.

14. Describe dietary supplementation recommendations for critically ill rabbit patients.

15. Describe proper intubation of a rabbit.

16. Describe common disease presentations of rabbits and treatment options.

REFERENCES

1. Donnelly TM. Basic anatomy, physiology and husbandry. In: Quesenberry KE, and Carpenter JW, eds. *Ferrets, rabbits and rodents: Clinical medicine and surgery,* 2nd ed. St. Louis, MO: Saunders/Elsevier; 2004:136–46.

2. Willsey AL, Cherry B, Rudd RJ, and Trimarchi CV. Rabies virus infection in a pet guinea pig and seven pet rabbits. *Journal of the American Veterinary Medical Association* 2005:227, 932–5.

3. Cheeke PR. *Rabbit feeding and nutrition.* Orlando, FL: Academic Press; 1987:15–33.

4. Brooks D. Nutrition and gastrointestinal physiology. In: Quesenberry KE, and Carpenter JW, eds. *Ferrets, rabbits and rodents: Clinical medicine and surgery,* 2nd ed. St. Louis, MO: Saunders/Elsevier; 2004:155–60.

5. Hromanik D. Application of Hay Science. *Exotic DVM* 2003;5.4:40–41.

6. Mader DR. Basic approach to veterinary care. In: Quesenberry KE, and Carpenter JW, eds. *Ferrets, rabbits and rodents: Clinical medicine and surgery,* 2nd ed. St. Louis, MO: Saunders/Elsevier; 2004:147–54.

7. Benson KG, and Paul-Murphy J. Clinical pathology of the domestic rabbit. In: Rupley AE, and Reavill DR, eds. *The vet clinics of North America, exotic animal practice, clinical pathology and sample collection.* Philadelphia: WB Saunders; 1999:539–51.

8. Johnson-Delaney CA, and Harrison LR. Rabbits. *Exotic companion medicine handbook for veterinarians.* Lake Worth, FL: Wingers Publishing; 1996:9–10.

9. Harkness JE, and Wagner JE. *The biology and medicine of rabbits and rodents,* 3rd ed. Philadelphia, PA: Lea & Febiger; 1989.

10. Harkness JE, and Wagner JE. *The biology and medicine of rabbits and rodents,* 4th ed. Philadelphia, PA: Lea & Febiger; 1995.

11. Quesenberry KE. Rabbits. In: Birchard SJ, and Sherding RG, eds. *Saunders manual of small animal practice.* Philadelphia: WB Saunders; 1994:1345–47.

12. Ramer JC, Paul-Murphy J, and Benson KG. Evaluating and stabilizing critically ill rabbits—Part II. *Compendium for Continuing Education* 1999;21:116–25.

13. Oxbow Pet Products, Critical Care™ for Herbivores Educational Brochure; 2003.

14. Hess L. Dermatologic diseases. In: Quesenberry KE, and Carpenter JW, eds. *Ferrets, rabbits and rodents: Clinical medicine and surgery,* 2nd ed. St. Louis, MO: Saunders/Elsevier; 2004:194–202.

15. Heard DJ. Anesthesia, analgesia and sedation for small mammals. In: Quesenberry, KE, and Carpenter, JW, eds. *Ferrets, rabbits and rodents: Clinical medicine and surgery,* 2nd ed. St. Louis, MO: Saunders/Elsevier; 2004:356–69.

16. Harcourt-Brown FM, ed. Rabbits. *Journal of Exotic Pet Medicine* 2007;16(3).

17. Capello V, and Lennox AM. Dentistry of exotic companion mammals. *Journal of Exotic Pet Medicine* 2008;17(2).

CHAPTER 5

Rodents

Guinea Pigs, Hamsters, Gerbils, Rats, and Mice

Information on the guinea pig and small pet rodent (hamsters, gerbils, rats, and mice) has been compiled into one chapter. Because there are many similarities in care, husbandry, diagnostic testing, and treatment for these animals, some information is true for all rodents, in which case it is described in just one area of the text, and readers are referred to that specific section. When information is unique to a specific species, that information is covered separately.

INTRODUCTION

GUINEA PIGS

Guinea pigs (*Cavia porcellus*) are native to the Andean highlands of north-central and northwestern South America.[1] Three main breeds are maintained as companion animals: (1) the English, or common, which is characterized by short, straight, fine hair; (2) the Abyssinian, with rough, wiry hair in rosettes or whorls; and (3) the Peruvian, with long, straight, silky hair (Figures 5.1A and 5.1B). Of all rodent species, guinea pigs might be the best choice for pets. They are usually nonaggressive, rarely bite, enjoy being held, and are long-lived in comparison with many other rodents.

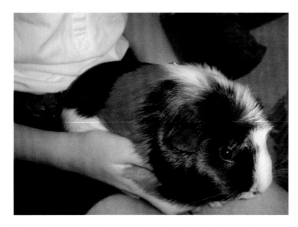

Figure 5.1A *Many different breeds of guinea pig can be purchased as pets. This photo shows a Tort and White.*

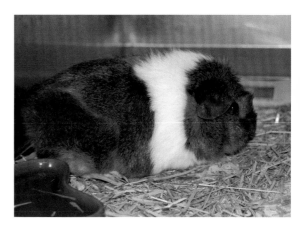

Figure 5.1B *This is a Red Dutch guinea pig.*

With the advent of commercial guinea pig diets and supplies from a large number of companies, it has never been easier to properly care for these rodents. Cavies (a common name for guinea pigs) belong to a group of animals that requires an external source of vitamin C. Often, the vitamin C is incorporated into the diet, but if the diet is deficient in the daily requirement of this essential vitamin, supplementation must be provided in the water or on the food. Vitamin C deficiency is one of the most common health problems treated by veterinarians. This information, along with basic dietary suggestions and husbandry techniques, should be provided to the owner during the cavy's first veterinary examination. To determine the health status of the patient and to answer basic questions, a technician should be familiar with baseline guinea pig physiologic information (Table 5.1).

As with other animals in the order Rodentia, guinea pigs have open-rooted teeth, which grow continuously; thus, they need a normal occlusive surface to wear properly and prevent overgrowth. It is common in cavies to have malocclusion of the cheek teeth, which causes enamel projections to rub against the tongue surface. This condition is commonly called "slobbers" by guinea pig owners, because the irritation promotes salivation and anorexia.

HAMSTERS

The golden or Syrian hamster (*Mesocricetus auratus*) is a very popular pet because of its small size and cute appearance, especially the teddy bear. The golden hamster is the most popular pet species of hamsters, but there are also Chinese, European, Hungarian, and Siberian dwarf hamsters. Although cute and small, these rodents can be territorial and aggressive, and they can bite their owners. Reduction of the animal's natural aggressive personality is usually achieved through routine handling. To reduce fighting between pet hamsters, animals should be housed in separate cages. All gender combinations will fight or succumb to immunosuppression initiated by psychological stress as a result of a dominant animal within the environment. Females that have given birth will often cannibalize their young if disturbed.

Hamsters are nocturnal animals and like to exercise during the night. If the exercise wheel is not oiled, the squeaking apparatus may disturb the owner. These animals are notorious for escap-

Table 5.1 **Guinea Pig Basic Information**[1]

GENERAL CATEGORY	CLASSIFICATION	PHYSIOLOGIC PARAMETERS/QUANTITY
Body Weight	Adult Male	900–1,200 g
	Adult Female	750–900 g
	Birth Weight	60–110 g
Temperature, Pulse, and Respiration	Rectal Body Temperature	101.5°–103°F
	Normal Heart Rate	230–380 beats/minute
	Normal Respiratory Rate	42–104 breaths/minute
Amounts of Food and Water	Daily Food Consumption	6 g/100 g body weight/day
	Daily Water Consumption	10 ml/100 g body weight/day
Age at Onset of Puberty and Breeding Life	Puberty, Male	9–10 weeks
	Puberty, Female	6 weeks
	Breeding Initiation, Male	3–4 months
	Breeding Initiation, Female	2–3 months
Female Reproductive Cycle	Estrous Cycle	15–17 days
	Estrus Duration	1–16 hours (avg. 8 hours)
	Gestation Length	59–72 days
	Litter Size	3–4 average

ing their enclosure. The owner must be made aware of the importance of purchasing an escape-proof cage with an appropriate screen top that can be fastened securely.

Veterinary technicians need to be aware of a few anatomical differences found in hamsters. (See the baseline hamster physical information listed in Table 5.2.[1]) The most prominent are the large cheek pouches that can store large pellets, seed, or bedding material. It is very common for hamsters to have full cheek pouches, which deform the face, but this is a normal behavior pattern for these animals. Male hamsters have two small, symmetrical black spots on the lateral flank region of the body. These are lateral flank sebaceous glands. The glands are testosterone dependent and are better developed in males than in females.[2] The only open-rooted teeth in small rodents, including hamsters, are the incisors.

To properly sex hamsters, rats, mice, and gerbils, the distance from the anus to the genital opening is measured. This distance in males is twice that of female animals.[2] Females have three openings in this area (urinary, genital, and anal), whereas males have two openings (urogenital and anal).[2] Male guinea pigs have a urethral opening between two large scrotal sacs cranial to the anus that when observed appear as an *i* from the anus. The dot on the *i* is the prepucal opening. The female guinea pig has a Y-shaped depression in the tissue cranial to the anus.

GERBILS

One of the friendliest small rodent pets is the Mongolian gerbil (*Meriones unguiculatus*) (Figures 5.2A and 5.2B). The most common color of pet gerbils is tannish brown (agouti), but other hair coat colors are available. If multiple animals are

Table 5.2 **Hamster Basic Information**[1]

GENERAL CATEGORY	CLASSIFICATION	PHYSIOLOGIC PARAMETERS/QUANTITY
Body Weight	Adult Male	85–130 g
	Adult Female	95–150 g
	Birth Weight	2 g
Temperature, Pulse, and Respiration	Rectal Body Temperature	99°–101°F
	Normal Heart Rate	250–500 beats/minute
	Normal Respiratory Rate	35–135 breaths/minute
Amounts of Food and Water	Daily Food Consumption	15 g/100 g body weight/day
	Daily Water Consumption	20 ml/100 g body weight/day
Age at Onset of Puberty and Breeding Life	Puberty, Male	45–75 days
	Breeding Initiation, Male	10–14 weeks
	Breeding Initiation, Female	6–10 weeks
Female Reproductive Cycle	Estrous Cycle	4 days (polyestrous)
	Gestation Length	15–18 days
	Litter Size	5–9 average

in the same enclosure with different hair coat colors, like-colored individuals will usually associate with each other.[1]

These animals are native to a very dry environment; therefore, they do not drink much water and produce little waste that would soil their environment. Owners should be encouraged to regularly clean the enclosure to maintain healthy animals in an artificial setting. Food, water, and husbandry management for gerbils is similar to that for other small rodents. (See the baseline gerbil physical information listed in Table 5.3.[2])

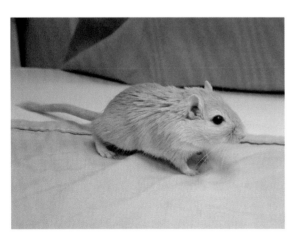

Figure 5.2A *Gerbils make excellent companion animals.*

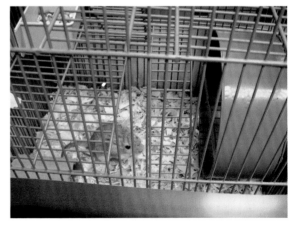

Figure 5.2B *Gerbil in a typical cage.*

Table 5.3 Gerbil Basic Information[1]

GENERAL CATEGORY	CLASSIFICATION	PHYSIOLOGIC PARAMETERS/QUANTITY
Body Weight	Adult Male	65–100 g
	Adult Female	55–85 g
	Birth Weight	2.5–3.5 g
Temperature, Pulse, and Respiration	Rectal Body Temperature	99°–101°F
	Normal Heart Rate	360 beats/minute
	Normal Respiratory Rate	90 breaths/minute
Amounts of Food and Water	Daily Food Consumption	5–8 g
	Daily Water Consumption	4 mL
Age at Breeding Initiation	Breeding Initiation, Male	70–85 days
	Breeding Initiation, Female	65–85 deays
Female Reproductive Cycle	Estrous Cycle	4 days (polyestrous)
	Gestation Length (nonlactating)	24–26 days
	Gestation Length (concurrent lactation)	27–48 days
	Litter Size	5–9 average

There is an androgen-dependent midventral scent gland on a gerbil's body. This scent gland should not be mistaken for an abnormal dermatologic lesion.

RATS

Rats, like mice, are common laboratory animals and are also propagated for reptile food. Unlike mice, rats have excellent pet characteristics that include a personable disposition and a charming intelligence. The common rat species maintained as a companion animal is *Rattus norvegicus*, with the white rat and hooded rat being the most common variations. Although rats have an excellent temperament for companionship, they can inflict a serious bite if provoked. Also, as with other animal species, humans can be allergic to their hair, skin dander, urine, and salivary proteins.[2] Rats are not as territorial as other rodent species and are very social. Food, water, and husbandry management is similar to that for other small rodents.

(Refer to the baseline rat physical information listed in Table 5.4.[1,2])

Rats are continuous, polyestrous rodents that should be bred in polygamous or monogamous setups because of the males' aggressive territoriality behavior.[1] When breeding rats in a polygamous ratio, there might be 1 male with 2–6 females. Females are removed from a polygamous cage prior to parturition. A monogamous pair is maintained together with the young until weaning.

MICE

Although not a common companion animal, mice (*Mus musculus*) are maintained in captive conditions as pets and for use as reptile food. The African pygmy mouse is a genus of mouse that is commonly maintained as a pet.[2] A number of behavioral and physical characteristics make mice undesirable pets, including aggressive, protective behavior, often resulting in painful bites to the owner; territorial

Table 5.4 **Rat Basic Information**[1]

GENERAL CATEGORY	CLASSIFICATION	PHYSIOLOGIC PARAMETERS/QUANTITY
Body Weight	Adult Male	450–520 g
	Adult Female	250–320 g
	Birth Weight	5–6 g
Temperature, Pulse, and Respiration	Rectal Body Temperature	99°–101°F
	Normal Heart Rate	250–450 beats/minute
	Normal Respiratory Rate	70–115 breaths/minute
Amounts of Food and Water	Daily Food Consumption	10 g/100 g body weight/day
	Daily Water Consumption	10–12 ml/100 g body weight/day
Age at Onset of Puberty and Breeding Life	Sexual Maturity, Male	65–110 days
	Sexual Maturity, Female	65–110 days
Female Reproductive Cycle	Estrous Cycle	4–5 days
	Gestation Length	21–23 days
	Litter Size	6–12 average

behavior that often results in severe injury to cage mates; potential human allergies to the hair and skin dander; and a strong, undesirable smell to the urine. Even with these undesirable characteristics, mice can be good pets for owners who are willing to work with the animals and accept their negative aspects. (See mouse basic information in Table 5.5.)

Mice are maintained in environments that are similar to those for other small rodents, but a thorough cage cleaning is required more often because of their smelly urine (Figure 5.3). Food, water, and husbandry management is similar to that for other small rodents listed in this chapter.

Mice, like rats, are continuous polyestrous rodents that should be bred in polygamous or monogamous setups, because of the males' aggressive, territorial behavior.[1] When breeding mice in a polygamous ratio, there might be 1 male with 2–6 females. Females are removed from a polygamous cage prior to parturition. A monogamous pair is maintained together with the young until weaning.

HUSBANDRY

Environmental Concerns

Guinea Pigs

Guinea pigs are commonly maintained in indoor cages. The general environment of the house will usually provide an adequate temperature range to maintain proper health and comfort. These animals are native to the Andean mountain range and are more sensitive to warmer temperatures than to cooler ones. Temperatures above 80°–85°F might cause heat-related death.[1]

A guinea pig enclosure should have 1 cubic foot of space per adult and be made out of wire mesh (0.5–1.5" spacing). Breeders should have twice the recommended adult floor space.[2] The cage should have an open top with sides at least 10" high and should also have a hiding box to provide security when needed.[1] Cavies are very susceptible to infectious pododermatitis, or "bumblefoot." A solid floor is preferred over a wire mesh floor to prevent bumblefoot and protect against limb and nail trauma. Other pets that might harm guinea

Table 5.5 **Mouse Basic Information**[1]

GENERAL CATEGORY	CLASSIFICATION	PHYSIOLOGIC PARAMETERS/QUANTITY
Body Weight	Adult Male	20–40 g
	Adult Female	25–40 g
	Birth Weight	0.8–2.0 g
Temperature, Pulse, and Respiration	Rectal Body Temperature	97°–100°F
	Normal Heart Rate	325–780 beats/minute
	Normal Respiratory Rate	60–220 breaths/minute
Amounts of Food and Water	Daily Food Consumption	15 g/100 g body weight/day
	Daily Water Consumption	15 ml/100 g body weight/day
Age at Onset of Puberty and Breeding Life	Sexual Maturity, Male	50 days
	Sexual Maturity, Female	50–60 days
Female Reproductive Cycle	Estrous Cycle	4–5 days
	Gestation Length	19–21 days
	Litter Size	10–12 average

pigs, such as dogs and cats, should be kept in an area that will prevent an attack and exposure to Bordetella spp. bacteria.

As with all rodents and pocket pets, guinea pigs' bedding must be changed on a regular basis, because feces, urine, food, and water soil the environment. Hardwood shavings, composite recycled paper materials, pellets, and shredded paper may be used as bedding material. Guinea pigs are also susceptible to submandibular abscesses, commonly called "lumps." These abscesses are caused by hay, straw, or woodchips that are eaten and puncture the gingival surface, seeding bacteria within the oral cavity. The bacterial infection migrates into the submandibular/cervical area, forming large abscesses. If a patient presents with these abscesses, the diet should be reviewed in order to help identify and eliminate the initiating cause of the problem.

Small Rodents

As discussed previously, hamsters commonly chew their way out of enclosures. It is important that the housing be "hamster-proof," or the animal could escape into the house. If a hamster does escape, the best way to capture it is to place food in the center of the room. Once it has been determined in which room the animal is hiding, the room should be sealed. Because hamsters are nocturnal animals, capturing them at night—in a dark room, with a flashlight—might work best. This technique will work for the capture of other small rodents and pocket pets as well.

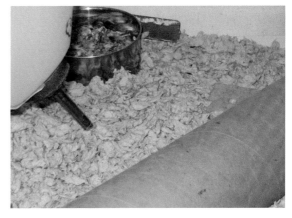

Figure 5.3 *Typical mouse cage, with recycled paper as a substrate.*

The recommended cage size for hamsters, mice, and gerbils is 20" × 20" × 6–10" high.[1] Owners should be informed that the cage should provide enough room for the animal to exercise and should contain an exercise wheel and a hiding box (Figures 5.4A and 5.4B). For proper ventilation, a screen top is recommended. Hardwood shavings, commercial recycled paper pellets (CareFresh; Absorption Corp., Ferndale, WA), and shredded papers are the primary substrate choices for rodent cages, with cleaning occurring one to two times a

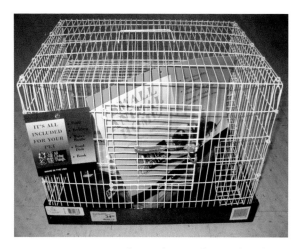

Figure 5.4A *A typical cage that can be purchased from a pet store.*

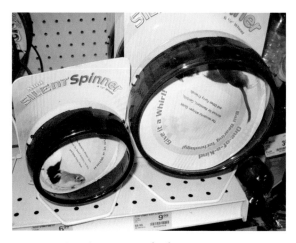

Figure 5.4B *An exercise wheel.*

week. If the plastic tube housing systems are used, routine cleaning of the sections, using hot water and a mild detergent, is called for. Ventilation is essential in all small-rodent housing to prevent irritation of the respiratory tract from the ammonia vapors generated by urine.

Nutrition
Guinea Pigs
A commercial guinea pig feed (20% crude protein and 16% fiber) is the best basic diet, along with free choice of timothy hay.[2] Many companies manufacture timothy hay guinea pig pellets, and this should be the base diet. Discourage owners from using any rodent diet that contains seed. The dietary source should be fresh and supplemented with ascorbic acid (vitamin C). If the diet is not fresh (within 30 days of milling date), there is a possibility that the vitamin content has degraded and is not adequate for the pet's daily requirements. Supplemental vitamin C will aid in the cavy's general health; it requires 7–10 mg/kg/day and, if pregnant, 20–30 mg/kg/day. Kale, cabbage, and oranges are very good dietary sources of vitamin C. Vitamin C tablets manufactured specifically for guinea pigs are available commercially through Oxbow Pet Products (Murdock, NE). Commercial vitamin C drops can be mixed into the sipper bottle water to provide additional vitamin C (Figure 5.5). Any vitamin C supplement that is added to the water must be reformulated and changed daily, because the half-life of vitamin C is only 24 hours in glass bottles of clean water.[1] Timothy hay, alfalfa cubes, small amounts of green vegetables, and apples are all treats that these animals eat on a regular basis.[2] Treats should be limited to 1–2 tablespoons over a 24-hour period, with the bulk of the dietary requirements coming from guinea pig chow.[2] Feeders and sipper tubes should be suspended on the side of the cage

to prevent fecal contamination and dumping of the contents onto the cage floor.

Small Rodents

The nutritional requirements for most small rodents are the same. A number of commercial hamster/rodent pellets are available (Figure 5.6). The formulas that contain at least 16% protein and 8% fiber provide for optimum health.[1,2] The owner should be informed that any seed-based rodent diet is unacceptable for health mainte-

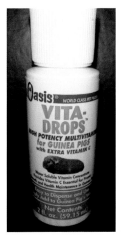

Figure 5.5 *Vitamin C supplement can be added to a guinea pig's drinking water.*

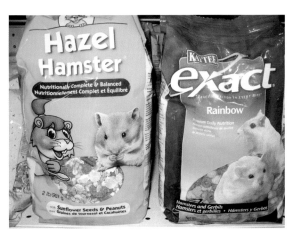

Figure 5.6 *Hamster food can be purchased as a pelleted diet or with a seed base. The recommended diet for hamsters is a pelleted diet.*

nance. Treats may be offered in the form of nuts, raisins, apples, and greens, at no more than ½ teaspoon per 24 hours.[1]

Sipper bottles and small food containers that fit on the side of the enclosure reduce spillage and urinary/fecal contamination. Water and feed containers should be cleaned daily and replenished with fresh contents.

Transport: All Rodents

There are a number of options for transporting small rodents. If the cage is small, it may be used, or there are a variety of small plastic and wire carriers suitable for these animals.

Grooming: All Rodents

The only small rodent that requires nail trimming on a regular basis is the guinea pig. Human toenail clippers can be used to trim the claws below the sensitive vascular "quick." On many guinea pig patients it is difficult to see exactly where the quick is; therefore, one should be conservative in the amount of nail removed. The rear nails are routinely longer than those on the front legs. The guinea pig should be properly restrained and if bleeding does occur, a silver nitrate–tipped cautery stick can be used to provide hemostasis.

Rats may have sharp claws that the owner asks to have cut. A very short trim, using human nail clippers, will adequately blunt the claws to reduce injury due to scratching in these animals.

HISTORY

GUINEA PIGS

The same basic background information is required for guinea pigs as for other animals that are examined at the veterinary clinic. How long the animal has been owned, where it was acquired, how often it is handled, and the character of the feces and urine are a few of the questions that should be asked for background information. Husbandry questions include where the animal is housed; whether it is allowed to roam unobserved in the house; cage location, type, size, material, substrate, furniture, and toys; how often the cage is cleaned; and the disinfectant used. When investigating the diet, it is important to ask owners if pellets are fed, how much, and also what the animal is actually eating. Supplemental offerings and frequency of feeding are very important data for the case workup. To round out the nutrition section, the technician should find out about the water supply, how often the water is changed, and how much the animal drinks on a daily basis. Because vitamin C is a required nutrient for guinea pigs, it is very important to ask about vitamin C supplementation and the age of the animal's food. Vitamin C will degrade over time and when exposed to extreme heat. Recently purchased food that has been stored properly is likely to have maintained the nutritious value of that vitamin.

Because animals can transmit diseases among one another, the technician's final questions should center on other pets in the household— if new animals have been added to the family or if the animals are housed together. Finally, a description of any previous problems and a complete chronological description of the presenting problem are needed to complete the history form.

SMALL RODENTS

The same questions used to obtain a history for guinea pig patients can be used for other small rodents and pocket pets. The history and physical examination information in the following rodent and pocket pet sections will not be repeated. It

is recommended that this section be referred to when examining these animals.

RESTRAINT

GUINEA PIGS

Guinea pigs should be restrained by grabbing the animal around the shoulders with one hand, lifting the animal up, and supporting the rear with the other hand (Figures 5.7A and 5.7B). The handler must be careful not to squeeze too hard with the hand around the neck and chest, because

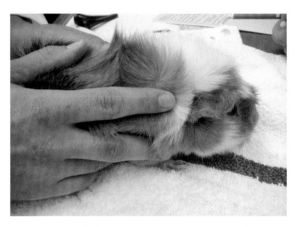

Figure 5.7A *When restraining a guinea pig, the animal must be supported in the rear.*

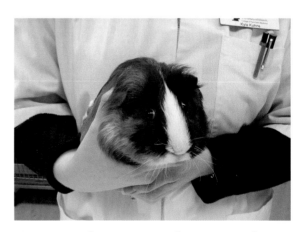

Figure 5.7B *Proper restraint of a guinea pig also requires a firm grasp around the shoulder and neck area.*

respiratory compromise could occur. To prevent respiratory distress, the handler should place the hand around the neck from the ventral aspect of the animal, while supporting the rear legs with the other hand.

HAMSTERS

Hamsters and other small rodents can be restrained by pinching the skin on the scruff. It is important to get a tight hold of the skin to prevent escape or injury. Hamsters' eyes can prolapse with a tight grip, but gentle pressure on the globe, pushing into the orbit, usually resolves the problem.

GERBILS

A gerbil should be restrained by cupping a hand over the animal's back and immobilizing its head between the forefinger and middle finger, with the thumb supporting the rear of the animal (Figure 5.8). **Never attempt to restrain a gerbil by its tail, because the skin is easily removed** (Figure 5.9).

RATS

To restrain a rat, the animal should be picked up with one hand placed over its back and rib cage, while restraining its head with the thumb and forefinger directly behind its jaws (Figure 5.10). The other hand grasps the tail, stabilizing the animal (Figure 5.11). As with other rodents, the skin on the dorsal cervical region can also be used to pick up rats.

MICE

To restrain a mouse, the tail should be grabbed with the thumb and forefinger, allowing the mouse to hold on to an object with its front feet. When the mouse securely attaches itself to an object, the other hand then grabs the dorsal skin

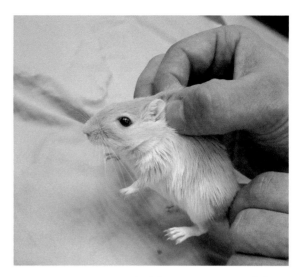

Figure 5.8 *Proper method for restraining a gerbil.*

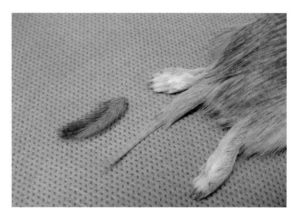

Figure 5.9 *A gerbil's tail should never be pulled, because as a defensive response, the skin will deglove.*

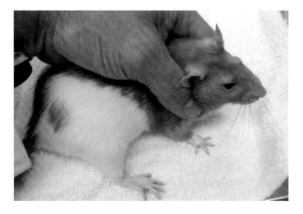

Figure 5.10 *The proper method for restraining a rat.*

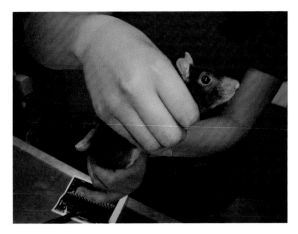

Figure 5.11 *A rat's body should be supported when it is being examined off a table.*

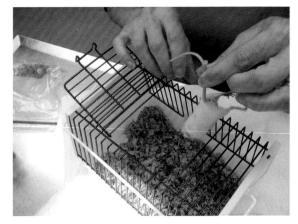

Figure 5.12A *Proper method for capturing and restraining a mouse. A mouse can be grabbed by the tail.*

in the cervical region, while keeping the tail in a firm grasp (Figures 5.12A, 5.12B, and 5.12C).

PHYSICAL EXAMINATION: ALL RODENTS

Prior to restraint, the veterinarian will observe the animal's attitude, activity, and posture. The next step is to weigh the animal in a basket on a digital gram scale. If possible, temperature, respiration, and pulse should be measured and any abnormalities in rate or character noted. The veterinarian will begin the physical examination at the head, looking for any abnormalities. Eyes, ears, and nares are observed, looking for discharge or inflammation. The oral cavity in guinea pigs is difficult to examine because of the small opening and tendency for the buccal mucosa to encroach toward the middle of the mouth. A small rabbit speculum or an otoscope can be used to examine the oral cavity and teeth (Figure 5.13). Mucous membranes help determine hydration status using capillary refill time and moisture. Body condition and abdominal palpation findings are important information to be obtained. Lymph nodes and limbs are palpated prior to examining the claws and plantar surface of each foot. It is not uncom-

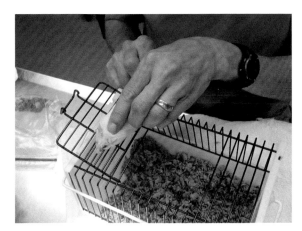

Figure 5.12B *Proper method for capturing and restraining a mouse.*

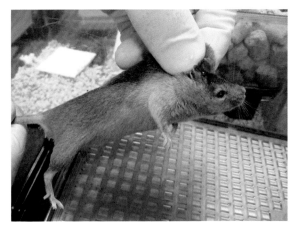

Figure 5.12C *Proper method for capturing and restraining a mouse.*

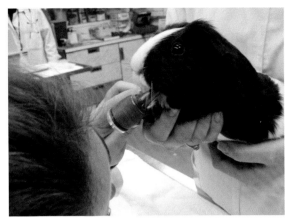

Figure 5.13 *An otoscope with a designated reusable plastic cone can be used to obtain a quick examination of the teeth of both guinea pigs and rabbits.*

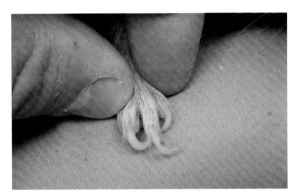

Figure 5.14 *Guinea pigs' claws should be trimmed on a regular basis.*

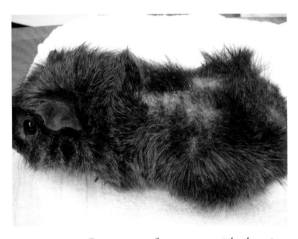

Figure 5.15 *Guinea pigs often present with alopecia, which might be associated with vitamin C deficiency and/or ectoparasite infestation.*

mon for guinea pigs to present with long claws (Figure 5.14). The patient should have a normal posture, be aware of its surroundings, and move properly. Any problems should be noted in the record. Finally, a dermatological exam considers hair coat quality, alopecia, external parasites, or any skin abnormalities (Figure 5.15). All abnormal findings are written in the record for case review, differential diagnosis determination, diagnostic testing, and treatment considerations.

DIAGNOSTIC SAMPLING

Blood Collection

Guinea Pigs

In guinea pigs and other pocket pets, blood collection can be quite difficult. Approximately 0.5–0.7 ml/100 grams of body weight can be safely removed from a non-anemic, healthy guinea pig.[3] For many small exotic mammal patients, including the guinea pig, the location of choice for blood collection is the cranial vena cava (see Figure 5.16). Owing to the location of the cranial vena cava and the size of other blood vessels, sedation or anesthetization of the guinea pig patient is recommended prior to performing the phlebotomy. To collect blood from the cranial vena cava, one should do the following:[4]

- Isolate the center of the cranial sternum and manubrium.
- Insert a 25- to 27-gauge needle to the right of the manubrium at a slight angle directed toward the opposite lateral body wall.
- Advance the needle only as negative pressure is applied. If there is not a "flash" of blood in the needle hub once the needle has been inserted, pull the needle almost out of the body cavity and redirect dorsally first, then if unsuccessful, ventrally until blood is observed in the syringe.

- Be sure not to advance the needle too far. In most patients the vessel is usually very close to the ventral surface under the cranial sternum.
- Maintain a consistent flow of blood once the cranial vena cava has been located.
- Finish collecting and then twist the needle when pulling it out of the body cavity.

The easiest veins to see are the lateral saphenous and cephalic, but they are very small and easily collapse when too much suction is used to collect blood. The fur should be clipped over the vein from which the blood will be taken and the surface prepared with alcohol. A small 25- or 26-gauge needle, usually placed on a 3 cc syringe, is recommended to collect the blood. The short jugular vein can be used, but it is difficult to find, and if the cranial vena cava is used in cavies for blood collection, it might lead to bleeding complications. The position to collect from the jugular vein is similar to the technique used for cats. Reference ranges for complete blood counts and serum chemistry panels are listed in Tables 5.6 and 5.7, respectively.[3]

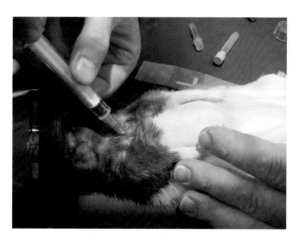

Figure 5.16 *Blood can be collected from the cranial vena cava of many small exotic mammals.*

Small Rodents

Although hamsters, gerbils, mice, and rats are very small animals, their blood must be collected and tested for diagnostic purposes. As described for the guinea pig, the cranial vena cava is the site of choice for collecting adequate volumes of blood for diagnostic testing on hamster patients. A safe amount of blood to draw from a noncritical ham-

Table 5.6 **Guinea Pig Complete Blood Count Reference Ranges**[3]

CELL TYPE	NORMAL RANGE
Erythrocytes	$3.2–8.0 \times 10^6/\mu l$
Hematocrit	32%–50%
Hemoglobin	10–17 g/dl
Leukocytes	$5.5–17.5 \times 10^3/\mu l$
Neutrophils	22%–48%
Lymphocytes	39%–72%
Eosinophils	0%–7%
Monocytes	1%–10%
Basophils	0%–2.7%
Platelets	$260–740 \times 10^3/\mu l$
Serum Protein	4.2–6.8 g/dl
Albumin	2.1–3.9 g/dl
Globulin	1.7–2.6 g/dl

Table 5.7 **Guinea Pig Serum Biochemistry Reference Ranges**[3]

ANALYTE	NORMAL RANGE
Serum Glucose	60–125 mg/dl
Blood Urea Nitrogen	9.0–31.5 mg/dl
Creatinine	0.6–2.2 mg/dl
Total Bilirubin	0–0.9 mg/dl
Cholesterol	16–43 mg/dl
Serum Calcium	8.2–12.0 mg/dl
Serum Phosphate	3.0–7.6 mg/dl
Alkaline Phosphatase	55–108 U/L
Alanine Aminotransferase (ALT)	25–59 U/L
Aspartate Aminotransferase (AST)	26–68 U/L

ster patient would be approximately 0.7 ml/100 grams of body weight. Clipping the hair and disinfecting the topical skin surface will properly prepare the blood collection sites. General anesthesia is a consideration whenever blood is being collected for diagnostic testing in these small animals. Usually, inducing the animal in a closed chamber and maintaining the patient in a mask will allow the technician plenty of time to collect the blood sample. Table 5.8 describes the technique used for retro-orbital blood collection in small rodents.

On smaller rodents, the saphenous vein or lateral vein of the tarsus can be used for multiple blood collections without the use of anesthesia. The patient must be properly immobilized in a restraint tube (35 cc syringe) with the leg extended and the skin held tight on the medial aspect of the thigh

using the thumb and forefinger. The taut skin on the lateral aspect of the thigh allows exposure of the saphenous vein. A 23-gauge needle is used to puncture the vein, and blood is collected in a microhematocrit tube as it flows from the vessel.[3]

The jugular vein and ear vessel can be used in larger rodents and pocket pets for blood collection. To collect blood from the jugular vein, a 3 cc syringe and 25-gauge needle are needed, whereas a microhematocrit tube is used to collect blood from the ear vessel. Blood samples obtained from nail and ear clips are not considered appropriate diagnostic samples. Cardiac puncture is recommended only for terminal cases, when the animal is maintained under general anesthesia, because of possible complications involving the lungs and heart vessels. Reference ranges for complete blood counts and serum chemistry panels for hamsters are listed in Tables 5.9 and 5.10, respectively.[1]

The collection of samples for diagnostic testing in gerbils is similar to the techniques used in other rodents. The reference ranges for complete blood counts and serum chemistry panels for gerbils are listed in Tables 5.11 and 5.12, respectively.[2,3]

The collection of samples for diagnostic testing in rats is similar to the techniques used with other rodents. The reference ranges for complete blood counts and serum chemistry panels for rats are listed in Tables 5.13 and 5.14, respectively.[2,3]

The collection of samples for diagnostic testing in mice is similar to techniques used for other rodents. The reference ranges for complete blood counts and serum chemistry ranges for mice are listed in Tables 5.15[1,2] and 5.16, respectively.

Bone Marrow Aspiration: All Rodents
Marrow samples can be obtained from the ilium, tibia, sternum, femur, or the bones of the proximal one-third of the tail.[4] Preparation of the

Table 5.8 Retro-Orbital Blood Collection[3]

1. Stabilize head at base of skull and point of jaw.
2. Occlusion of the jugular vein may distend the venous plexus.
3. Retract the dorsal lid of the eye with the index finger.
4. Collection:
   → *Hamsters*—a microcapillary tube or small-bore Pasteur pipette is inserted midway along the superior border of the eye and advanced to the plexus located posterior to the globe.[4]
   → *Mice and Gerbils*—a microcapillary tube or small-bore Pasteur pipette is inserted at the medial canthus.
   → *Rats*—the middorsal approach, similar to that used with hamsters, is considered the most direct access to the dorsal anastomotic vein.
5. Once the tube is placed in the correct position, the tube can be gently rotated until the conjunctiva is punctured and the orbital venous plexus is penetrated.
6. The tube is filled by capillary action.
7. Slight pressure may be placed over the eye to aid in hemostasis after the bleeding.
8. 0.5 ml may be collected from an adult mouse or gerbil.

Table 5.9 **Hamster Complete Blood Count Reference Ranges**[1]

CELL TYPE	NORMAL RANGE
Erythrocytes	5.0–10 x 10^6/µl
Hematocrit	36%–55%
Hemoglobin	10–16 g/dl
Leukocytes	6.3–8.9 x 10^3/µl
Neutrophils	10%–42%
Lymphocytes	50%–95%
Eosinophils	0%–4.5%
Monocytes	0%–3.0%
Basophils	0%–1.0%
Platelets	200–500 x 10^3/µl
Serum Protein	5.9–6.5 g/dl
Albumin	2.63–4.10 g/dl
Globulin	2.7–4.2 g/dl

Table 5.11 **Gerbil Complete Blood Count Reference Ranges**[2,3]

CELL TYPE	REFERENCE RANGE
Erythrocytes	7.0–10 x 10^6/µl
Hematocrit	41%–52%
Hemoglobin	12.1–16.9 g/dl
Leukocytes	4.3–21.6 x 10^3/µl
Neutrophils	5%–34%
Lymphocytes	60%–95%
Eosinophils	0%–4.0%
Monocytes	0%–3.0%
Basophils	0%–1.0%
Platelets	400–600 x 10^6/µl
Serum Protein	4.3–12.5 g/dl
Albumin	1.8–5.5 g/dl
Globulin	1.6–6.0 g/dl

Table 5.10 **Hamster Serum Biochemistry Reference Ranges**[1]

ANALYTE	NORMAL RANGE
Serum Glucose	60–150 mg/dl
Blood Urea Nitrogen	10.0–25.0 mg/dl
Creatinine	0.92–0.99 mg/dl
Total Bilirubin	0.25–0.60 mg/dl
Cholesterol	25–135 mg/dl
Serum Calcium	5.0–12.0 mg/dl
Serum Phosphate	3.4–8.2 mg/dl
Alkaline Phosphatase	3.2–30.5 U/L
Alanine Aminotransferase (ALT)	11.6–35.9 U/L
Aspartate Aminotransferase (AST)	37.6–168.0 U/L

Table 5.12 **Gerbil Serum Biochemistry Reference Ranges**[2,3]

ANALYTE	REFERENCE RANGE
Serum Glucose	50–135 mg/dl
Blood Urea Nitrogen	17.0–27.0 mg/dl
Creatinine	0.5–1.47 mg/dl
Total Bilirubin	0.2–0.6 mg/dl
Cholesterol	90–150 mg/dl
Serum Calcium	3.7–6.2 mg/dl
Serum Phosphate	3.7–7.0 mg/dl

samples is consistent with that of other mammalian patients. (See "Bone Marrow Aspiration" in Chapter 4 on rabbits.)

Urine Collection: All Rodents

When the patient is hospitalized, a standard rodent cage (without substrate) can be used to collect urine and feces. For small rodents, the sample can also be collected by placing the animal in an unsealed ziplock bag, which often will cause it to urinate. For guinea pigs and larger pocket pets, a standard cystocentesis procedure can be used to collect urine directly from the bladder.

Microbiology: All Rodents

Guinea pigs are susceptible to *Bordetella bronchiseptica* and *Streptococcus pneumonia* respiratory bacterial infections. It is best to prevent these respiratory infections by separating other pets (e.g., dogs, cats, rabbits) from guinea pigs. *Staphylococcus*

Table 5.13 Rat Complete Blood Count Reference Ranges[2,3]

CELL TYPE	NORMAL RANGE
Erythrocytes	5.4–8.5 x 10^6/µl
Hematocrit	37%–49%
Hemoglobin	11.5–16 g/dl
Leukocytes	6.6–12.6 x 10^3/µl
Neutrophils	6–17%
Lymphocytes	9–34%
Eosinophils	0–6%
Monocytes	0–5%
Basophils	0–1.5%
Platelets	450–885 x 10^3/µl
Serum Protein	5.6–7.6 g/dl
Albumin	3.8–4.8 g/dl
Globulin	1.8–3.0 g/dl

Table 5.15 Mouse Complete Blood Count Reference Ranges[1,2,3]

CELL TYPE	REFERENCE RANGE
Erythrocytes	7.0–12.5 x 10^6/µl
Hematocrit	36%–49%
Hemoglobin	10.2–18 mg/dl
Leukocytes	6.0–15.0 x 10^3/µl
Neutrophils	10%–40%
Lymphocytes	55%–95%
Eosinophils	0%–4.0%
Monocytes	0.1%–3.5%
Basophils	0.0%–0.3%
Platelets	60–1,200 x 10^6/µl
Serum Protein	3.5–7.2 g/dl
Albumin	2.5–4.8 g/dl
Globulin	1.8–3.0 g/dl

Table 5.14 Rat Serum Biochemistry Reference Ranges[2,3]

ANALYTE	REFERENCE RANGE
Serum Glucose	50–135 mg/dl
Blood Urea Nitrogen	15.0–21.0 mg/dl
Creatinine	0.2–0.8 mg/dl
Total Bilirubin	0.20–0.55 mg/dl
Cholesterol	40–130 mg/dl
Serum Calcium	7.2–13.9 mg/dl
Serum Phosphate	3.11–11.0 mg/dl
Alkaline Phosphatase	56.8–128 U/L
Alanine Aminotransferase (ALT)	17.5–30.2 U/L
Aspartate Aminotransferase (AST)	45.7–80.8 U/L

Table 5.16 Mouse Serum Biochemistry Reference Ranges[1,2,3]

ANALYTE	REFERENCE RANGE
Serum Glucose	62–175 gm/dl
Blood Urea Nitrogen	12–28 mg/dl
Creatinine	0.3–1.0 mg/dl
Total Bilirubin	0.1–0.9 mg/dl
Cholesterol	26–82 mg/dl
Serum Calcium	3.12–8.5 mg/dl
Serum Phosphate	2.3–9.2 mg/dl

aureus is the major causative agent found in infectious pododermatitis lesions. *Streptococcus zooepidemicus* and *Streptobacillus moniliformis* are common isolates of infections affecting the cervical lymph nodes, commonly called "lumps." Routine culture techniques should be used to isolate and identify the bacterial organism causing a disease. Bacterial infections also cause disease in other pet rodent species. The specific bacte-rial diseases that are of great concern, including mycoplasma in rats and mice and *Lawsonia intracellularis* in hamsters, are discussed in greater detail in the "Health Maintenance and Disease" section later in this chapter.

Radiology: All Rodents

Radiology techniques for guinea pigs and other pocket pets are similar to those used on rabbits. Please refer to Chapter 4 for radiology techniques needed for guinea pigs and pocket pets.

Fecal Examination and Anal Tape Test: Small Rodents

Routine fecal parasite evaluations should be performed on small rodents when presented for a health examination or an abnormal stool. Common protozoal organisms that can be detected using a direct fecal examination include *Giardia* spp., cryptosporidiosis, and *Spironucleus muris*.[3] *Hymenolepis diminuta* is a tapeworm that can cause constipation in hamsters.[3] This tapeworm can be detected during a fecal examination, at which time the owner must be informed that it is a zoonotic parasite.

Rodent pinworms, specifically *Syphacia muris* and *Syphacia obvelata*, are commonly diagnosed using the sticky side of clear cellophane tape to make an impression of the anus. The sticky surface will pick up the banana-shaped pinworm eggs, which can then be observed under a microscope.

Parasitology

External Parasites

Guinea Pigs

Guinea pigs can be infested by mites, lice, and fleas. The most significant ectoparasite is the sarcoptic mite, *Trixacarus caviae*.[3] Guinea pigs infested with *T. caviae* have intense itching episodes that result in hair loss and skin lesions, primarily involving the thighs and back.[3] Treatment of guinea pigs diagnosed with *T. caviae* is difficult, because the environment and the animal must be treated at the same time. Pet owners should be advised to clean the enclosure at least twice a week during the treatment period, and all toys and bedding material should be removed. It is also important to discuss the zoonotic potential of *T. caviae* with the owner. During the treatment phase, the owner should wear latex gloves, and exposure to other family members and pets should be limited during the recovery period. Once the guinea pig has been treated and no mites remain, new toys should be purchased.

Lice and mites, including *T. caviae*, can be treated with imidacloprid and moxidectin (Advantage Multi for cats [orange], Bayer HealthCare, Shawnee Mission, KS, 0.1 ml/kg topically, every 30 days for 3 treatments) or ivermectin (Ivomec, Merck & Co., Inc, West Point, PA, 0.5 mg/kg SC, and repeat in 10 days. Unfortunately, *T. caviae* and other guinea pig parasites are becoming resistant to ivermectin treatment alone, so 4–5 treatments of ivermectin (10 days apart) are needed, with the owner cleaning the environment twice a week. To aid in treatment of difficult mite and lice infestations, lime sulfur dip (2.5% solution, apply once per week for 4–6 weeks) is also prescribed as an adjunct therapy. The combined treatment protocol is usually effective.

Guinea pigs are exposed to ectoparasites through direct contact. Most of the animals that are affected are recent purchases from a pet store. If fleas are a problem, a pyrethrin-based cat flea powder is effective, especially after the environment is treated and the patient has been bathed. As with rabbits, newer antiparasitic medications appear effective in treating guinea pigs that present with ectoparasites. Imidacloprid and moxidectin (Advantage Multi for cats 9 weeks of age and 5.1–9.0 lbs, topical solution, Bayer HealthCare LLC, Animal Health Division, Shawnee Mission, KS) can be used to treat guinea pigs diagnosed with fleas, mites, or lice at a dose of 0.1 ml/kg once every 30 days for 3 treatments. As with other treatments, it is very important that the owner maintain a clean environment for the patient with regular cleaning of the cage, at least 2 times a week, while it is on the medication protocol.

Small Rodents

Three species of mites are found in hamsters: *Demodex criceti*, *Demodex aurati*, and *Notoedres* spp.[6] Imidacloprid and moxidectin (Advantage Multi for cats 9 weeks of age and 5.1–9 lbs, topical solution, Bayer HealthCare LLC, Animal Health Division, Shawnee Mission, KS) can be used to treat the *Demodex* spp. hamster mites at a dose of 1 drop topically once a week. *Notoedres* spp. are found around the hairless areas of the body: nose, ears, feet, and genitals.[6] *Spleorodens clethrionomys*, the nasal mite, and *Ornithonyssus bacoti*, the tropical rat mite, can also infest hamsters.[6] Diagnosis of ectoparasites in small rodents is similar to that in other species listed in this text. A skin scraping of the affected area will usually yield the parasite that needs to be treated.

Ivermectin is the drug of choice for ectoparasites in small mammals and pocket pets. Topical spot applications of amitraz, using a cotton-tipped applicator, work the best on very small mammals diagnosed with *Demodex* spp.

Gerbils are generally healthy animals; consequently, they are not very susceptible to parasite infestations. If parasites are suspected, follow the instructions for diagnostic testing used in other small rodents. *Demodex* spp., causing clinical dermatological lesions, including alopecia, have been reported.[4] Parasites are not a problem in healthy animals, and underlying causes of immunosuppression must be investigated if they are diagnosed. The same dose of imidacloprid and moxidectin topical solution described for hamsters can be used for gerbils diagnosed with *Demodex* spp.

Specific parasites identified in rats include the dwarf tapeworm (*Hymenolepis nana*), pinworms (*Syphacia muris*), nematodes (specifically *Trichosomoides crassicauda*), *Giardia muris*, and the following ectoparasites: *Ornithonyssus bacoti* (tropical rat mite), *Radfordia ensifera* (rat fur mite), *Demodex nanus*, *Polyplax spinulosa* (spined rat louse), and fleas. Diagnosis and treatment are similar to those recommended for mice, although the dosages and duration will differ. The dose of imidacloprid and moxidectin topical solution for rats is 1 drop topically once a month to treat external parasites.

A number of parasites have been identified in mice. *Hymenolepis nana* (dwarf tapeworm) and *Cysticercus fasciolaris* (larval stage of the cat tapeworm) can be isolated from these small rodents. The dwarf tapeworm is often found in young mice that are dead or in mice that present with severe gastroenteritis (resulting in diarrhea). Diagnosis of the dwarf tapeworm can be made with a fecal flotation exam or by finding the tapeworms in the small intestine at necropsy. Dwarf tapeworm can be treated with praziquantal.

Syphacia oblevata are commensal oxyurid nematodes that feed on bacteria that inhabit the intestinal tract of mice.[6] Although nonpathogenic in most cases, an overwhelming number can cause severe irritation of the terminal gastrointestinal tract. These nematode parasites can be diagnosed using transparent tape and applying it to the rectal area. After removing the tape from the affected rectal area, it can be placed on a slide and the ova viewed under a microscope. Ivermectin and fenbendazole have been used effectively in treating this parasite in mice.[6]

Giardia muris is a common protozoal parasite that affects mice. This organism can be seen using a direct fecal examination. Metronidazole is the treatment of choice for *Giardia* infections in small rodents.

Ectoparasitism in mice is a presentation that clinicians often see and diagnose. *Myobia musculi, Myocoptes musculinis, Radfordia affinis,* and *Psoregates* simplex are all mice fur mites that can cause severe self-mutilation and hair loss (Figure 5.17).

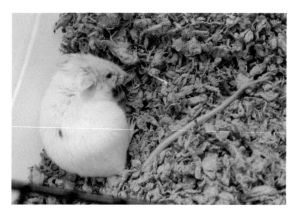

Figure 5.17 *Mice are susceptible to ectoparasites and often present with alopecia.*

Polyplax serrata, the house mouse louse, can cause anemia, pruritus, dermatitis, and death.[6] Diagnosis of ectoparasites in mice is similar to that in other companion animal species. Treatment of ectoparasites can be accomplished with ivermectin and topical mitacide. As with those of other rodent species, there appears to be an increasing resistance to ivermectin by ectoparasites that affect mice. The dose to treat mice ectoparasites with imidacloprid and moxidectin topical solution) is 1 drop once every 30 days.

Internal Parasites

Guinea Pigs

Not many internal parasites of consequence are commonly diagnosed in pet guinea pigs. *Cryptosporidium wrairi* is a protozoal diarrhea that infects the small intestine and can cause death.[5] Clinical signs are consistent with other gastrointestinal illnesses, including diarrhea, anorexia, and weight loss. This infection is rare, but possibly zoonotic. There is no effective treatment for guinea pigs with this disease.

Small Rodents

Hymenolepis nana, the dwarf tapeworm, can cause constipation in hamsters. Diagnosis can be made by finding individual eggs with polar bodies during fecal examination, or by finding the whole worm within the lumen of the small intestine during necropsy.[6]

As mentioned earlier, this is a zoonotic parasite and proper precautions should be taken regarding hygiene to prevent exposure after handling the animal. Recommended treatment for *H. nana* is praziquantel (Droncit, Bayer HealthCare LLC, Animal Health Division, Shawnee Mission, KS, 5–10 mg/kg IM or SC).

THERAPEUTICS: ALL RODENTS

This section will include the therapeutic issues for all small mammals and pocket pets. The size of these patients contributes to the difficulty in properly administering therapeutic medication. The scruff of the neck and caudal flank are the subcutaneous sites that can be used to administer medication or fluids.[7] The semitendinosus, triceps, or epaxial muscles are commonly used for intramuscular injections, whereas intraperitoneal injections are used in extremely small species.[7] On larger rodents and pocket pets, intravenous injections can be given in the cephalic, saphenous, or jugular vein.[7] Intraosseous catheters are much easier to administer in these small animals than intravenous catheters. The tibial plateau and the greater trochanter are the sites of choice for intraosseous catheter placement in pocket pets.[7]

Although many methods can be used to administer medication in small mammals, oral treatment (using a dropper or tuberculin syringe) is the easiest and least stressful to the patient. Medication can be added to the food or water, but often the patient is anorexic, which means that the medicated food/water is not palatable. Hence, the patient will not self-treat.

SURGICAL AND ANESTHETIC ASSISTANCE: ALL RODENTS

Inducing and maintaining guinea pigs, other small rodents, and pocket pets under anesthesia can be very challenging. There are still concerns and differences in anesthetic protocol because of these animals' small size, but in general, isoflurane anesthesia is a safe agent when used on a relatively healthy surgical candidate.

An induction chamber is used to induce the patients and then they are maintained under gas anesthesia using a face mask (Figures 5.18, 5.19, and 5.20). Although it might be possible to intubate a larger rodent or pocket pet, it is very difficult under most conditions.[8] Guinea pigs will have elevated fluid accumulation around the glottis if it is irritated during intubation. The elevated fluid will increase the difficulty of intubating the animal and could result in aspiration or apnea. In most cases a guinea pig can be maintained for a procedure in which general anesthesia is required by using a face mask.

Guinea pigs have a tendency to regurgitate gastric contents when under general anesthesia; therefore, it is recommended to fast these animals at least 2–4 hours prior to surgery.[8] To guard against aspiration of stomach contents in a patient that is not intubated, place the head and neck in a position slightly higher than the body.

Table 5.17 provides guidelines for surgical preparation and assistance in surgical procedures on small exotic animals.[9]

Premedication and sedation doses for rodents are listed in Table 5.18. If the surgeon wants to perform the procedure under injectable general anesthesia, the doses are listed in Table 5.19. Analgesia is important for patient recovery and should be administered prior to, during, and after surgery, depending on the case presentation and

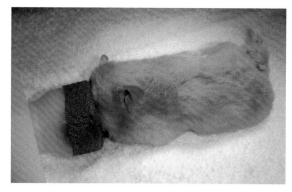

Figure 5.18 *Hamsters as well as other exotic small mammals are often maintained on gas anesthesia by using a face mask.*

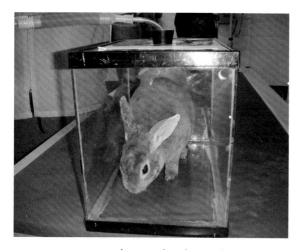

Figure 5.19 *An induction chamber is often used to induce exotic small mammals for general gas anesthesia.*

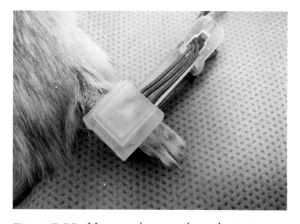

Figure 5.20 *Mouse under general anesthesia, in preparation for surgery.*

Table 5.17 Basic Surgery Guidelines for Rodents and Pocket Pets[9]

1. Obtain accurate body weight.

2. Know the appropriate preoperative fasting interval.

3. Properly dose and administer medication.

4. Minimize stress through premedication or minimal handling.

5. Administer oxygen when using only injection anesthesia.

6. Prevent hypothermia by using external heat sources.

7. Provide fluid therapy and maintain hemostasis during surgery.

procedure being performed. In Table 5.20, analgesic drug doses are listed for small animals.

Rat Intubation

Although rats are often maintained on general anesthesia with a face mask, if needed they can be intubated. A speculum (Hallowell Engineering and Manufacturing Corp., Pittsfield, MA) has been developed specifically to intubate rats and a smaller one for mice. The rat patient is premedicated with midazolam (1–2 mg/kg IM) and buprenorphine (0.02–0.05 mg/kg SC) prior to the intubation procedure. Once sedated, the patient

Table 5.18 Premedication and Sedation Drug Doses for Rodents[9]

DRUG	GUINEA PIG	RAT	MOUSE	HAMSTER	GERBIL
Acepromazine	0.5–1.5	0.5–2.5	0.5–2.5	0.5–5.0	0
Diazepam	1.0–5.0	3.0–5.0	3.0–5.0	3.0–5.0	3.0–5.0
Midazolam	1.0–2.0	1.0–2.0	1.0–2.0	1.0–2.0	1.0–2.0
Xylazine*	5.0–10.0	10.0–15.0	10.0–15.0	8.0–10.0	5.0–10.0
Atropine	0.05	0.05	0.05	0.05	0.05

*Xylazine has a reversal agent, Yohimine (0.2 mg/kg IV).
All doses are mg/kg and should be given IM or SC.

Table 5.19 Injectable Anesthesia in Rodents[9]

DRUG	GUINEA PIG	RAT	MOUSE	HAMSTER	GERBIL
Acepromazine/ Ketamine	0.5–1.0 20–50	2.5–5.0 50–150	2.5–5.0 50–150	2.5–5.0 50–150	0 0
Xylazine/ Ketamine	3.0–5.0 20–40	5 90	5.0–10.0 50–200	5.0–10.0 50–150	2.0–3.0 50–70
Diazepam/ Ketamine	3.0–5.0 20–40	3.0–5.0 40–100	3.0–5.0 40–150	5 40–150	3.0–5.0 40–150
Tiletamine/ Zolazepam	20–40	50–80	50–80	50–80	50–80

All doses are mg/kg and should be given IM.

Table 5.20   **Analgesic Doses for Rodents**

DRUG	GUINEA PIG	RAT	MOUSE	HAMSTER	GERBIL
Butorphanol	2 (q2h–4h)	2 (q2h–4h)	1.0–5.0 (q2h–4h)	1.0–5.0 (q2h–4h)	1.0–5.0 (q2h–4h)
Buprenorphine	0.005 (q8h–12h)	0.05–0.1 (q8h–12h)	0.05–0.1 (q8h–12h)	0.05–0.1 (q8h–12h)	0.05–0.1 (q8h–12h)

All doses are mg/kg and should be given SC or IM.

is placed in ventral recumbency with the head elevated. With a pair of hemostats, the tongue is retracted, allowing for visualization of the glottis with the aid of the rat speculum. A drop of lidocaine is then placed on the glottis using a catheter sheath, after which one should wait approximately 60 seconds prior to the intubation attempt. For most adult rats a soft 16- to 20-gauge catheter sheath can be used, through which a stiff piece of fishing line is passed to act as a guide. The tongue should be retracted again and the glottis visualized using the speculum attached to an otoscope head. Insert the fishing line into the trachea, remove the speculum, and feed the endotracheal tube through the fishing line into the trachea. Be careful not to bend the very flexible catheter sheath that is now serving as an endotracheal tube. The endotracheal tube can then be tied in place and verified through the use of positive pressure ventilation. Similar placement of an endotracheal tube can be performed on a mouse.

HEALTH MAINTENANCE AND DISEASE

GUINEA PIGS
Scurvy
Guinea pigs lack the ability to endogenously synthesize ascorbic acid. Therefore, to maintain proper health, it is essential that a dietary supplement of vitamin C be provided. Common signs associated with vitamin C deficiency include hemorrhage in the joints and gingiva, malocclusion, rough hair coat, alopecia, anorexia, lameness, and bruxism. The appropriate vitamin C supplementation for guinea pigs is 15–25 mg/day, and for pregnant animals 30 mg/day.[6] Vitamin C can be ingested in the food and water or on the food as a supplement. Fresh cabbage, kale, and oranges are sources of supplemental vitamin C.[6]

"Bumblefoot"
"Bumblefoot," or infectious pododermatitis, is usually the result of footpad trauma progressing into a chronic *Staphylococcus aureus* infection.[6] The initiating cause of many bumblefoot infections is inadequate caging substrate, particularly wire-bottom cages and abrasive bedding material. Owners must be informed of the guarded prognosis in resolving these foot infections. Surgical debridement, topical and systemic antibiotic treatment, and bandaging of the affected feet are required to improve the chances of recovery. To prevent recurrence, the owner should be advised to change the substrate and floor of the cage into a solid floor with nonabrasive bedding.

"Lumps"
Lumps is a common term given to a disease of the cervical lymph nodes that results in abscessation owing to a *Streptococcus zooepidemicus* infection (Figures 5.21A and 5.21B). *S. zooepidemicus* is part of the normal flora of guinea pig conjunctival

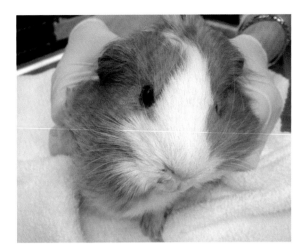

Figure 5.21A *A common disease presentation of guinea pigs is submandibular abscessation.*

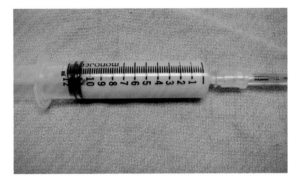

Figure 5.21B *Aspirated purulent material collected from a submandibular abscess.*

and nasal mucosa.[6] Once the oral mucosa has been compromised, usually by poor-quality hay, the bacteria travel through the bloodstream into the cervical lymph nodes. Complete surgical excision of the affected lymph nodes is recommended for treating the disease. The owner should be informed of the disease process and measures taken to prevent recurrence, including stress reduction and a quality diet.

Malocclusion

Guinea pigs have open-rooted incisors, premolars, and molars. Open-rooted teeth grow continuously and, if the teeth are not properly aligned, malocclusion will occur—resulting in overgrowth of the affected teeth. All of the teeth previously mentioned can become overgrown, resulting in anorexia and hypersalivation. The teeth should be trimmed on a regular basis to prevent the inability to eat and trauma to the tongue and buccal surface. General anesthesia is recommended for trimming the molars and premolars, although the incisors can be trimmed using regular restraint. Vitamin C deficiency has been implicated as a possible contributor to the disease process owing to the breakdown of collagen formation in the tooth socket, causing instability that leads to malocclusion.

Antibiotic-Associated Enterotoxemia

When treating guinea pigs with antibiotics, it must be remembered that their normal gastrointestinal flora are predominantly Gram-positive organisms.[6] Classes of drugs that include penicillin and aminoglycosides will kill the normal gastrointestinal flora, causing an overgrowth of *Clostridium difficile*.[6] **Never prescribe antibiotics for a guinea pig patient unless there is a reference for its use in this species.** Other antibiotics that are recommended for use in guinea pigs should be monitored during the treatment period. If there is any evidence of the patient becoming anorexic or having diarrhea, the medication should be discontinued and the patient rechecked for drug-induced gastroenteritis. Placing the patient on a probiotic or yogurt supplement while it is being treated with antibiotics might be helpful.

HAMSTERS

This section will review the common hamster diseases seen in veterinary practice. An overview of etiology, treatment, and prevention will follow a brief description of the disease presentation.

"Wet-Tail"

Diarrhea and gastrointestinal disorders in hamsters have been given a common name by the medical community and general public: "wet-tail." A number of conditions and bacterial organisms can contribute to this condition, but the primary organisms implicated in this disorder are different for young and adult animals.

In young hamsters (3–10 weeks old) proliferative ileitis is commonly caused by *Lawsonia intracellularis*.[7] This disease must be treated aggressively with fluid therapy, antibiotics, and force-feeding. One of the recommended antibiotic regimes is enrofloxacin (10 mg/kg PO q12h for 5–7 days).[7] Fluid therapy is very important to combat electrolyte imbalances caused by diarrhea, dehydration, and anorexia. An electrolyte and glucose injection, at a dose of 40–60 ml/kg SC q24h, should help maintain fluid and electrolyte levels within the body.[7] Force-feeding a finely ground mixture of one-half fruits and vegetables and one-half hamster pellets, at a dose of 20–30 ml/kg q24h PO, will increase the caloric intake and energy level of the patient.[7]

When an improper antibiotic is selected to treat adult hamsters that present with diarrhea, normal flora can be killed, resulting in overgrowth of *Clostridium difficile*. Penicillin, lincomycin, and bacitracin are all antibiotic choices that will contribute to the death of normal gut flora in hamsters, leading to enterotoxemia.[7]

Tyzzer's disease, caused by the bacterium *Clostridium piliforme*, brings about significant gastrointestinal illness in hamsters and gerbils, but not in rats and mice.[7] Tyzzer's disease is commonly transmitted between animals in displays and holding areas. This gastrointestinal bacterial infection primarily affects immunosuppressed, stressed animals.

Neoplasia

The average life span of a hamster is 2 years. The short life span and aging process increase the prevalence of tumors in these small rodents. If an animal is more than 18 months of age, neoplastic disease should be considered as a differential diagnosis, especially if an asymmetrical mass is present. Treatment is removal of the affected tissue, if possible, to increase the quality of life for the small rodent.

Ocular System

Hamsters might present with one or both eyes protruding from the socket(s). If the animal is grabbed too tightly on the back of the neck, the eyes will start to bulge out of the sockets. If the eyes do prolapse from the socket, the eye and ocular area should be moistened with ophthalmic wash and lubricant (the lid margins retracted) and the globe gently returned to its normal anatomical location. The animal should then be maintained on antibiotic ophthalmic treatment for a week to 10 days.[7] If the problem recurs, a tarsorrhaphy or enucleation may be indicated.

Trauma

If two or more hamsters are housed together in the same cage, it is not uncommon for bite wounds to occur (Figure 5.22). These wounds often become infected and should be treated by shaving the hair around the wound, culture of the affected area, flushing with a dilute antimicrobial solution, then treating with a topical antibiotic along with systemic antibiotic therapy.

GERBILS
"Sore Nose"

"Sore nose" in gerbils is a disease condition thought to be caused by an increased secretion of porphyrins.[5] The harderian gland secretes porphyrins, which act as a primary skin irritant around the nasal opening. The irritated skin area is susceptible to secondary bacterial infections caused by *Staphylococcus* spp. Treating the resulting infectious dermatitis and reducing stress to the animal will usually resolve the problem (Figure 5.23).

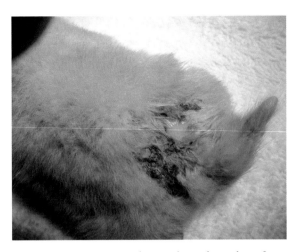

Figure 5.22 *Hamsters that are housed together often fight and may develop bite wound abscesses.*

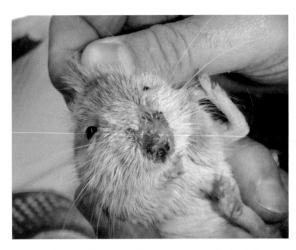

Figure 5.23 *"Sore nose" is a common clinical disease presentation of gerbils.*

Epileptiform Seizures

At around 2 months of age, 20%–40% of gerbils develop epileptiform seizures.[5] There is no treatment for the seizures, which usually last for a few minutes but do not appear to leave any permanent physical damage. As the animal ages, the seizure activity declines in severity and occurrence.

RATS

Bacterial and Viral Infections

Staphylococcus aureus is the most common cause of ulcerative dermatitis in rats.[7] *Mycoplasma pulmonis, Streptococcus pneumoniae, Corynebacterium kutscheri,* Sendai virus, and cilia-associated respiratory bacillus have been isolated and identified as infectious agents causing rat respiratory disease. With respiratory pathogens, clinical signs can vary from mild dyspnea to severe pneumonia and death. The treatment of mycoplasmosis in rats is similar to that described for infected mice in the next section.

Tumors

Rats are very susceptible to tumors, most likely because of the animals' average life expectancy of approximately 3 years and their physiologic predisposition. The most common subcutaneous tumor in rats is the fibroadenoma of the mammary tissue (Figure 5.24).[7] Mammary tumors can reach very large sizes and affect both males and females. To reduce the incidence of fibroadenomas, ovariohysterectomies are advocated at an early age in female rats. Whereas mammary tumors in mice are almost always malignant, rat mammary tumors are usually localized and respond to surgical resection (Figure 5.25).

Sialodacryoadenitis Virus

This virus is a cornavirus that affects the cervical salivary glands and sometimes the lacrimal glands of the eye. The cervical lymph nodes can become enlarged, and the eyes might protrude if the lacrimal gland(s) are affected. There is no treatment for this highly contagious disease.

MICE

Barbering

Barbering is a condition in which a cagemate bites fur from the affected area to the skin without caus-

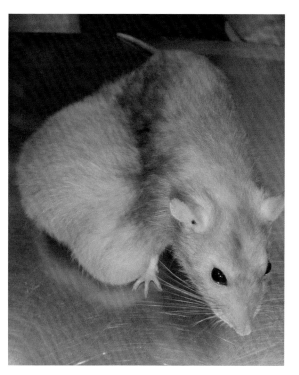

Figure 5.24 *Mammary tumors are commonly diagnosed in older female rats.*

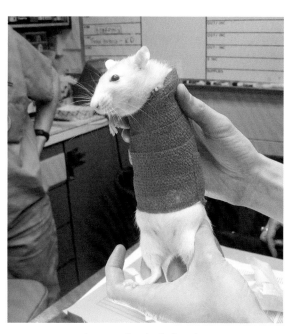

Figure 5.25 *A rat with a body bandage to prevent self-trauma to a surgical site that involved the removal of a mammary tumor.*

ing any dermatological damage. This condition is usually caused by stress induced by overcrowding or because of the establishment of a hierarchy within the group.

Tumors

As with many small rodents, mammary tumors are a common presentation in older female mice. The most common mammary tumor found in mice is the adenocarcinoma.[7]

Bacterial and Viral Infections

Bacterial infections associated with dermatitis lesions and subcutaneous abscesses in mice are commonly caused by *Staphylococcus aureus*, *Pasteurella pneumontropica*, and *Streptococcus pyogenes*.[7] Acute and chronic respiratory infections can be caused by Sendai virus or *Mycoplasma pulmonis*, but are most commonly associated with Sendai virus, from which adults survive but neonates often die. Chronic respiratory infections—with clinical signs of pneumonia, suppurative rhinitis, and occasionally otitis media—might be the result of a *M. pulmonis* infection. Both infections should be treated using supportive care, although mycoplasmosis can be treated specifically with enrofloxacin in combination with doxycycline hyclate for 7 days.[7]

ZOONOTIC DISEASES: GUINEA PIGS

There are not many zoonotic diseases associated with guinea pigs. The zoonotic diseases that could cause problems are rarely transmitted to human caretakers. *Trixacarus caviae*, or the guinea pig sarcoptic mite, may be the most problematic. When guinea pigs are being treated for a mite infestation, owners should take precautions against exposure.

Guinea pig dermatophyte, or "ringworm" infections, can be transmitted to humans. Dermatophyte infections, particularly *Trichophyton mentagrophytes*, do not commonly affect guinea pigs; but if diagnosed, environmental cleaning and patient treatment are required to resolve the disease condition. Again, owners should be instructed to use caution to prevent exposure and possible contamination.

SELF-STUDY QUESTIONS

1. Which rodent requires vitamin C supplementation, and how is this vitamin provided to prevent a deficiency?

2. How are rodents sexed?

3. What are the dietary recommendations for rodents?

4. What are the husbandry requirements for pet rodents?

5. Describe nutritional recommendations for each rodent species commonly kept as a companion animal.

6. How would you properly restrain a rodent patient for a physical examination?

7. Describe how to perform a physical examination on rodent patients.

8. How and where is blood collected from each rodent species for diagnostic sampling?

9. What are the proper procedures for collecting bone marrow and urine from rodent patients?

10. What are the common pathogenic organisms cultured from rodents?

11. What is the anal tape test? Why is it used?

12. Describe common external parasites diagnosed in pet rodents and recommended treatment options.

13. How are rodents sedated, induced, and maintained on general anesthesia? Describe how rats are intubated.

14. Describe common rodent disease presentations and treatment options.

REFERENCES

Guinea Pig

1. Harkness JE. *Pet rodents: A guide for practitioners*. Lakewood, CO: AAHA Press; 1997.
2. Johnson-Delaney CA, and Harrison LR. *Guinea pigs. Exotic companion medicine handbook for veterinarians*. Lake Worth, FL: Wingers Publishing; 1996:1–20.
3. Quesenberry KE, Donnelly TM, and Hillyer EV. Biology, husbandry and clinical techniques of guinea pigs and chinchillas. In: Quesenberry, KE, and Carpenter, JW, eds. *Ferrets, rabbits and rodents: Clinical medicine and surgery*, 2nd ed. St. Louis, MO: Saunders/Elsevier; 2004:232–44.
4. Cualiffe-Beamer T, and Les E. The laboratory mouse. In: Poole TB, ed. *The UFAW handbook on the care and management of laboratory animals*. Essex: Longman Scientific & Technical;1994:290–91.
5. Chrisp CE, Suckow MA, Fayer R, et al. Comparison of the host ranges and antigenicity of *Cryptosporidium parvum* and *Cryptosporidium wrairi* from guinea pigs. *J Protozool* 1992;39:406–49.
6. O'Rourke DP. Disease problems of guinea pigs. In: Quesenberry KE, and Carpenter JW, eds. *Ferrets, rabbits and rodents: Clinical medicine and surgery*, 2nd ed. St. Louis, MO: Saunders/Elsevier; 2004:245–54.
7. Adamcak A, and Otten B. Rodent therapeutics. *Vet Clinics of North America. Exotic Animal Practice*. January 2000;3:221–35.
8. Bennett RA. Soft tissue surgery. In: Quesenberry KE, and Carpenter JW, eds. *Ferrets, rabbits and rodents: Clinical medicine and surgery*, 2nd ed. St. Louis, MO: Saunders/Elsevier; 2004:316–29.
9. Heard DJ. Anesthesia, analgesia and sedation for small mammals. In: Quesenberry KE, and Carpenter JW, eds. *Ferrets, rabbits and rodents: Clinical medicine and surgery*, 2nd ed. St. Louis, MO: Saunders/Elsevier; 2004:356–69.

Hamster, Rat, and Mouse

1. Johnson-Delaney CA, and Harrison LR. *Small rodent: Exotic companion medicine handbook for veterinarians*. Lake Worth, FL: Wingers Publishing 1996:48–61.
2. Harkness JE. *Pet rodents: A guide for practitioners*. Lakewood, CO: AAHA Press; 1997:27–30.
3. McClure DE. Clinical pathology and sample collection in the laboratory rodent. *Vet Clinics of North America. Exotic Animal Practice* (September 1999);2:565–90.
4. Silverman J. Biomethodology. In: Vantloosier GL Jr., and McPherson EW, eds. *Laboratory hamsters*. Orlando, FL: Academic Press; 1987:70–94.
5. Bihun C, and Bauck L. Small rodents, basic anatomy, physiology, and clinical techniques. In: Quesenberry KE, and Carpenter JW, eds. *Ferrets, rabbits and rodents: Clinical medicine and surgery*, 2nd ed. St. Louis, MO: Saunders/Elsevier; 2004:286–98.
6. Morrisey JK. Parasites of ferrets, rabbits and rodents. *Seminar on Avian Exotic Pet Medicine* 1996;5:106–14.
7. Donelly TM. Disease problems of small rodents. In: Quesenberry KE, and Carpenter JW, eds. *Ferrets, rabbits and rodents: Clinical medicine and surgery*, 2nd ed. St. Louis, MO: Saunders/Elsevier; 2004:299–315.

Gerbil

1. Wong R, Gray-Allan P, Chifa C, and Alfred B. Social preference of female gerbils (*Meriones unguiculatus*) as influenced by coat color of males. *Behavioral Neural Biology* 1990;54: 184–90.

2. Johnson-Delaney CA, and Harrison LR. *Small rodents: Exotic companion medicine handbook for veterinarians.* Lake Worth, FL: Wingers Publishing; 1996:38–46.

3. Bihun C, and Bauck L. Small rodents, basic anatomy, physiology, and clinical techniques. In: Quesenberry KE, and Carpenter JW, eds. *Ferrets, rabbits and rodents: Clinical medicine and surgery,* 2nd ed. St. Louis, MO: Saunders/Elsevier; 2004:286–98.

4. Morrisey JK. Parasites of ferrets, rabbits and rodents. *Seminar on Avian Exotic Pet Medicine* 1996;5(2):106–14.

5. Donelly TM. Disease problems of small rodents. In: Quesenberry KE, and Carpenter JW, eds. *Ferrets, rabbits and rodents: Clinical medicine and surgery,* 2nd ed. St. Louis, MO: Saunders/Elsevier; 2004:299–315.

CHAPTER 6

Hedgehogs

INTRODUCTION

Hedgehogs are shy, nocturnal mammals from the order Insectivora. Although these animals are known primarily for their sharp quills, there are many other fascinating characteristics about them. In the United States, the most common hedgehog pet species is the white-bellied, four-toed African or African pygmy hedgehog (*Atelerix albiventris*).[1] These animals were originally imported two to three decades ago, but are now captive bred in large numbers. Although they have not yet garnered the popularity of other small exotic mammals (e.g., rabbits and guinea pigs), they have certainly found a niche among pet owners.

Anatomy and Physiology

The most obvious anatomic peculiarity associated with hedgehogs is their quills (Figure 6.1). Although these quills are a useful antipredator tool in the wild, they make the job of veterinary personnel charged with examining them challenging. When aggravated, the classic response of a hedgehog is to "ball up." Because of their unique anatomy, they are capable of completely tucking in their short limbs and forming an impenetrable "ball of quills." Fortunately, as these animals age and are handled, they become more agreeable to examination. In cases when they don't, general anesthesia can be used to limit the effect of the quills.

The quills of hedgehogs are not barbed, but do come to a sharp point (Figure 6.2). There is also a misconception that they can inject venom. Although hedgehog quills are not venomous, it is not uncommon for hedgehogs to "anoint" their quills with saliva, which can introduce bacterial pathogens into puncture wounds of would-be predators or unprotected handlers. When hedgehogs are not on alert, they lay their quills down, and touching them is analogous to petting rigid hair; however, any time hedgehogs become

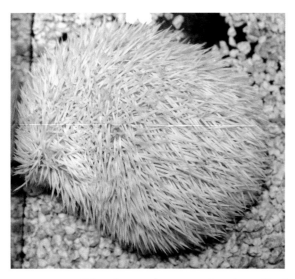

Figure 6.1 *Although it might appear that the quills of an African hedgehog cover their entire body, in actuality they cover only their dorsum.*

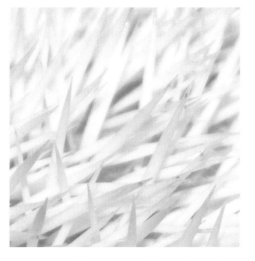

Figure 6.2 *This close-up of the quills reinforces how sharp they are at their point. Veterinary personnel working with these animals should wear appropriate leather gloves to minimize the likelihood of injuring themselves or the animal (e.g., by dropping the animal).*

defensive, they can erect their quills, using a combination of muscles to create a protective barrier. The primary muscle groups associated with control over the quills are the front dorsalis, caudodorsal, and panniculus carnosus orbicularis. Because most hedgehogs consider a visit to the veterinary hospital a negative experience, veterinary personnel working with hedgehogs should wear leather gloves (e.g., welder's or gardening gloves) to reduce the likelihood of being injured. Hypersensitivity reactions to hedgehog quills have been documented.

Hedgehogs are well suited for a terrestrial existence. They have long snouts that they use, similar to pigs, for rooting out grubs and vegetation (Figure 6.3). The eyes of hedgehogs are small, dark (or pink in leucistic or albino animals), and set back. They appear to rely more on their sense of smell than on their vision. Hedgehogs have short hair–covered ears. It is not uncommon for them to have crusts or splints in the edges of their ears. Although at times this finding is associated with a mite infestation, at other times it appears to be related to low environmental humidity. These animals should be maintained in 30%–50% humidity to limit the potential for dry skin. The teeth of hedgehogs have closed roots, so dental conditions should be managed like those of a dog or cat. Their dental pattern is: incisors 3/2, canine 1/1, premolars 3/2, and molars 3/3. Their incisors are normally slightly procumbent and have a wide gap.

Sexing hedgehogs is straightforward. Males have an obvious prepuce, but no scrotum. They also have open inguinal rings, which allow them to move their testicles between the inguinal region and abdomen. Females have an obvious vulva that is cranial but close to the anus. The gestation of hedgehogs is approximately 35 days. Although these animals can become sexually mature before

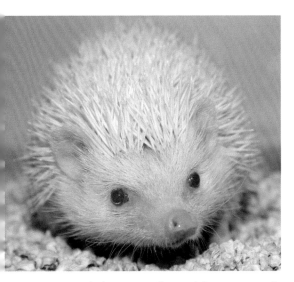

Figure 6.3 *Hedgehogs are well suited for a terrestrial existence. Note the long snout for rooting, the short legs, and the deep-set eyes.*

6 months, it is recommended to delay breeding until after 6 months to minimize problems with dystocia.

The average longevity for hedgehogs is 3–5 years. Although these animals should be capable of living 6–10 years, many succumb to cancer much earlier. Captive hedgehogs appear to have a high prevalence of neoplasia compared with other species.[2,3]

Hedgehogs have some interesting behaviors that can be confusing to those with limited experience with these animals. A hedgehog, when presented with a new object, might perform a ritual called self-anointing. The animal first licks the object, then begins to hypersalivate. This frothy saliva is then rubbed on its skin and spines; the purpose of this ritual is unknown.[3] Some people have confused this with rabies, but this is a normal behavior elicited under certain conditions.

Hedgehogs are territorial, as are most small mammals; therefore, close monitoring for fighting is required when a new animal is introduced to a group within an enclosure. Males are typically solitary, but do maintain harems. As with other animals, it is important for the technician to know the normal physiologic values in order to assess the patient's health status. In Table 6.1,[2] a list of common physiologic data used to interpret a physical examination can be found.

HUSBANDRY

Environmental Concerns

Pet hedgehogs can be maintained in the environmental temperatures favored by human inhabitants of the house (70°–78°F). Cold environmental temperatures (<65°F) can induce brumation (a type of hibernation) in hedgehogs. This can lead to reduced metabolism and increased likelihood of opportunistic infections. Sustained warm temperatures

Table 6.1 **Hedgehog Basic Information**[2]

GENERAL CATEGORY	CLASSIFICATION	PHYSIOLOGIC PARAMETERS/QUANTITY
Average Life Span		3–5 years
Body Weight	Adult Male	500–600 g
	Adult Female	250–400 g
	Birth Weight	Average 10 g
Temperature	Rectal Body Temperature	97°–100°F
Female Reproductive Cycle	Gestation Length	34–37 days
	Litter Size	3 average

(>88°F) can lead to heat stress, which can be fatal. Owners should be informed that if they live in environments where the ambient temperature is higher or lower than that considered acceptable for a hedgehog, they might need to provide supplemental heat or cooling for their pet.

The preferred housing for these small, spiny animals is a glass-sided enclosure with a commercial screen top that can be secured with tabs or screws. The "hedgehog house" should have enough floor surface area to include a small hiding box, a specific hedgehog exercise wheel (wire wheels are dangerous), and a pan or shallow dish for swimming. Plastic-sided cages with appropriately sized wire bars (not too large, or they will allow escape or injury) can also be used. The cage substrate of choice is shredded newspaper or a pelleted paper product. Woodchips, ground corncob, ground walnut shell, and cloth towels are not recommended for hedgehog cage flooring, because these materials might be inappropriately ingested or cause string strangulation of the limbs. Instruct the client to clean the enclosure and substrate regularly, because glass tanks have poor ventilation, and a buildup of urine and fecal material can lead to respiratory problems.

Nutrition

Hedgehogs need fresh water daily. Although they can learn to drink from sipper tubes, a small shallow dish might be preferred as a water container. These animals are naturally insectivores/omnivores, and their diet should reflect their dietary wants and nutritional needs. Commercial pelleted hedgehog diets can be used, but they should be used in combination with vegetables, fruits, and insects. When insects are offered, they should be "gut loaded" to maximize their nutritional value. It is important to read the labels of commercial hedgehog diets. These products are not regulated, and there can be extreme differences in the quality of the foods. For example, one commercial product has 15% protein and another has 35% protein. This is a >100% difference in protein. Hedgehogs fed one of these diets might be provided too much protein, depending on what else is in their diet, and the animal fed the lower-protein diet may not receive sufficient protein. Because hedgehogs are omnivores, like humans, diversity in their diet is best. A recommended diet for adult hedgehogs is provided in Table 6.2, and should be followed if a commercial diet is not available. Hedgehogs are capable of digesting chitin and have a relatively low metabolism. Advise owners to avoid high-fat, soft, or high-sugar foods to avoid obesity, a common problem in hedgehogs.

Transport

Hedgehogs can be transported in their enclosure, if small enough, or carriers suitable for small mammals (e.g., guinea pigs, rats).

Grooming

Hedgehogs may develop long claws that require routine trimming. If the claws need to be trimmed, the same technique as described for a rat (Chapter 5) can be used. In most cases the hedgehog will need to be sedated. An alternative method for an alert hedgehog is to place the animal on a screen and trim the claws as they extend through the mesh.

HISTORY

A thorough history is essential to making an appropriate diagnosis for any exotic animal case, because many of the problems identified in exotic animals are directly related to inappropriate hus-

Table 6.2 **Hedgehog Daily Diet**[2]

---

1. 3 heaping teaspoons high-quality cat/kitten chow

2. 1 heaping teaspoon fruit/vegetable mix
   Finely chop all ingredients and mix together:
   → ½ teaspoon leafy dark greens (spinach, kale, leaf lettuce)
   → ¼ teaspoon diced carrot, ¼ teaspoon diced apple,
   → ¼ teaspoon diced banana, ¼ teaspoon diced grape or raisin
   → ¼ teaspoon vitamin/mineral powder (e.g., Vionate)

3. 6 small mealworms or 1–2 crickets

---

bandry. A veterinary technician should first collect the signalment, including age and sex of the hedgehog. Knowledge of the animal's age and sex can be useful when developing a differential diagnosis list. For example, an adult intact female hedgehog may be more likely to suffer from a reproductive neoplasia than a young, immature animal.

After defining the signalment, the history should focus on collecting background information, including where the animal was acquired, length of time owned, if the owner has other pets or hedgehogs, if he or she recently acquired another hedgehog, and the interaction between the owner and the pet. This information should provide the technician with an initial understanding of the client's knowledge of the pet hedgehog.

The next set of questions should focus on how the animal is managed at home (husbandry), including whether the animal is housed indoors or outdoors, if it has supervised or unsupervised run of the house, cage size and material, cage location in the house, whether animals are housed singly or together, substrate used in the cage, how often the cage is cleaned and type of disinfectant, whether a litter pan is used, and types of cage furniture (e.g., shelter). Questions about the animal's nutrition are also important

and should include types of food (e.g., commercial, live foods), brand, amount fed, frequency, supplements, water source, and how often the food and water are changed.

Finally, questions should focus on the animal's current health status and include past medical history, current presenting problem, and duration of complaint. Although it is natural to want to focus on the problem at hand, a great deal of information could be overlooked if the technician doesn't collect the history using a thorough and systematic approach.

RESTRAINT

The spines on these small mammals make restraint difficult. The animal handler should wear lightweight leather gloves (gardening or work gloves) to prevent injury to the technician or veterinarian examining the patient. Some hedgehogs are docile enough to be examined without "balling up," but there is always a possibility that they will become frightened and curl, causing pain to the handler. Most hedgehog patients need to be anesthetized with isoflurane or sevoflurane to facilitate the physical examination process. General anesthesia is quick and, in most cases, reduces stress to the animal and handler. The patient is induced in an induction chamber or large mask and maintained using an appropriately sized mask to fit over its snout. If the hedgehog will be kept under anesthesia for an extended time, it should be intubated. In some cases, it is preferable to give injectable preanesthetics to induce or extend anesthesia. A list of appropriate preanesthetics can be found in Table 6.3.

Other methods have been used to uncurl and examine these animals without using general anesthesia: (1) Rocking back and forth while holding the animal in ventral recumbency a few inches over

Table 6.3 Injectable Anesthetic Agents Used in Hedgehogs[4]

DRUG	ROUTE	DOSAGE
Ketamine	IM	5–20 mg/kg
Ketamine and Diazepam	IM	5–20 mg/kg (Ketamine) 0.5–2.0 mg/kg (Diazepam)
Ketamine and Xylazine	IM	10–20 mg/kg (Ketamine) 2 mg/kg (Xylazine)

the table; as the head extends from the curl, put one thumb on the back of the neck and the other on the back to encourage uncurling. (2) Stroke the rump spines in a circular pattern or backward motion. (3) Hold the animal facedown over the examination area. The hedgehog can be "scruffed" by holding the spined skin for restraint. These physical handling techniques are not recommended unless the animal is very ill or docile.

PHYSICAL EXAMINATION

The animal must be properly restrained. It is important that the technician or veterinarian be able to examine the entire animal without concern about being stuck by quills. A complete physical examination will be performed on each hedgehog patient that enters the clinic. The questions used to obtain the clinical history and physical examination procedures for hedgehogs are similar to those used for other small mammals. It is recommended that the examination begin with the nose, eyes, and ears. There should be no nasal discharge and the nose should be moist. The eyes should be clear and free of discharge. Positioning of the eyes should be noted, because severely dehydrated hedgehogs (>8%) will have sunken eyes. The corneas should be transparent. If there are any concerns about corneal ulcers, a fluorescein stain should be performed. The anterior chamber can be examined by using a direct light source. Hedgehogs have small globes and pupils, which make fundic exams difficult, even with mydriatics. The ears might have cerumen (earwax), which should be removed and examined for the presence of ear mites.

The oral cavity should be moist and pink. Examine the teeth for excess tartar. Because neoplasia is so common in hedgehogs (e.g., squamous cell carcinoma), it is important to look for masses in the oral cavity or any crusting around this area. The integument and spines should be examined closely. Any masses should be examined further, using fine needle aspirates and cytology or biopsy. Crusts and quill loss are common with dermatologic diseases such as mite infestations or ringworm. Again, if these types of lesions are seen on the examination, they should be noted and further evaluated using appropriate diagnostic tests (e.g., skin scrape and cytology and dermatophyte culture, respectively).

The areas where the submandibular, prescapular, axillary, lumbar, and popliteal lymph nodes are located should be palpated. In healthy hedgehogs, the lymph nodes will be small and not palpable. Abdominal palpation should include all four abdominal quadrants. Internal anatomy of hedgehogs is similar to that of other domestic pets, so veterinary technicians can rely on their experience with those species to determine what is normal or abnormal. The limbs should be palpated for any abnormal structures or crepitus. Examine the nails closely. Because hedgehogs are held on soft substrates in captivity, their nails tend to grow and curl under or around the foot-pads. Check the body temperature of a hedgehog using a plastic (not glass) thermometer. Hedgehog body temperatures are typically 97°–100°F.

Finally, auscult the hedgehog. Heart and respiratory rates are typically 160–220 and 30–40, respectively. Of course, the stress associated with travel to the clinic and the examination itself can alter these numbers.

DIAGNOSTIC SAMPLING

Blood Collection
Using a 1 or 3 cc syringe with a ¼" 26-gauge needle, blood samples can be collected from the superficial veins, including the lateral saphenous and cephalic veins. However, it is best to reserve the cephalic vein for intravenous catheter placement. For larger volumes of blood, the jugular vein, cranial vena cava, and femoral veins can be used. The cranial vena cava is the preferred venipuncture site for hedgehogs, because most of their other vessels are small and surrounded by subcutaneous fat. The cranial vena cava can be approached from either the right or left side of the thoracic inlet. A 3 cc syringe with a ⅝", 26- or 25-gauge needle can be used to collect the sample. The venipuncture site should be aseptically prepared using standard techniques. The needle should be inserted at the level of the first rib and manubrium (sternum) (Figures 6.4 and 6.5). The vessel is not typically

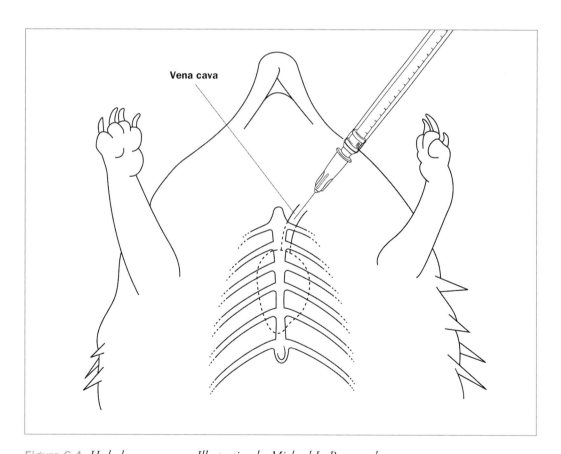

Figure 6.4 *Hedgehog vena cava. Illustration by Michael L. Broussard.*

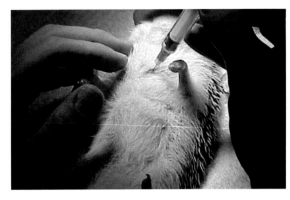

Figure 6.5 *The cranial vena cava is an excellent site for collecting blood samples from hedgehogs.*

Table 6.4 **Hedgehog Complete Blood Count Reference Ranges**

CELL TYPE	NORMAL RANGE
Erythrocytes	$4.4–6.0 \times 10^6/\mu l$
Hematocrit	28%–38%
Hemoglobin	9.9–13.1 g/dl
Leukocytes	$5.8–21.0 \times 10^3/\mu l$
Neutrophils	49%–70%
Lymphocytes	22%–38%
Eosinophils	2%–11%
Monocytes	0%
Basophils	0%–5%
Platelets	$200–412 \times 10^3/\mu l$
Serum Protein	5.3–6.3 g/dl
Albumin	3.4–3.6 g/dl

Table 6.5 **Hedgehog Serum Biochemistry Reference Ranges**

ANALYTE	REFERENCE RANGE
Serum Glucose	81.5–116.1 mg/dl
Blood Urea Nitrogen	21.3–32.9 mg/dl
Creatinine	0.2–0.4 mg/dl
Total Bilirubin	0–0.1 mg/dl
Serum Calcium	9.5–10.9 mg/dl
Serum Phosphorus	4.7–6.5 mg/dl
Alanine Aminotransferase (ALT)	39.7–68.9 IU/L

very deep, and it is unlikely you will need to insert the needle more than 0.25 cm into the chest. Blood for diagnostic sampling is best obtained from an anesthetized hedgehog rather than from one that is being manually restrained. Reference ranges for complete blood counts and serum chemistry panels are listed in Tables 6.4 and 6.5, respectively.[5]

Bone Marrow Aspiration

This is not a common procedure for hedgehog patients. Methods that have been described for other small animals (e.g., dogs, cats) should be used for hedgehogs while taking into account the relative size of their anatomical structures. A spinal needle should be used to access the marrow cavity of hedgehog bones (tibia or femur). The spinal needle has a stylet inside the cannula of the needle that will prevent plugging with bone and/or cartilage.

Microbiology

Microbiological samples can be obtained from hedgehog patients as with other small animals. Since the normal flora of hedgehog anatomical areas/body systems (e.g., reproductive, gastrointestinal, integument) have not been determined, critical assessment of the microbial isolates relative to the disease condition of the patient is highly recommended. Microbiological assessments of hedgehog disease conditions are as important as with other small-animal patients.

Urinalysis

Urinalysis can provide important insight into the general well-being of a hedgehog. Urine can be collected by cystocentesis, catheterization, or free catch.[4] Abnormal findings in hedgehog urine include white blood cells, neoplastic cells, and crystalluria.[4] Because these animals are omnivores, their urine should be screened using references for dogs.

Radiology

Other diagnostic procedures that need to be performed on hedgehogs are done in a manner similar to those used for other small mammals. Radiographs, for example, should be done under anesthesia. This will ensure that the animals are motionless and positioned in a manner so that desired organ systems/structures can be evaluated. A minimum of two survey radiographs should be collected from each animal. Radiographic interpretation is similar to that for domestic pets, although the quills can become superimposed over important soft tissues if the animal is not positioned correctly (Figures 6.6A and 6.6B).

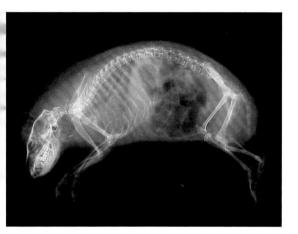

Figure 6.6A *Lateral radiograph of a hedgehog. Note the ileus in the small intestine. This animal had gastrointestinal disease associated with a neoplastic condition and an opportunistic bacterial infection.*

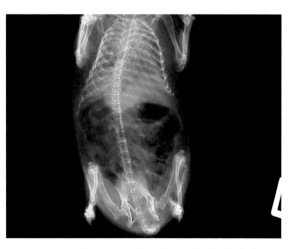

Figure 6.6B *Dorsoventral radiograph of a hedgehog.*

Parasitology

External Parasites

A common clinical presentation is quill loss owing to *Caparinia tripilis*, the common mange mite of hedgehogs.[6] Pruritus, quill loss, and hyperkeratosis are commonly associated with a quill mite infestation. Diagnosis can be made through skin scrapings of the affected area. Treatment can be achieved using ivermectin (0.2–0.4 mg/kg orally or subcutaneously every 10–14 days for 2 or 3 treatments); however, resistance can occur and higher doses may be necessary. Selamectin can also be used to treat hedgehogs with mite infestations. For an effective treatment, owners should be made aware that they must clean the environment at least every two days to prevent reinfestation.

Other mite species, including *Chorioptes* spp., fleas, and ticks, are also external parasites that might be found on hedgehogs.[5] Treatment and prevention of mites are similar to those used with other small mammals.

Internal Parasites

Routine fecal flotation and direct fecal parasite examinations are used to diagnose internal parasites. *Isospora eriniacei* and *Eimeria rastegaiv* are the common coccidian parasites identified in hedgehogs.[4] To treat coccidia, sulfadimethoxine is recommended (2 to 20 mg/kg, orally, daily for 2–5 days, skip 5 days and repeat).[4] Ponazuril (20 to 30 mg/kg, orally, every other day for 3 treatments), a coccidiocide, can also be used to eliminate coccidians.

Commonly identified nematode species include the lungworm (*Crenosoma striatum*), intestinal nematodes (*Capillaria erinacei*), tapeworms (*Hymenolepis erinacei*), and flukes (*Brachylaemus erinacei*). The treatment of choice for nematodes is fenbendazole (10–25 mg/kg orally) or ivermectin (0.2 mg/kg subcutaneously or orally).[4] Cestodes should be treated with praziquantel (7 mg/kg subcutaneously or orally) and might require additional treatments to fully resolve.[4] These parasites are less commonly seen now that the majority of hedgehogs are bred in captivity.

THERAPEUTICS

Because hedgehogs are covered with spines and go into a defensive posture when upset, treatment can be difficult. Oral medications that are flavored to be palatable are the recommended treatment of choice. The patient readily accepts this type of treatment without stress and trauma. If subcutaneous injections are used, tissue absorption can be affected by the thick fat layer under the skin. For this reason, subcutaneous injections should be given ventrally, where the fat layer is less dense.

Because hedgehog veins are short and small, an intraosseous catheter placed in the proximal femur or proximal tibia is recommended for critical patients. The approach is through the trochanteric fossa in the femur or off the tibial tuberosity with the tibia. A 1.5", 20- or 22-gauge spinal needle can be used to insert the catheter.[7]

SURGICAL AND ANESTHETIC ASSISTANCE

Hedgehogs require general anesthesia for a thorough physical examination or for a surgical procedure. These animals have a tendency to salivate excessively while under general anesthesia; therefore, premedication with atropine, 0.01–0.04 mg/kg intramuscularly, should be administered, especially if a face mask is used for the procedure.

Although there a variety of anesthetic agents (e.g., ketamine, dexmedetomidine, propofol, buprenorphine, butorphanol) that can be used for hedgehogs, inhalant anesthetics are by far the most commonly used. Injectable anesthetics can be used to preanesthetize the animal or in situations when an inhalant anesthetic is not available. For procedures that will induce pain, an appropriate analgesic protocol should be established.

Hedgehogs should be fasted for a minimum of 12 hours prior to an anesthetic procedure, although special precautions should be taken (e.g., IV dextrose) for an animal susceptible to a hypoglycemic episode (e.g., chronic disease, starvation). A water source can be left with the hedgehog up to the time of the procedure. Hedgehogs should be maintained on a water-recirculating heating pad during any anesthetic procedure and recovered in a warmed environment to prevent hypothermia, which can lead to torpor in these animals.

For short procedures, such as venipuncture or radiography, inhalant anesthetics can be used to facilitate sample collection. Hedgehogs can be placed in an induction chamber and anesthetized. Inducing anesthesia via face mask at 5% isoflurane or 8% sevoflurane expedites the process of getting the animal through the sedation phase, which is the time when they struggle. Once the hedgehog has lost its righting reflex, it can be maintained at 1%–2% isoflurane or 2%–3% sevoflurane. Anesthetized hedgehogs should be intubated to gain control over their respiration. Hedgehogs can be intubated using a 1.0–3.5 mm OD endotracheal tube, depending on their size. A laryngoscope can be used to increase visualization of the airway. The animal should be monitored closely during the procedure using appropriate equipment (e.g., Doppler, pulse oximeter, and EKG).

Surgical preparation of the hedgehog should follow the same protocols described for dogs and cats. The surgical site should be shaved using a standard grooming clipper at a slow, cautious speed to prevent clipper burn and tearing of the skin. The shaved area should be uniform and provide the surgeon ample room to perform the surgery without the risk of contamination. If an approach over the dorsum is required, the quills can be individually plucked. The surgical site should be aseptically prepared, using a surgical scrub and warmed sterile saline. Avoid using alcohol to prepare the surgical site because it can result in significant heat loss. The surgical site should be covered with a sterile drape until the surgeon begins. The surgical instruments used to perform surgery on dogs and cats can be used for hedgehogs as well.

HEALTH MAINTENANCE AND DISEASE

Neoplasia

Neoplasia is by far the most common disease presentation in hedgehogs. These animals are susceptible to many of the same types of neoplasias reported in domestic pets, including osteosarcoma, squamous cell carcinoma, lymphosarcoma, neurofibromas, adenocarcinomas, and leukemia. Because there are many neoplastic diseases that affect hedgehogs, any abnormal mass should be biopsied for disease determination. Some internal neoplasias can present as nonspecific diseases, so all sick hedgehogs should have a complete diagnostic workup. As with other animal species, the older the animal, the more predisposed it is to neoplastic disease. Hedgehogs are considered geriatric when they reach 3 years of age.

Dermatomycoses

Fungal organisms that are often identified as infecting hedgehogs are *Trichophyton mentagrophytes, T. erinacei,* and *Microsporum* spp.[5] These organisms can be diagnosed as a single infection or a concurrent infection with a mite infestation. Diagnosis is established by culturing spines from the affected areas in DTM media. Systemic treatment of oral griseofulvin is recommended at 30–40 mg/kg once daily for 30 days.[5] Lime sulfur dip and enilconazole are nonteratogenic alternatives that have a better therapeutic window.

Respiratory Disease

Bordetella bronchiseptica, Pasteurella multocida, and *Corynebacterium pneumonia* have been identified as respiratory pathogens affecting hedgehogs. Routine diagnostics to identify the causative agent of the respiratory disease are required for proper treatment. Treatment for severe respiratory disease includes antibiotics (based on culture and sensitivity of the causative agent), supportive fluid therapy, oxygen therapy, and nebulization.[4]

Neurologic Disease

Hedgehogs are susceptible to a demyelinating paralysis. The etiology of this disease is not known; however, it typically occurs in young adult animals (18–24 months of age). Affected animals have a progressive ascending ataxia. Over time the hedgehogs lose weight and become unable to move. This disease appears always to be fatal. Animals presenting with these clinical signs should be given a thorough workup. It is likely at some point in the near future that an etiology will be identified if enough cases are thoroughly evaluated.

Cardiac Disease

Hedgehogs are susceptible to developing cardiomyopathy. Affected animals often present with a history of lethargy, general weakness (especially in the hind limbs), coughing, and exercise intolerance. A thorough examination, including radiographs and echocardiography, is necessary to make a diagnosis. These diagnostic tests are important to characterize the type of cardiomyopathy (hypertrophic vs. dilatative). A final diagnosis is necessary to select treatment. Treatment should follow standards used for domestic pets.

Gastrointestinal Disease

Being omnivores, hedgehogs typically harbor the same types of microflora seen in dogs. In general, it is expected that their microflora is a combination of Gram-positive and Gram-negative aerobes and facultative anaerobes. Hedgehogs with gastrointestinal disease typically present with a history of anorexia and diarrhea. A thorough workup similar to that done for domestic pets should be performed in these cases. A number of potential opportunistic bacteria can cause disease, including *Pseudomonas* spp., *E. coli*, and *Salmonella* spp. There has also been at least one report of cryptosporidiosis in an African hedgehog.[8] This parasite can infect the lower small intestine and large intestine, causing severe pathology. *Cryptosporidium* spp. are difficult to diagnose because of their small size, so if they are being considered in a differential list, it is important to submit fecal samples for acid fast staining and immunofluorescent antibody testing. This disease is difficult to eradicate; most cases either self-clear or the animals succumb to the disease.

ZOONOTIC DISEASES

There are few reports of zoonotic diseases associated with African hedgehogs. One of special concern is *Salmonella* spp. It is not known whether hedgehogs normally harbor *Salmonella* spp. as an indigenous component of their microflora, as reptiles do, but based on the previous reports of *Salmonella* Tilene being isolated from hedgehogs and human caretakers, it is likely that these animals can naturally harbor this pathogen.[9,10] Since that time, salmonellosis associated with different serotypes has been reported.[11] Clients should be made aware of the potential zoonotic risk associated with these animals, and given recommendations for practicing routine disinfection. Recommend that they clean hedgehog cages and equipment with 10% bleach, allowing for at least 10 minutes of contact between the bleach and the equipment. It is important to remove all organic material before applying the bleach, to limit the potential for deactivation.

The finding of cryptosporidiosis in a juvenile hedgehog is important. Animals harboring *Cryptosporidium parvum* can pose a special health risk to humans, especially young, geriatric, or immunocompromised individuals.[8]

Dermatomycosis is a potential zoonotic disease that has been associated with hedgehogs.[11] This disease is common to many exotic small mammals, so it should come as no surprise that hedgehogs can serve as a source of infection to humans. Affected animals develop typical dry, scaly skin. Because these animals can be asymptomatic, it is important to consider their potential role when a human case occurs in a household.

SELF-STUDY QUESTIONS

1. How do you determine the sex of a hedgehog?

2. How long do hedgehogs live? What is the primary disease process affecting their longevity?

3. What is an appropriate environmental temperature for hedgehogs?

4. What type of enclosure is best for a hedgehog?

5. What type of diet is best for a hedgehog?

6. Describe the techniques used to perform restraint and a physical examination on a hedgehog patient.

7. What are some common venipuncture sites in hedgehogs?

8. Name two common ectoparasites of hedgehogs.

9. Why is it difficult to deliver medications to hedgehogs?

10. Name three potential zoonotic agents associated with hedgehogs.

REFERENCES

1. Smith AJ. Husbandry and nutrition of hedgehogs. *Vet Clinics of North America (Exotic Animal Practice)* 1999;2(1):127–41.
2. Johnson-Delaney C, Harrison LR. *Hedgehogs: Exotic companion medicine handbook for veterinarians.* Lake Worth, FL: Wingers Publishing; 1996:1–14.
3. Hoefer HL. Hedgehogs. *Vet Clinics of North America (Small Animal Practice)* 1994;24(1): 113–20.
4. Larsen RS, Carpenter JW. Husbandry and medical management of African hedgehogs. *Veterinary Medicine* (October 1999): 877–88.
5. Ness RD. Clinical pathology and sample collection of exotic small mammals. *Vet Clinics of North America (Exotic Animal Practice)* 1999; 2(3):591–620.
6. Gerson L, Boever WJ. Acariasis (*Caparinia* spp.) in hedgehogs (*Erinaceus* spp.): Diagnosis and treatment. *Journal of Zoo Animal Medicine* 1983;14:17–19.
7. Brown SA, and Rosenthal KL. *Self-assessment color review of small mammals.* Ames: Iowa State University Press; 1997:14–15.
8. Graczyk TK, Cranfield MR, Dunning C, Strandberg JD. Fatal cryptosporidiosis in a juvenile captive African hedgehog (*Atelerix albiventris*). *Journal of Parasitology* 1998;84: 178–80.
9. Centers for Disease Control and Prevention. African pygmy hedgehog–associated salmonellosis—Washington, 1994. *Morbidity and Mortality Weekly* 1995;44:462–3.
10. Craig C, Styliadis S, Woodward D, Werker D. African pygmy hedgehog–associated *Salmonella* Tilene in Canada. *Canada Communicable Disease Report* 1997;23:129–31.
11. Riley PY, and Chomel BB. Hedgehog zoonoses. *Emerging Infectious Diseases* 2005;11:1–5.

CHAPTER 7

Sugar Gliders

INTRODUCTION

The sugar or honey glider (*Petaurus breviceps*) is a marsupial that is native to New Guinea and Australia (Figure 7.1). It is about the size of a North American flying squirrel, generally gray with a black stripe running along the dorsal surface from the nose to the base of the tail. These animals have some control of the tail, which can be used as a rudder during gliding or for carrying nest material up a tree. The second and third digits of each hind foot are partially fused, forming a "hair comb," which is used for grooming their soft fur (Figure 7.2).

Male sugar gliders have three scent glands: one on top of the head (which forms a bald spot upon maturation), another on the chest (causing an orange or rusty discoloration of fur in that area), and one in the anal area. When stressed or frightened, both sexes can secrete a white oily substance from three paracloacal glands.[1] The testicles are located in a furry pouch in the midventral, and a bifurcated penis is ventral to the base of the tail (Figure 7.3). Male sugar gliders reach sexual maturity about 12–15 months after they leave the pouch.[1] The penis has a distal bifurcation and extends from the prepuce located near the base of the tail. The urethra terminates at the proximal aspect of the penis, not the distal bifurcation.[1]

The female has a pouch, or marsupium, located on the ventral aspect of the body where the young are raised as well as being the location of their largest scent gland. Female sugar gliders do not have the bald scent gland (on top of the head) that is found on males of this species (Figure 7.4).

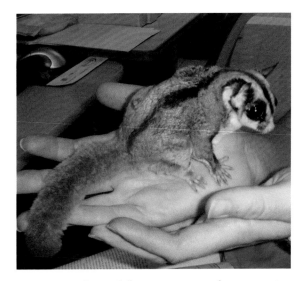

Figure 7.1 *Sugar gliders are maintained as companion animals. Photograph courtesy of Javier Nevarez, DVM.*

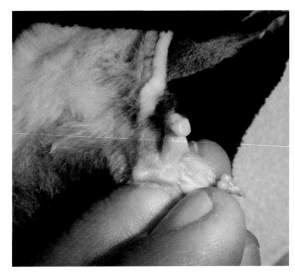

Figure 7.2 *Modified sugar glider claw, which is used as a grooming tool. Photograph courtesy of Javier Nevarez, DVM.*

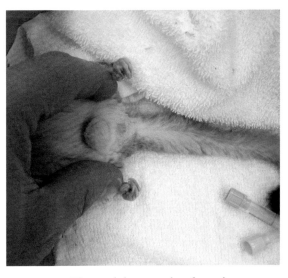

Figure 7.3 *The pendulous testicles of a male sugar glider.*

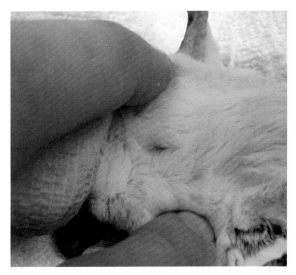

Figure 7.4 *Scent glands of a sugar glider are also found on the cranial ventral body wall.*

Sexual maturity of female sugar gliders is reached at approximately 8–12 months after they leave the pouch.[1] Once sexually mature, they cycle every 29 days.[1]

Sugar gliders groom themselves on a regular basis and will use saliva generated from sneez-ing into their paws to brush their hair coat.[1] This sneezing should not be confused with a disease condition.[1] Sugar glider sounds have been classi-fied as crabbing, barking, chirping, and hissing.[1] The noises are similar to their identifying terms but are emitted based on different conditions.

Table 7.1 **Sugar Glider Basic Information[1]**

GENERAL CATEGORY	CLASSIFICATION	PHYSIOLOGIC PARAMETER/QUANTITY
Body Weight	Adult Male	113–170 g
	Adult Female	85–142 g
	Birth Weight	0.19 g
Temperature	Rectal Body Temperature	97.2°F
Female Reproductive Cycle	Sexual Maturity	8–12 months
	Gestation Length	15–17 days
	Litter size	1–2 average
	Pouch Emergence	60–70 days
	Weaning Age	110–120 days
	Averge Life Span (captive)	12–15 years
Heart Rate		200–300 beats/minute
Respiratory Rate		16–40 breaths/minute
Food Consumption		15%–20% body weight
Male Sexual Maturity		12–15 months

Crabbing, a loud irritating noise, is produced when the animal is frightened or believes it is in danger. Barking is an apparent form of communication, whereas chirping is a low purring sound made when the animal is content.[1] As mentioned earlier, the hissing or sneezing sound is made when the sugar glider is generating saliva for grooming and should not be considered a disease condition. Sugar gliders are nocturnal animals, as evidenced by their extremely large eyes. Because these animals are awake at night, they have a tendency to bark—especially the males during a full moon. Leaving a light on in an adjacent room will help reduce this bothersome behavior early in the morning. As it is with other animals, it is important for the technician to know the normal physiologic values in order to assess the patient's health status (See Table 7.1).

These animals are extremely sensitive to pesticides, cedar shavings, branches from toxic trees, and bright direct light (either artificial or sunlight). Dogs and cats should be kept at a distance, and strict supervision must be maintained when sugar gliders are handled by small children or released from their enclosure.

HUSBANDRY

Cage dimensions for adult sugar gliders should be at least 18" × 18" × 24" with the size of the wire openings not more than 0.5–1.0". The cage size recommended for 1–2 young sugar gliders (joeys) that are less than 5 months out of the pouch is 20" × 30".[1] The smaller cage size encourages exercise, reduces stress, and promotes bonding for young animals.[1] Any cage material that meets the specified dimensions will work, but polyvinyl chloride–coated stainless steel wire mesh is recommended. To prevent trauma, the owner must be advised to be sure no protruding wires or openings are found within the enclosure, with the rectangular cage openings being no larger than 0.5" × 1".[1]

Young joeys require a nesting cloth that cannot be pulled apart and is easily washable for sleeping, warmth, and security. The nesting cloth, along with a suspended heat lamp, will help reduce the incidence of hypothermia in young sugar gliders. A pine box approximately 6" × 8" × 6" is needed for adult animals to sleep in during the day. This box can be a premanufactured bird nesting box. Shredded paper makes an excellent nontoxic box substrate. Old towels or cloth can unravel, leaving loose strings to choke the animal or strangulate a foot or tail. Tree branches need to be included in the enclosure for the animal to climb on during its play and exercise time. The branches can be obtained from nontoxic species of hardwood trees (e.g., maple, hickory, manzanita). The ambient temperature range that should be provided for sugar gliders is 75°–80°F.[1]

Toys manufactured for rodents will provide entertainment and exercise for sugar gliders and are recommended. Although sugar gliders are relatively clean and odor-free, owners should be aware that the cage will develop an unpleasant smell if not cleaned about twice a week because of accumulation of food and excreta.

Nutrition

Sugar gliders are messy eaters; therefore, placing their food in a separate container within the enclosure that they can crawl into to eat will keep the food and surrounding substrate clean. Two food dishes and a sipper bottle should be used to feed and provide water for sugar gliders. Because sugar gliders appear sensitive to chlorinated water, owners should provide bottled or filtered water in the sipper bottle and change it daily.[1] One food dish is used for dry food, and the other is for moist food. The recommended daily diet for a sugar glider should be 15%–20% of the animal's body weight.[1] The diet should include a sugar glider pellet (NutriMax, VetsPride, Nashville, TN; Glider-R-Chow, PocketPets, Cape

Coral, FL) as 75% of overall diet (i.e., 30–60 g/day/animal), a calcium-based multivitamin, and fresh fruits and vegetables.[1] Calcium-based multivitamin supplements (Glide-A-Mins, PocketPets, Cape Coral, FL) should be applied as indicated on the container instructions or sprinkled lightly on fruits and vegetables every other day.[1] No more than 25% of the diet should be fresh fruits and vegetables.

As mentioned previously, a separate "dining" area established in a container will keep the enclosure free of food debris that results from the messy feeding habits of these animals. Any fruits and vegetables left at the end of the day should be removed and the dining container cleaned prior to the next day's meal. To help young sugar gliders adapt to a pellet diet, a fruit sauce (e.g., apple) can be placed on top of the offering. Treats can be given periodically, but only those manufactured for sugar gliders are recommended.

Grooming

Sugar glider nails can be trimmed using human nail clippers in a similar manner to that described for rats (Chapter 5). Owners must be aware that the trimming of nails may reduce their pet's ability to climb.

HISTORY

The same basic background information is required for sugar gliders as for other animals that are examined at the veterinary clinic. How long the animal has been owned, where it was acquired, how often it is handled, and the character of the feces and urine are a few of the questions that should be asked for background information. Husbandry questions include where the animal is housed; whether it is allowed to roam unobserved in the house; cage location, type, size, material, substrate, furniture, and toys; and how often the cage is cleaned and the disinfectant used. When investigating the diet, it is important for the technician to ask if commercial products/table foods are fed, how much, and also what the animal is actually eating. The same needs to be asked regarding live (prey) foods (e.g., mealworms). Supplemental offerings and frequency of feeding are very important data for the case workup. To round out the nutrition information, the technician should find out about the water supply, how often the water is changed, and how much the animal drinks on a daily basis.

Because diseases are transmissible between animals, the final questions should center on other pets in the household: if new animals have been added to the family or if the animals are housed together. Finally, a description of any previous problems and a complete chronological description of the presenting problem are needed to complete the history form.

RESTRAINT

Sugar gliders are restrained by holding the head between the thumb and middle finger and resting the index finger on top of the head.[1] The body will then lie in the palm of the restrainer's hand. Isoflurane anesthesia is the agent of choice for general anesthesia of these small marsupials. Placing the patient in an induction chamber using 5% isoflurane with 1.5 L flow of oxygen will allow the animal to become anesthetized with minimal stress. The animal can then be maintained on approximately 2%–3% isoflurane, using a face mask and 1.5 L flow of oxygen.

PHYSICAL EXAMINATION

The animal must be properly restrained. It is important that the veterinarian be able to exam-ine the entire animal without stress to the patient or veterinarian. A complete physical examination will be performed on each sugar glider patient that enters the clinic. The physical examination procedures for sugar gliders are similar to those used for other small mammals.

DIAGNOSTIC SAMPLING

Blood Collection
Recommended sites for blood collection, which is best accomplished under general anesthesia, are the jugular vein, cranial vena cava, and medial tibial artery.[1] Blood volumes of up to 1% of the animal's body weight can be safely collected using a 1 cc syringe and a 26-gauge needle. Reference ranges for complete blood counts and serum chemistry panels are listed in Tables 7.2 and 7.3, respectively.[1] The technique used to collect blood from the cranial vena cava is described in Chapter 5 in the "Guinea Pig" section. When collecting blood from a sugar glider patient, only 0.9% of an animal's body weight in grams can be safely removed.[1] The amount of blood collected will depend on the condition of the patient.

Bone Marrow Aspiration
This is not a common procedure performed on sugar glider patients. Methods that have been described for other small animals (e.g., dogs, cats) should be used for sugar gliders while taking into account the relative size of their anatomical structures. A spinal needle should be used to access the marrow cavity of sugar glider bones. The spinal needle will have a stylet inside the cannula that will prevent plugging with bone and/or cartilage.

Microbiology
Microbiological samples can be obtained from sugar glider patients as with other small animals.

Table 7.2 **Sugar Glider Complete Blood Count Reference Ranges**[1]

CELL TYPE	REFERENCE RANGE
Erythrocytes	$7.0–8.8 \times 10^6/\mu l$
Hematocrit	39.7–47.7%
Hemoglobin	13.9–17.1 g/dl
Leukocytes	$2.1–8.5 \times 10^3/\mu l$
Neutrophils	$0.2–2.4 \times 10^3/\mu l$
Lymphocytes	$1.6–6.0 \times 10^3/\mu l$
Eosinophils	$0.04–0.16 \times 10^3/\mu l$
Monocytes	$0–3.0 \times 10^3/\mu l$
Platelets	$602–904 \times 10^3/\mu l$

Table 7.3 **Sugar Glider Serum Biochemistry Reference Ranges**[1,2,3]

ANALYTE	REFERENCE RANGE
Serum Glucose	152–171 mg/dl
Blood Urea Nitrogen	15–18 mg/dl
Creatinine	0.6–0.8 mg/dl
Total Bilirubin	0.1–0.7 mg/dl
Serum Calcium	8.7–9.1 mg/dl
Serum Phosphorous	5.0–6.0 mg/dl
Alanine Aminotransferase (ALT)	96–136 IU/L
Aspartate Aminotransferase (AST)	54–99 IU/L
Alkaline Phosphatase	89–115 IU/L
Creatinine Phosphokinase	1,080–1,636 IU/L
Sodium	138–143 mEq/L
Potassium	4–5 mEQ/L
Chloride	105–108 mEq/L
Cholesterol	111–123 mg/dl
Magnesium	1–2 mEq/L
Amylase	2,117–3,350 IU/L
Total Protein	6.74–7 g/dl
Albumin	3.12–4.64 g/dl
Globulin	2.9–3.1 g/dl

Since the normal flora of sugar glider anatomical areas/body systems (e.g., reproductive, gastrointestinal, integument) have not been determined, critical assessment of the microbial isolates relative to the disease condition of the patient is highly recommended. Microbiological assessment of sugar glider disease conditions is as important as with other small animal patients.

Urinalysis

The analysis of urine can provide important insight into disease presentations such as cystitis, hematuria, and stranguria. Urine can be collected by cystocentesis (ventral percutaneous approach) or free catch on a smooth metal or plastic tray.

Radiology

Radiographic images are obtained in a manner similar to that used with other small mammals. With most sugar glider cases, quality radiographic images require the patient to be placed under general anesthesia. This will ensure that the animal is motionless and positioned in a manner whereby desired organ systems/structures can be evaluated. A minimum of two survey radiographs should be obtained from each patient. Radiographic interpretation is similar to that for domestic pets.

Injection Sites

Intravenous injection sites on sugar gliders include the cephalic and lateral saphenous veins. Quadriceps, biceps, and cervical epaxial muscles are commonly used as intramuscular injection sites. Administration of subcutaneous therapeutic agents is performed along the dorsal midline between the scapulas. Subcutaneous fluids can be administered at approximately 2% of the body weight every 8–12 hours.[1]

Other diagnostic procedures performed on sugar gliders are done in a manner similar to those used on other small mammals.

Parasitology

Internal Parasites

Although common in wild sugar gliders, parasites are not commonly diagnosed in captive-bred animals. *Coccidia* and *Giardia* spp. have been identified in animals raised in captivity.[2]

Sulfadimethoxine is recommended for treatment of coccidia, and metronidazole is the drug of choice for *Giardia* spp. infections.

THERAPEUTICS

The most effective route to administer up to 10% of the patient's body weight in replacement fluids is via an intraosseous catheter. The proximal tibia is the recommended location for placing the 24-gauge introsseous catheter in a sugar glider. Fluid administration should follow the same parameters as those for a similarly sized mammal. This includes estimating dehydration deficit, daily fluid maintenance requirements, and interosseous fluid administration in the proximal femur. The selection of fluid product to use is dependent on the patient's physiologic status and disease diagnosis. Subcutaneous fluid administration is best achieved along the dorsum. Sugar gliders are small animals, and all precautions used for other animals of their size should be taken into consideration prior to, during, and after surgery. The surgical candidate should be fasted for 4 hours prior to the initiation of the procedure.[1] Care in providing external heat, hemostasis, and fluid therapy during surgery is essential for a successful completion and an uneventful recovery.

SURGICAL AND ANESTHETIC ASSISTANCE

An induction chamber using isoflurane or sevoflurane as the anesthetic agent is recommended for sugar gliders. Once the patient is induced, a face mask or 1 mm endotracheal tube is used to administer the flow during the procedure. Sugar gliders can develop apnea during induction, but careful monitoring of the heart rate will help determine the overall condition of the patient until it is fully induced and begins breathing on its own. If the heart rate begins to decrease significantly, stop the procedure and wake up the animal. Surgical preparation of sugar gliders is similar to that for other small mammals.

HEALTH MAINTENANCE AND DISEASE

Nutritional Osteodystrophy

The most common disease seen in captive-bred sugar gliders is nutritional osteodystrophy.[1] Animals that present with severe depression and hind limb paralysis will radiographically reveal osteoporosis and pathologic fractures.[1] Treatment consists of cage rest, supplemental calcium (initial treatment: calcium gluconate 100 mg/kg subcutaneous administration every 12 hours for 3–5 days, followed by calcium glubionate 150 mg/kg orally every 24 hours as needed), vitamin D3, and diet modification.[1] A preventive diet should contain approximately 1% calcium, 0.5% phosphorus, and 1,500 IU/kg vitamin D3 on a dry-weight basis.[1] Poor nutrition can also lead to obesity, emaciation, and constipation in sugar gliders.

Pasteurella Multocida

Pasteurella multocida has been identified in sugar glider deaths that resulted from generalized organ and subcutaneous abscessation.[1] Prevention starts with keeping sugar gliders away from rabbits that might be subclinical carriers of this bacterial organism. The treatment of choice is enrofloxicin.

Table 7.4 **Dosages of Common Therapeutic Agents Used for Sugar Gliders**[1,2,3]

DRUG	DOSAGE	COMMENTS
*Antimicrobials**		
Amoxicillin	30 mg/kg PO, IM q24h x 14 days	
Amoxicillin/Clavulanic acid	12.5 mg/kg PO divided q24h	
Ciprofloxacin	10 mg/kg PO q12h x 7–10 days	
Clindamycin	5–11 mg/kg PO	Higher dose for osteomyelitis
Enrofloxacin	5 mg/kg PO q12h	
Itraconazole	5–10 mg/kg PO q12h	
Trimethoprim/Sulfamethoxazole	15 mg/kg PO q12h x 7–10 days	
Antiparasitic Medication		
Fenbendazole	20–50 mg/kg PO q24h x 3 days	Repeat in 14 days
Ivermectin	0.2 mg/kg PO, SC	Repeat in 10–14 days
Metronidazole	25 mg/kg PO q12h x 7–10 days	
Selamectin	6–18 mg/kg topically	Repeat every 30 days
Analgesics		
Buprenorphine	0.01–0.03 mg/kg IM	
Butorphanol	0.1–0.5 mg/kg IM q6–8h	
Diazepam	0.5–1.0 mg/kg IM 1.0–2.0 mg/kg PO	Treat seizure activity
Meloxicam	0.1–0.2 mg/kg PO q12h	
Other Therapeutic Agents		
Atropine	0.01–0.02 mg/kg SC, IM	
Bismuth subsalicylate	1 ml/kg PO q8–12h x 5–7 days	
Calcium glubionate	150 mg/kg PO q24h	
Calcium gluconate	100 mg/kg SC q12h x 3–5 days	Diluted in saline to 10 mg/ml
Cisapride	0.25 mg/kg q8–24h PO, IM	Use with stool softener
Dexamethasone	Anti-inflammatory: 0.1–0.6 mg/kg SC, IM, IV Shock: 0.5–2.0 mg/kg SC, IM, IV	
Diphenhydramine	0.5–2.0 mg/kg PO, SC q8–12h	
Enalapril	0.5 mg/kg	
Furosemide	2–4 mg/kg	
Metoclopramide	0.05 mg/kg PO, SC q8h	
Sulfadimethoxine	10 mg/kg PO q12h x 7–10 days	
Vitamin A	500–5,000 IU/kg IM	
Vitamin B complex	0.02–0.2 ml/kg SC, IM	
Vitamin E	10 IU/kg SQ	

*For compounding oral formulations tutti frutti and other fruit flavors recommended.
IM: intramuscular; IV: intravenous; PO: *per os* (oral); SC: subcutaneous.

Other Diseases

Sugar gliders can present with many disease conditions, like other small exotic mammals. These include gastrointestinal, urinary tract, respiratory, ocular, traumatic, toxicosis, reproductive, and dental disease.[1] For self-mutilating animals, fluoxetin (1–5 mg/kg orally every 8 hours) has been used with some success, with the dose being increased depending on treatment response. A listing of common sugar glider therapeutic agents and dosages is found in Table 7.4.

SELF-STUDY QUESTIONS

1. What are the second and third digits on each hind foot used for?

2. What are scent glands, and where are they located?

3. Describe the external anatomy of both male and female sugar gliders.

4. What are the husbandry and dietary recommendations for sugar gliders?

5. What is the proper procedure for restraining a sugar glider?

6. Describe the techniques used to perform a physical examination on a sugar glider.

7. How is blood collected from a sugar glider?

8. Where are the injection sites located?

9. Describe the therapeutic options for sugar gliders.

10. How are sugar gliders anesthetized?

REFERENCES

1. Brust DM. Sugar gliders: A complete veterinary care guide. Association of Sugar Glider Veterinarians. http://www.sugarglidervetinfo.com/default.html. Veterinary Interactive Publications;(2009).
2. Pye G, and Carpenter JW. A guide to medicine and surgery in sugar gliders. *Vet Medicine* (October 1999):891–904.
3. Ness RD. Clinical pathology and sample collection of exotic small mammals. *Vet Clinics of North America (Exotic Animal Practice)* 1999; 2(3):591–620.

CHAPTER 8

Fish

INTRODUCTION

The popularity of ornamental fish dates back more than 2,000 years in China. In the United States, interest in ornamental fish rose during the 1940s with the advent of aviation and the importation of fish from around the world. The advancement of aquarium technologies, such as filtration and nutrition, has enabled this hobby to continue to flourish today. In 2001, at the time of the first edition of this text, the American Veterinary Medical Association market research statistics for pet ownership in the United States estimated there were more than 6,000 fish per 1,000 households. In its most recent survey (2007), the number of fish per 1,000 households has increased by 50%, with more than 9,000 fish per household. As numbers of the animals continue to rise, there will be increased demand for veterinarians and veterinary technicians to provide medical and surgical care for these animals.

Most ornamental fish are maintained in aquariums within the home, although the popularity of outdoor ponds continues to rise. Historically, ornamental fish were considered replaceable pets; however, as the value of these animals has risen, pet owners have sought the advice of veterinary professionals to manage their valuable collections. Another contributing factor to the change in the human-animal bond as it relates to fish is associated with the longevity of these animals. Improved husbandry (e.g., filtration, water treatment methods) and nutrition have helped maximize longevity in fish. Fish that historically were short-lived (1–2 years) in the past are now being kept alive for significantly longer periods (4–6 years). Goldfish and koi are known to live well into their 20s and 40s, respectively. As these animals live longer and owners become attached to their pets, veterinarians and their technicians will be expected to give the same high-quality care that they provide for other domestic species.

Changes in the availability of medications (e.g., antibiotics) for treating fish are also expected to increase the reliance of aquarists on veterinarians. In the United States, "prescription only" antibiotics (e.g., tetracyclines, ampicillin, erythromycin, metronidazole) and antiparasitics (e.g., praziquantel, fenbendazole) for treating fish have been sold for decades over the counter at local pet retail stores. Because the federal government was concerned that humans were buying their prescription medications at their local pet retailer because of cost, they made manufacturers of these drugs change their products from tablet to powder form. Although one can appreciate the government's attempts to prevent citizens from purchasing lesser-quality antibiotics, it is unlikely that altering the product's form will be sufficient, if price is more important to the consumer. This fact, in combination with increased concerns about appropriate disposal of antibiotics and antibiotic resistance in bacteria, may lead to further restrictions that will result in veterinarians being the primary source for these drugs for aquarists.

Taxonomy

Fish represent the largest group of vertebrates, with over 25,000 different species, 50 orders, and 445 families. While the majority of fish found in the world are from marine environments (61%), freshwater fish tend to be presented more commonly to the veterinary hospital, especially koi (*Cyprinus carpio*) and goldfish (*Carassius auratus*). Within this class of animals there is a high degree of anatomic and physiologic variation. For veterinary personnel, this presents a real challenge when working with these animals. Fortunately, there are closer to 250 species commonly found in the pet trade, which still represents the largest group of vertebrates found in captivity. Develop-

ing an understanding of the taxonomy of these animals, along with basic anatomic and physiologic differences among these species, is essential to our success with managing them in captivity.

Anatomy and Physiology

Technicians should develop a basic understanding of anatomy prior to working with an animal species. A background knowledge of anatomy will prove beneficial when collecting diagnostic samples or administering therapeutics. The focus of this chapter will be on teleosts or bony fishes.

Fish are covered with a mucous coat that is produced by cells in their integument. This mucous coat serves as the first line of defense against pathogenic organisms, such as bacteria, fungi, and viruses. This is an important component of their innate immune system, which fish heavily rely on because the other components of their immune system (cell-mediated and humoral components) are more primitive than those of other vertebrates. The mucous barrier contains various-sized proteins (e.g., immunoglobulins) that bind these pathogens and prevent invasion. If this protective barrier is penetrated, fish must rely on their humoral and cell-mediated defenses; however, whereas mammals have at least five different types of antibodies, fish have only one (IgM). It is for this reason that veterinarians and veterinary technicians need to use caution when handling fish, to minimize any damage to the protective mucous barrier and skin. Fish that present to a veterinary hospital with an increased white-gray slime covering need to be evaluated to determine the underlying cause of the increased mucus appearance (see "Diagnostic Sampling" later in the chapter). Fish should be handled only when necessary to prevent damaging this protective barrier; it is preferable to anesthetize fish for examination and diagnostic tests to minimize any damage to the integument and mucous barrier that might occur in alert fish when they struggle.

The scales of a fish are located in the dermis and provide protection over the musculature. Several types of scales are found on teleosts, including ganoid, cycloid, and ctenoid. The ganoid and cycloid scales are found on the more primitive species of teleosts, whereas the ctenoid scales are found on the more evolutionary advanced fish. The scales serve as a protective armor, and damage to or loss of the scales might result in introduction of opportunistic infections. Handling should be minimized to avoid traumatizing the scales.

Teleosts typically have two sets of paired fins, the pectoral and pelvic fins, and three unpaired fins: the dorsal, anal, and caudal fins (Figure 8.1). Some fish can have two dorsal fins. There are also some groups (e.g., salmonids, characins, and catfishes) of fish that have an additional small adipose fin between their dorsal fin and caudal fin. Fins are used for steering, balancing, and braking. Certain species have modified fins to adapt

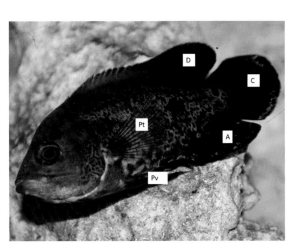

Figure 8.1 *Fish have both paired (pectoral [Pt] and pelvic [Pv]) unpaired fins (dorsal [D], caudal [C], and anal [A]). These structures function in locomotion and steering. Injuries to the fins can lead to opportunistic infection, difficulty in acquiring food, and increased stress from bullying by other fish.*

to certain niches. For example, the anal fin of the knifefish is a large single fin located on the ventrum of the animal and serves as the primary source of locomotion. Spines might be associated with some fins and serve as a defense mechanism. The lionfish (*Pterois volitans*) produces venom that can be injected into a potential predator, causing significant pain and discomfort. Knowledge of the species that produce venom is essential to prevent injury to the handler. Fish can damage their spines when captured in a net. To prevent this, fish can be scooped into a plastic cup or bucket to facilitate removal from an aquarium.

Gills are the primary respiratory organs of most fish, although certain species use accessory organs to aid in the absorption of oxygen. Gills serve to absorb oxygen, excrete waste products (e.g., ammonia and carbon dioxide), and regulate ion and water balance. It is important to note that, unlike other vertebrates that excrete end products of protein catabolism (e.g., uric acid or urea nitrogen) through the kidneys, fish excrete these products through the gills. Therefore, damage to the gills from infectious diseases or poor water quality can exacerbate problems for fish because of their inability to release systemic toxins. Teleosts have four pairs of gills, and the gills are located under the operculi (gill plates) in the branchial chambers. The gills are attached to a bony gill arch, and each gill comprises primary and secondary lamellae. The secondary lamella is the site of gas exchange. Exposure to parasites and toxic compounds, such as ammonia, results in the excessive production of mucus, which can impede gas exchange (see "Diagnostic Sampling"). Fish possess a two-chambered heart: a single atrium and a ventricle. The heart is located ventral to the pharynx and cranial to the liver. Unoxygenated blood is pumped from the heart to the gills, where it is oxygenated and distributed to the rest of the body. Fish possess two portal systems, a renal portal system that drains the caudal musculature and a hepatic portal system that drains venous blood from the digestive tract.

The lateral line is a mechanosensory structure that is used by fish to monitor changes in sound waves and water pressure. The lateral line originates on the head, around the eyes and nares, and extends along the lateral body wall. Certain groups of marine fish, including tangs, angelfish, and freshwater fish (e.g., cichlids) maintained in captivity, can develop head and lateral line erosions (Figure 8.2A and 8.2B). The specific etiologies for this syndrome have not been elucidated, but dietary deficiency, water quality, and infectious diseases are all suspected.

The digestive tracts of fish vary depending on their feeding strategy. Herbivorous fish have a much longer digestive tract than omnivorous and carnivorous fish. This relates primarily to an increased demand for time to maximize the extraction of nutrients from cellulose-based products. In many cases, segments of the bowel are tightly coiled to conserve space within the coelomic cavity. The stomach is absent in some species, such as the goldfish and carp. Pyloric cecae are found in some species of fish, which secrete digestive enzymes and increase the absorptive surface area of the digestive tract. The number of pyloric cecae can be used in fish identification to differentiate certain species. Fish possess a large liver that is located in the cranial area of the body cavity. The normal color of the liver should be red-brown; however, yellow, fatty livers are a common finding at necropsy. This is often the result of diets rich in fats and protein.

The swim bladder is a unique structure found in fish. In some species, such as the lungfish, the swim bladder serves as a respiratory organ; however, in most fish, the swim bladder serves to

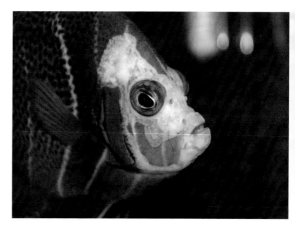

Figure 8.2A *A marine Koran angelfish (*Pomacanthus semiciculatus*) with severe head and lateral line erosions.*

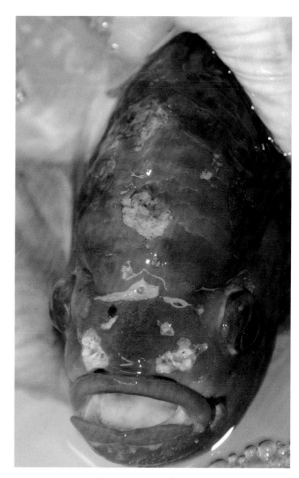

Figure 8.2B *A freshwater cichlid (oscar;* Astronotus ocellatus*) with severe head and lateral line erosions. Note the full thickness erosions into the dermis.*

maintain the buoyancy of the fish. There are two different types of swim bladders: physostomous and physoclistous. Physostomous swim bladders have a duct that connects the swim bladder to the esophagus. Air in the swim bladder is controlled via gas flow through this duct. Physoclistous swim bladders do not have a connecting duct, but instead have airflow regulation through the blood supply (*rete mirabile*). The swim bladder is located in the dorsal coelomic cavity; the only structure more dorsal is the kidney. Fish that have problems with their swim bladder frequently present with buoyancy issues (e.g., floating on the surface or sunk to the bottom).

Fish possess a single kidney that is divided into an anterior and a posterior segment. The kidney is located retrocoelomically in the dorsal body wall. The kidney functions primarily as an osmoregulatory and hematopoietic organ. The anterior kidney and the interstitium of the posterior segment serve as the primary sites for blood cell and immunoglobulin production; fish do not possess bone marrow. The posterior kidney primarily regulates electrolyte and urine output. Fish that are found in a saltwater or hypertonic environment tend to lose water and absorb salts. To prevent dehydration, these fish must drink water and excrete excess electrolytes, such as sodium and chloride, through the kidney and gills. Fish that live in a freshwater or hypotonic environment constantly absorb water by osmosis. To prevent overhydration, freshwater fish excrete large volumes of dilute urine. This physiology is important to consider when developing treatment plans for fish. Fish from a saltwater environment are more likely to ingest medications (e.g., antibiotics) that are placed in the water, whereas freshwater fish are less likely to do the same because they don't "drink the water." Not considering this during the treatment plan can lead to less effective results with freshwater fish.

Determining the sex of a fish depends on whether the animal is sexually dimorphic or not. For example, in some livebearers, males have a gonopodium, which serves as an intromittent organ (e.g., penis). The gonopodium is located on the anal fin and lies parallel to the body. In other fish, males develop specific colors or structures (e.g., growths on their head or fins) during the breeding season that help separate the sexes. During this period, females often develop a round abdomen because of the increased size of their ovaries. Because there are more than 25,000 different species of fish, it is not possible to learn/know all of the intricacies of determining sex in fish, so it is best to research the methods for the species presenting at your hospital. In cases when sex of the fish needs to be determined, endoscopic sexing can be done.

Fish possess a defense mechanism—composed of free and fixed phagocytic macrophages located in the spleen, heart, and kidney—that filters foreign material from the blood. The erythrocytes of fish are oval-shaped with a centrally located nucleus. When using a Wright-Giemsa or Diff-Quik stain, the cytoplasm has a pale pink/orange color and the nucleus a deep purple color.

Thrombocytes have a small nucleus and a spindle-shaped cell. Typically, the cytoplasm of a thrombocyte is clear. These cells are analogous to platelets in mammals and are responsible for blood clotting. In some fish, these cells can be difficult to discern from small lymphocytes. Because of their "sticky" nature, the cytoplasmic membranes of thrombocytes tend to get stuck on a slide and deform when a blood smear is made. This is generally a sufficient finding to separate a thrombocyte from a well-formed, round lymphocyte.

Fish leukocytes can be divided into the same two basic groups seen in higher vertebrates: agranular and granular. Agranular leukocytes include the lymphocyte and monocyte, whereas granular leukocytes include the neutrophil/heterophil and eosinophil. Neutrophil and heterophil are often used interchangeably in fish based on the staining characteristics of the cells. In either case, these cells lack some of the enzymatic capacity of higher vertebrates.

Lymphocytes are the most common cell type in fish and are morphologically similar to those in mammals, with an acentric nucleus, high nuclear to cytoplasmic ratio, and blue cytoplasm. Fish produce both T and B lymphocytes, and the cell size can vary from small to large. Lymphocytes are important in producing antibodies and modulating the cell-mediated immune response.

Monocytes are the largest leukocyte and have a pale blue-gray cytoplasm and a higher cytoplasmic to nuclear ratio than lymphocytes. These cells play an important role in phagocytizing foreign material and presenting antigen to lymphocytes for antibody production. They are also commonly associated with chronic inflammatory responses. Large lymphocytes can be difficult to discern from monocytes; however, if you compare nuclear to cytoplasmic ratios between the cells, it should be possible to separate them.

Neutrophils/heterophils possess rod-shaped granules and are weakly phagocytic. These cells are associated with the acute inflammatory response and stress leukograms. Eosinophils exist in some species of fish, but their function is unclear. It is likely that they play some role in controlling/managing parasites in fish. The existence of basophils is controversial. An example of common fish white blood cells can be found in Figures 8.3A–D.

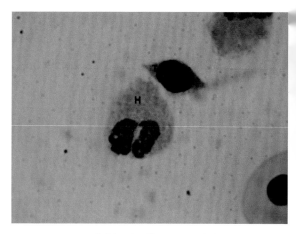

Figure 8.3A *Fish blood cells. Heterophil (H), thrombocyte (T).*

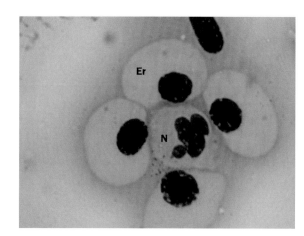

Figure 8.3B *Fish blood cells. Neutrophil (N), erythrocyte (Er).*

HUSBANDRY

Environmental Concerns

Aquarium

Fish are housed primarily in glass or acrylic tanks. The primary differences between these tanks are that glass weighs more than acrylic, acrylic scratches more easily, and acrylic tanks are available in a wider range of sizes and shapes. When dealing with larger glass tanks, the weight of the structure should be included with the water weight when deciding

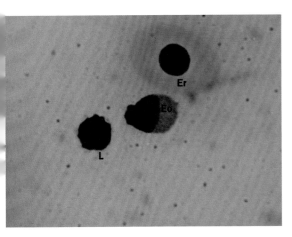

Figure 8.3C *Fish blood cells. Eosinophil (Eo), lymphocyte (L), erythrocyte (Er).*

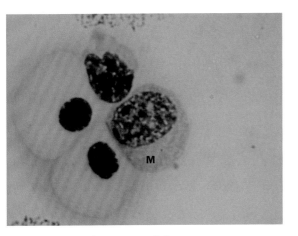

Figure 8.3D *Fish monocyte (M).*

whether a stand or floor joist has sufficient strength to support the system. Acrylic tanks are typically more popular with marine fish enthusiasts. When making recommendations to clients regarding the most appropriate size and shape of a tank, it is important to take into consideration the types of fish an individual expects to maintain and the aesthetic appeal of the aquarium as a piece of furniture. For example, freshwater angelfish should be maintained in an aquarium with vertical height to prevent cramping of their tall dorsal and anal fins.

Water weighs approximately 8 pounds per gallon. The weight of a large aquarium can place significant stress on a floor. A pet owner should be advised to assess the structural integrity of a floor prior to placing a large aquarium in the home. An aquarium should be placed on a secure, level stand.

Fish are primarily considered ectotherms, or "cold-blooded," and are dependent on their environmental temperature to regulate their core body temperature. To maintain the overall health of these animals, they should be housed at a constant environmental temperature. A commercially available aquarium heater can be used to establish an appropriate temperature. Freshwater tropical species should have a water temperature of 76° to 78°F. Certain species (e.g., Discus: *Symphysodon aequifasciatus*) might require higher temperatures (82°–86°F) to stimulate their reproductive cycle. Freshwater coldwater species (e.g., goldfish and koi) should be maintained at 65° to 68°F. Marine tropical species tolerate temperatures of 74° to 78°F. Fish that are maintained at low temperatures will develop hypothermia; this can lead to a reduction in the overall metabolism and immune function of the fish, making them less active and more susceptible to chronic infections. Fish maintained at excessive temperatures often become hyperthermic and die. Outdoor pond fish can develop hyperthermia in certain climates, and owners should be advised to provide them with appropriate shade.

The selection of a substrate for an aquarium should be based on the types of fish being placed in the system, whether live or plastic plants will be used, and the aesthetics of the system. Gravel size is important when working with fish that are aggressive feeders or "gravel sifters." Problems are commonly seen with large, predatory fish that are aggressive feeders and consume gravel when hunting prey. In some cases, they consume sufficient gravel to cause a foreign body obstruction in the stomach or small intestine/stomach interface. Affected animals typically present with anorexia, and a diagnosis can be made using survey radiographs. If there is a complete obstruction, surgery to remove the foreign material is required. Fish that are "gravel sifters" occasionally ingest gravel that can lead to an obstruction, but this is rare. Gravel size and depth are an important consideration for live plants. Some plants will die if they do not have sufficient substrate depth to establish roots, whereas others will perish if their roots are buried too deeply. The aesthetic component is really a decision to be made based on preference; however, to minimize the potential for problems, gravel should be of a sufficient depth to maintain live plants, if desired, and plants should be large enough that they can't be ingested.

Live plants have their own following among aquarists. Although live plants can add oxygen to the water, remove carbon dioxide and nitrates, and add beauty, they can also introduce disease. Many live plants are infested with snails (gastropods). These unwanted visitors can harbor a variety of bacterial and parasitic disease agents. Clients should be made aware of this and educated about the importance of inspecting their plants before adding them to an aquarium or pretreating the plants with a commercial anti-gastropod product.

Lighting is an important consideration for aquariums. Fish are built to be exposed to light cycles common to their origin. For example, fish at the equator are used to a more standard light cycle than those found near the poles, where light duration increases or decreases between seasons. In captivity, it is easiest to manage fish on a 12-hour light and 12-hour dark cycle. A variety of lights are available for aquariums. In general, the most recommended variety is a high-quality fluorescent light. The primary benefits to the fish come from the provision of well-defined visible light. This is especially important for fish bred in captivity, because it maximizes their color and allows for standard breeding rituals to occur. The infrared or heat component of artificial light is not required if a heating element is provided. It is preferred to use a heating element to stabilize temperature rather than light, because temperature can fluctuate when the light is turned on and off. Ultraviolet B radiation is not considered important for fish because it does not penetrate water very deeply, although there have been no studies evaluating its effect on fish.

Filtration

In nature, waste products produced by fish, plants, and other sources are carried away by flowing water, reducing the potential dangers to fish. In the home aquarium or pond, wastes and toxins can accumulate, leading to a dangerous situation for fish. Filtration is the key to maintaining healthy water for fish in an aquarium or pond. There are three primary types of filtration, including mechanical, biologic, and chemical (Figures 8.4A, 8.4B, and 8.4C). The different types of filtration work independently of one another, but should be used in combination to maximize water quality.

Mechanical Filtration. Mechanical filtration removes organic debris from the water by passing it through a filter material, such as floss, fiber, or a paper cartridge. The amount of work that this type of filter can perform depends on the type and (pore) size of the filter material and the motor or pump that is moving the water past the filter material. A densely packed fiber or small pore size in the paper cartridge will restrict the size of waste that can pass. Maintenance of these filters involves cleaning or replacement of the floss or cartridge.

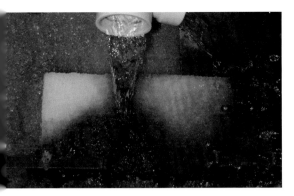

Figure 8.4A *Three types of filtration are used in most filtrations systems: mechanical, chemical, and biological. In this filter, the synthetic pads serve as the mechanical filter.*

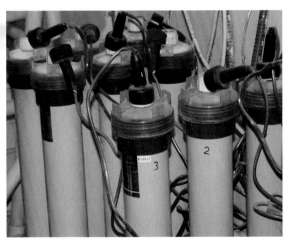

Figure 8.4B *Ultraviolet radiation serves as a chemical filter.*

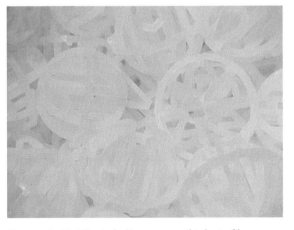

Figure 8.4C *Plastic balls serve as a biologic filter.*

The air pressure exerted by the pump will also affect a mechanical filter. The faster the pump pushes water past the filter material, the faster it will clog. Mechanical filtration is very useful in both the home aquarium and outdoor pond. This type of filtration is best used with other types of filtration (chemical and biologic) to improve the overall quality of water in the system. However, for a combination filter to be most effective, the mechanical filter needs to be placed in line before the chemical or biologic filter; this will prevent obstructions from forming in the chemical and biologic filters. Mechanical filtration should always be used with a sand filter or bead filter. The mechanical filter will protect the sand or bead filter by removing large particulate matter, which might otherwise clog the biologic filter. Mechanical filtration does have limitations and is not effective for trapping finite particles or chemicals.

Biologic Filtration. Biologic filtration relies on bacteria to take toxic compounds and make them less toxic (e.g., *Nitrosomonas* spp. oxidizes ammonia to nitrite and *Nitrobacter* spp. oxidizes nitrite to nitrate; *Nitrospira* spp. also plays a role in this process). This type of filtration is the most common form used in the home aquarium and outdoor pond. While the water and surfaces of the tank serve as sites for bacteria to grow and function, several different types of commercial biologic filters are available that enable the bacteria to become colonized, including undergravel filters, bio-wheels, sand or bead filters, and wet-dry filters. A biologic filter should be selected based on the size of the aquarium (gallons of water), number of fish (density), and frequency of feeding.

Nitrogen is a component of protein. When fish are fed, they take protein from the diet and convert it to energy and waste product. The waste product is converted into ammonia and excreted from the gills. Leftover food in an aquarium also degrades into ammonia. In an aquarium, ammonia levels can build to dangerous levels for fish, leading to illness or death. Ammonia is an irritant to the gills and skin of fish. Fish suffering from ammonia toxicity might become tachypneic, gasp at the surface, try to jump out of the aquarium, or rub against rocks and plants.

Total ammonia-nitrogen (TAN) is divided into two forms, ionized (NH_4+) and un-ionized (NH_3). The un-ionized form is more toxic than the ionized form.[1] The quantity and form of ammonia found in water are dependent on biologic, chemical, and physical factors.[2] Biologic factors include the number of fish, the amount of food offered, live plants, and so on. Chemical factors include pH and alkalinity. When the pH is low, or acidic, the majority of ammonia in the water is ionized, whereas when the pH is high, or basic, the un-ionized or more toxic form is common. Temperature affects the amount of each form of ammonia in the water; as water temperature increases, the amount of un-ionized ammonia also increases.

Several factors can affect the function of a biologic filter, including water temperature, water oxygen content, and drugs/therapeutics. In outdoor ponds when the water temperature drops below 65°F, nitrite is not converted into nitrate as rapidly because *Nitrobacter* bacteria do not tolerate the cold. Owners should be advised to closely monitor nitrite and nitrate levels during those times when the water temperature might drop. To prevent excess work for the biologic filter, owners should stop or reduce the amount of food being offered to the fish. All of the bacteria essential to the biologic filter need oxygen (aerobic conditions). In the home aquarium, oxygen levels are often adequate; however, in outdoor ponds, oxygen levels can become depleted, depending on the time of day or season. (See "Oxygen" under "Water Quality.") To prevent a problem with

oxygen depletion, owners should aerate the water with a fountain or airstone during the times when a problem might occur.

Antibiotics can have negative effects on biologic filters. These types of compounds are routinely used to empirically treat aquariums and ponds; however, they are not specific and kill beneficial bacteria and pathogens alike. If there is concern about the biologic filter, it is recommended to shut off the biologic filter to protect the bacteria essential to its function.

A biologic filter requires time to become established. The amount of time depends on the temperature of the water and the organic load on the system. For example, a system maintained at 23°C takes 4–6 weeks to become established. Commercial microbial products are available that claim to expedite the establishment of the microflora. Unfortunately, there is no hard evidence to support using these products. Water samples, filter pads, or aquarium substrates from established systems have also been used to seed a tank. However, the addition of these products might also lead to the introduction of pathogens.

Chemical Filtration. A number of different types of chemical filters are available in the pet trade. Chemical filtration refers to those filters that remove toxic compounds by binding them or converting them into nontoxic substances. The original form of chemical filtration was activated carbon. Carbon can bind a number of different substances (nonspecific). When the binding sites are full, they no longer act as filters and will need to be replaced or cleaned. Placing the carbon in vinegar (acetic acid) will acidify it and break the bonds with any chemicals that have formed, allowing it to be reused in the tank after being rinsed thoroughly. Other forms of chemical filtration are more specific, such as the resins that bind only ammonia. Other forms of chemical filtration, such as ultraviolet sterilizers and protein skimmers, alter or trap compounds. Ultraviolet sterilizers expose compounds to short-wavelength light, altering their form and rendering them harmless. Protein skimmers trap protein in bubbles so that they can be separated from the water and removed. Chemical filtration, in combination with mechanical and biologic filtration, can improve water quality dramatically, creating a healthy environment for fish.

Ultraviolet (UV) sterilizers can be used to control certain pathogens and algae. A UV sterilizer has a UV bulb encased in a waterproof sheath within a cylinder. As water passes through the cylinder, the water is exposed to ultraviolet light, which can alter the DNA or RNA of a microorganism. The amount of time that it takes for the water to pass the bulb and the bulb wattage determine the effectiveness of the UV sterilizer. A low-wattage bulb in a short cylinder will have little effect on pathogens. These systems have also been used with great success at controlling pathogens and algae in outdoor ponds.

Water Quality

Water quality is very important to the health of a fish, and poor water quality can prove fatal. Two types of systems can be used: open and closed. In open water systems, the water in the aquarium is continually replenished using a freshwater source. A person who lives by the ocean might collect seawater for a home marine aquarium, although this is not recommended because of the potential contaminants in the water. Open water systems are rarely used because they are labor-intensive and require regular exchange of the entire system. The majority of home aquariums use closed recirculating systems, which recirculate the same water over and over again using a filter. In the closed system, freshwater is added only after evaporation or at the time of a water change.

Ammonia, Nitrite, and Nitrate. Ammonia is produced in fish as an end product of protein catabolism and is excreted directly across the gills into the aquatic medium. Ammonia is also derived from feces, uneaten food, and decaying organic matter. Ammonia nitrogen can occur in two forms: ammonium (NH_4+) and ammonia (NH_3). Ammonia is the more toxic form to fish.[1] The relative concentration of each form varies with water pH and temperature.[2]

Ammonia is soluble in water, and minimal amounts are lost through evaporation. In a closed system, such as an aquarium or backyard pond, ammonia levels can build up to toxic quantities (>1 ppm). Even low levels of ammonia can be toxic to the gills and skin, resulting in increased susceptibility to infection. (See "Diagnostic Sampling.") Owners should be advised to closely monitor ammonia levels in new systems or systems that contain a large number of fish. Ammonia should be tested weekly using a standardized commercial test kit, which is available at local pet retailers. In an established system, the ammonia level should be zero. If the ammonia level begins to rise, then the system should be reevaluated. Overfeeding and overstocking an aquarium can overburden the biologic filter. Severe temperature fluctuations and insufficient oxygen levels can also result in a significant loss of the biological filter. This is especially common in ponds that have significant summer algal blooms. New systems require time to become established, and new fish should be added gradually to prevent an overload of the biologic filter.

Because ammonia is a common waste product produced by fish and excessive decaying food, most problems can be prevented by limiting the stocking numbers in an aquarium and by offering only the quantity of food that the fish will consume within a 2- to 5-minute period. In cases when ammonia levels are creating problems, the first recommendation technicians should give their clients is to remove 25%–50% of the water from the system and replace it with fresh, dechlorinated water. There are commercial products available that can chelate the ammonia source, but they are only a temporary solution. The primary cause of the elevated ammonia level must be diagnosed and corrected.

Ammonia is a colorless, odorless substance that can cause significant mortality in a home aquarium. Most inexperienced aquarists tend to single out infectious diseases when they experience fish losses; however, poor water quality (e.g., excessive ammonia or nitrite) is often a primary or secondary cause of mortality in these animals, and water should be tested on a regular basis.

The nitrogen cycle eliminates ammonia by converting it into less toxic compounds. Ammonia is initially oxidized to nitrite (NO_2) by bacteria (*Nitrosomonas* spp. and *Nitrospira* spp.) within the aquatic system. Nitrite is also toxic to fish and can be rapidly absorbed across the gills. Affected animals develop a methemoglobinemia and have characteristic "brown-blood," gasp for air at the water surface, and die suddenly. Nitrite levels in an aquatic system might rise soon after treatment of the water with antibacterial compounds or a reduction in water temperature. Antibiotics added to the water are nonselective and will kill both pathogenic and commensal organisms. These compounds can kill enough bacteria associated with the biologic filter to prevent the oxidation of ammonia and nitrite. *Nitrosomonas* spp. will recolonize before *Nitrobacter* spp., so ammonia levels should be expected to decrease before nitrites. *Nitrobacter* spp. are more sensitive to temperature fluctuations than *Nitrosomonas* spp.; therefore, elevated nitrite levels are often detected soon after a reduction in water temperature. Nitrite levels

less than 0.5 ppm are generally regarded as safe; levels less than 3.0 ppm are associated with stress and can predispose fish to opportunistic infection; levels greater than 5 ppm are considered toxic.

When fish show clinical signs associated with nitrite toxicity, they should be removed from the toxic water and placed into a fresh, dechlorinated, well-oxygenated system. Fish with methemoglobinemia have reduced oxygen carrying capacity and require well-oxygenated water. This can be accomplished by placing into the hospital tank a fine-mist airstone that creates a break in water surface tension, increasing water oxygen levels. A significant water change (25%–50%) should be made in the original aquarium or pond and the biologic filter reestablished.

In the nitrogen cycle, nitrite is further oxidized to nitrate (NO_3) by *Nitrobacter* spp. and *Nitrospira* spp. Reports of nitrate toxicity are rare in fresh- and saltwater fish, but elevated levels can be stressful and predispose the animals to opportunistic pathogens. Nitrate is used by plants and algae as a food source. Nitrate can be removed from an aquatic system by performing regular water changes.

"New Tank" Syndrome. "New tank" syndrome is a common problem reported by beginner/novice aquarists who overload a newly established biologic filter. "New tank" syndrome occurs primarily when fish are overstocked in a new aquarium. The high density of fish creates a high ammonia load on the new system. This is often coupled with overfeeding, which leads to additional organic load on the system and a rise in ammonia levels. In most cases, the owners report acute death of the fish and the clinical signs are consistent with ammonia and nitrite toxicity. These problems can be prevented if the new owner is patient and realizes the importance of providing a break-in period for the filter (4–6 weeks). Owners should be made aware that fish should be stocked gradually, usually 1–2 fish per week. A standard rule of thumb for freshwater stocking density is 1–1.5" of fish per gallon of water, whereas in saltwater systems the stocking density should be 2–2.5" of fish per gallon of water. With the advent of new filtration systems, stocking densities will continue to increase; however, if the filter becomes compromised or fails, the results would be disastrous.

Oxygen. Fish acquire free oxygen directly from the water. Oxygen diffuses into water at the surface when the surface tension of the water is broken. The amount of available or dissolved oxygen (DO) within the system can be measured using special equipment. In most cases, a DO >5 ppm is sufficient to maintain fish. In most home aquariums, there is sufficient DO.

Oxygen depletion is a major concern in outdoor ponds during the summer months. During the day, plants produce their own food (photosynthesis) by taking carbon dioxide from the water and using energy produced by the sun. As plants make their food, they release oxygen into the water. During the night when plants or algae cannot undergo photosynthesis, they actually consume oxygen. In ponds with a large number of plants or phytoplankton, oxygen levels in the water can fall to dangerously low levels for the fish. Another factor that can affect oxygen levels in water is temperature. Oxygen is lost to the atmosphere more rapidly in warm water than in cold water. The use of aerators or fountains, especially at night, will help maintain adequate levels of oxygen in a pond.

Water pH. The pH of water is calculated as the negative logarithm of hydrogen ions. In simplest terms, pH can be divided into three categories: acid, neutral, and basic. The range of pH values fits on a scale of 1–14. Values below 7.0 represent acidic water, values between 7.0 and 7.9 are neutral, and values above 8.0 are basic. The pH in most aquariums and ponds should fall between 6.5 and 8.5. In the extreme ranges (<4 or >10), water would be so acidic or basic that it would burn the fish. This means that the difference between 7.0 and 8.0 is much more significant than you might expect, because the pH values are based on a logarithmic scale. Therefore, if the pH is allowed to fluctuate, fish will become stressed and more susceptible to disease.

The pH of natural bodies of water varies based on the substrate, watershed, and other environmental factors. Fish from Central and South America thrive in water that is neutral or slightly acidic, whereas fish from Africa and Asia thrive better in neutral to alkaline water.

Water should always be tested prior to replacement in an aquarium. A number of factors can affect the pH in an aquarium or pond, including the biologic filter, fish density, vegetation, and algae. Biologic filtration actually produces acid when ammonia is converted into nitrite. If the water has a low buffering capacity and the aquarium or pond biologic filter is converting a large amount of ammonia, the pH could become very acidic. Fish produce carbon dioxide (CO_2) as a waste product. When an aquarium or pond is heavily stocked with fish, the amount of CO_2 can build up in the water. Carbon dioxide promotes acid production and can actually decrease the pH (acidic). Plants and phytoplankton (algae), which use photosynthesis during the day to make energy, use CO_2 as their primary substrate. However, at night, plants and algae use oxygen (like fish) and expel CO_2 as a waste product. In a system with a large amount of plants and phytoplankton, the pH can drop to a dangerously low level. Fish die-off in ponds is often associated with high CO_2, low pH, and low oxygen levels. When plants or fish die, they also release compounds that can lower the pH. To prevent this from becoming a problem, owners should be advised always to remove dead fish or plants immediately.

Chlorine. Chlorine is a gas that is added to our municipal water supplies to protect us from bacteria and other harmful organisms. Unfortunately, chlorine is toxic to fish. When a fish is placed in chlorinated water, the chlorine crosses the gills and blocks the fish's ability to absorb oxygen, which causes suffocation. This whole process can take minutes to hours, depending on the amount of chlorine in the water. Sodium thiosulfate can be added to tap water to neutralize chlorine, immediately making the water safe for fish. Municipal water supplies add variable amounts of chlorine at different times of the year, depending on the source of water. If owners have questions about the timing or amounts of chlorine that are added, they should be advised to call their local water company. They should always test the water before replacing it in the aquarium or pond to ensure that the chlorine has been removed.

Chloramine. Chloramines are also routinely added to municipal water supplies for sterilization purposes. Chloramines are formed by combining chlorine with ammonia. Commercial dechlorinators can be added to tap water to neutralize chlorine; however, the ammonia will remain in the water. Ammonia is toxic to fish and can prove fatal to fish at levels higher than 1 ppm. A functional biologic filter will convert the ammonia to nitrate.

Hardness. Hardness is a measure of the amount of divalent cations, primarily calcium and magnesium, in the water. In natural waters, the divalent ions are derived from limestone, salts, and soils. The normal range for hardness in freshwater systems is 0–250 mg/L, whereas in saltwater systems the total hardness can exceed 10,000 mg/L.[3] Calcium and magnesium play an intricate role in water quality conditions. Calcium appears to protect fish that are exposed to a low pH or elevated ammonia by altering osmoregulatory functions.[3] Calcium and magnesium are essential to growth and development of young fish.[4] Calcium and magnesium can also protect fish from heavy metal exposure by competing for gill absorption sites. Copper is routinely used to treat ectoparasites on fish. Calcium and magnesium will compete with the copper for absorption sites, reducing the effectiveness of the copper. Distilled water should never be used to replenish water in an aquarium, because it is deficient in these essential cations.

Alkalinity. In natural water systems such as lakes, fish are exposed to a relatively stable pH because of buffers. The most common buffers in aquatic systems are bicarbonate (HCO_3) and carbonate (CO_3^{2-}). Other buffers that can occur in water in lesser amounts are hydroxide ($OH-$), silicates, phosphates, and borates. The quantity of buffers within a system depends on location. Some municipal water supplies contain minuscule amounts of buffers, whereas others might have large quantities of buffers. Commercial buffers can be added to an aquarium or pond to increase the total alkalinity in the system, creating a more stable pH.

Total alkalinity also plays an important role in the chemistry of potential toxins such as lead, zinc, and copper. Heavy metals are absorbed from the water by the gills and are fatal to fish. Bicarbonate and carbonate can actually bind the heavy metals, rendering them harmless. This is important to remember when treating fish with nonchelated copper. If the alkalinity is high, the unchelated copper can be bound and rendered useless.

Monitoring Water Quality. For new tanks, owners should test water weekly for ammonia, nitrite, nitrate, pH, alkalinity, and hardness. If problems occur, they should test the water more frequently, and allow 4–6 weeks for the biologic filter to become established. Owners should be advised to add only 1 or 2 fish at a time so that the biologic filter is not overloaded. They should always test new water for the previously mentioned parameters and for chlorine and chloramine before replacing it in the aquarium or pond.

For established tanks, 10%–20% of the water should be replaced every 1–3 weeks. Frequency of water change will depend on the load on the system (i.e., size of aquarium, number of fish, amount of food offered). A small aquarium will need more frequent changes than a large aquarium. By closely monitoring the water (ammonia, nitrite, nitrate, pH, alkalinity, and hardness), owners will be able to determine when it needs to be changed. Before replacing the water, owners should be sure to test it for the same parameters, as well as for chlorine and chloramine.

Nutrition

A variety of commercially available fish foods are available in the pet retail trade (Figure 8.5). Many of these diets are specifically formulated to meet the needs of particular fish, including herbivores, omnivores, and carnivores. It is important for veterinarians and veterinary technicians to learn to read the labels of foods offered to their patients, so that they can give owners sound advice regarding what should and should not be recommended. In general, carnivorous fish should be offered diets with the highest protein (>50%), followed by omnivores (40%–50%) and herbivores (30%–40%). The inverse is true as it relates to fiber. Commercial fish foods are sold in flake and pelleted rations. In certain fish, especially ornamental goldfish, the ingestion of floating pellets has been associated with buoyancy problems (Figure 8.6). Fish that develop such problems should be offered sinking pellets. In addition, feeding

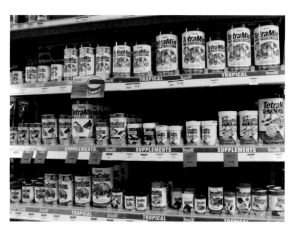

Figure 8.5 *A wide variety of commercial fish food is available at local pet retailers. It is important to read labels carefully to ensure that a particular group of fish is provided the most appropriate diet.*

cooked, squashed peas has also been found to have positive benefits for fish with swim bladder disease. It is not known why this dietary supplement works, but it is suspected to be associated with changes in gas-producing bacteria. Obesity is a common problem identified in captive ornamental fish because of a combination of high-fat, high-protein commercial diets and restricted exercise (aquarium size). Restricted feeding and providing the largest swimming area possible will reduce the potentially life-threatening problems associated with obesity. Live foods are routinely offered to carnivorous fish to balance commercial food preparations and to increase exercise levels. Live foods can transmit disease and should be purchased only from a reputable dealer. Another benefit of live foods is that they provide enrichment for fish and force them to practice normal hunting behaviors.

Transport

Fish should be transported in a plastic sealed container, which should be used exclusively to transport fish and never reused to carry human food items.

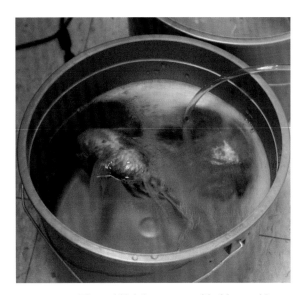

Figure 8.6 *This goldfish has a swim bladder problem. Feeding floating pellets to some fish can lead to increased ingestion of air, which can affect buoyancy.*

The container should be cleaned with warm, soapy water and rinsed thoroughly after each use. Bleach should never be used to clean the container. The water used to transport the animal should come from the home aquarium. A separate container of aquarium water should also be brought to the veterinary hospital—in case of spillage, for water quality testing, and as a source for recovery from anesthesia. The fish should be transported immediately to the veterinary hospital. Special precautions should be made during the winter and summer to prevent water temperature fluctuations, such as preheating and -cooling the transport automobile in the winter and summer, respectively. Signs of transport stress may not be apparent for several days after the move, so owners should be advised to monitor the animals closely for 3–5 days post-transport.[5]

HISTORY

A thorough history is key to developing a diagnostic and therapeutic plan. Four key areas must be addressed in the history: the owner's general knowledge, the aquarium environment, the water, and the fish. Questions regarding the owner's general knowledge of aquarium management should include length of aquarium ownership/experience, number of aquariums they own, where the fish were obtained, time spent viewing the fish, and weekly maintenance program.

The history of the aquarium environment should include questions about tank volume, tank placement, tank top, lighting, heating, filtration, substrate, and aquarium decorations (e.g., plants, rocks, logs, and toys). It is important for the technician to ask about tank volume, because it allows him or her to determine the relative stocking density of the aquarium. The placement of the tank within the home might provide insight into problems associated with algal overgrowth (e.g., direct sunlight exposure) or toxins (e.g., cleaning sprays). Some fish owners do not cover their aquariums with a top. Tanks without tops experience faster evaporation and are more prone to fish loss because of jumping.

A number of different lighting systems are available for the home aquarium. Owners should be asked whether they have fluorescent or incandescent lighting, the bulb wattage, and the amount of time the lighting remains on during the day. Incandescent lights produce radiant heat and are associated with increased water temperatures. Fluorescent lighting, especially full-spectrum lighting, is preferred for live aquatic plant systems.

Most aquariums are heated with thermostatically controlled heaters. Questions regarding heater usage (yes or no), type, and wattage size should be asked. Owners should also be asked if they use a thermometer and, if so, the temperature in the aquarium. Fish are poikilotherms and must be provided an appropriate environmental temperature.

Because there are a number of different types of filters, questions should be asked to determine type of filter, length of usage, and owner's general knowledge of filtration. Information should be ascertained regarding aquarium decorations, such as plants, rocks, logs, and toys. The addition of new live plants might introduce disease.

Most fish-owning clients have a limited knowledge of water chemistry; therefore, veterinary technicians must be patient with their clients when taking a history of water quality. Questions must be asked regarding the source of the water, how often the water is changed, and water quality tests that have been performed. Veterinary hospitals that work with ornamental fish should have water quality test kits and should perform the appropriate water tests during the visit.

The final history questions should focus on the fish. Questions regarding types of fish, number of fish, and length of ownership are all important. Many infectious disease cases are the direct result of adding new, unquarantined fish. Types of other aquatic organisms, such as snails, must also be addressed because these animals can also introduce disease. Owners should be asked whether the fish are eating and if any abnormal behaviors have been noted, such as whirling, inverted swimming, jumping, tachypnea, or lethargy. The final questions should address the number of affected fish, specific lesions, and duration of the presenting disease.

PHYSICAL EXAMINATION

A fish physical examination will be performed in two stages: a hands-off examination and a hands-on examination. The hands-off examination should be done while the fish is in its transport container. Observe the fish for abnormalities in behavior, breathing, locomotion, and attitude. Because fish are typically anesthetized for the hands-on component of the examination, abnormalities in breathing, locomotion, and mentation might not be seen. Any abnormal findings should be recorded prior to a hands-on examination.

A fish can be captured with a net or a gloved hand, or it can be scooped into a plastic cup or bucket. Animals in a large aquarium must be caught with a net. Netting a fish can be a very traumatic experience. It is best to reduce the lighting in the room when capturing a fish to prevent it from swimming into the tank walls and injuring itself. Once the fish is captured, it should be transferred into a bucket with water collected from the primary aquarium.

A hands-on physical examination of a fish should be performed in a thorough and rapid manner (Figure 8.7). The veterinarian will wear examination gloves to minimize the potential spread of zoonotic pathogens through open cuts on his or her hands and to protect the fish skin from the oils found on human hands. Generally, a fish is anesthetized for a physical examination and diagnostic tests are collected at the same time. Tricaine methane sulfonate is the anesthetic of choice (see "Diagnostic Handling"). If the fish is already moribund, anesthesia can be skipped. The physical examination should be performed out of water to improve visualization of the animal. The fish should be replaced into the water bucket every 30–45 seconds during the procedure to allow it to respire and to rewet the gills and body. The fish should be cupped in the hand with minimal restraint, because the protective mucous layer and scales can be damaged from minor manipulation.

Handlers should have a basic knowledge of the fish they are working with to prevent injury to themselves and other hospital staff. Many ornamental fish have spines associated with their fins, which can cause pain upon puncture and become a source of

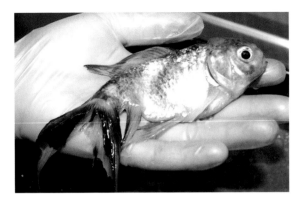

Figure 8.7 *A hands-on examination of a fish should be done using the same thorough protocol used for domestic pets. Never go directly to an abnormality, but instead start at the head and work through the fish, being sure to examine all systems. Anesthetizing the patient for the examination reduces the stress on the fish and gives the examiner additional time to examine the fish.*

infection to the handler. There are also a number of ornamental fish, such as the lionfish, that can inject venom; they should be handled only by professionals. In most cases, anesthetizing fish is preferred to ensure safety of the animals and the handler.

When performing the hands-on physical examination, the following structures should be evaluated:

- *Nares*: They should be clear and not eroded. These are blind pockets in most fish.
- *Eyes*: The corneal surfaces should be clear. A fluoroscein stain can be done to check for corneal ulcers. The anterior chamber should be clear of red and white blood cells. Lenticular dislocation is common with trauma and should be evaluated. Fundic examinations are difficult in fish.
- *Mouth*: The mouth should be clear of discharge. The maxillae and mandibles should be freely movable. Dislocation is common in some species. Water should move freely through the oral cavity and out the opercula.

- *Opercula and gills*: The opercula should move freely during normal respiration. When the opercla are lifted, the gills should be bright red. Excessive mucus and free hemorrhage are abnormalities that require additional examination/testing.
- *Body condition*: The muscling over the head, neck, and spine should be evaluated. Any prominence of the skull or spine is an indication of poor body condition.
- *Skin*: The integument should be inspected for lost scales, hemorrhage, abscesses/granulomas, and excessive mucus.
- *Fins*: The pectoral, pelvic, anal, caudal, dorsal, and adipose (if present) fins should be inspected for excessive mucus, hemorrhage, and tears. Any erosions noted on the fins should be documented.
- *Abdominal cavity*: The abdominal cavity (location of the viscera) should be palpated to determine if there are any firm masses or free fluid (ascites).
- *Anus/Urogenital openings*: Most teleosts have a separate anus as the terminus of the gastrointestinal tract and a urogenital opening as the terminus of the excretory and reproductive tracts. Examine these openings for any discharge or prolapse of tissues.

DIAGNOSTIC SAMPLING

Fish have evolved to mask their illness. Although this protects against predation under natural conditions, it can make the job of the veterinarian and veterinary technician more difficult. Because of this defense mechanism, it is important for veterinary professionals to pursue appropriate diagnostic tests to determine underlying causes of disease. The purpose of this section is to review common diagnostics used to characterize the disease status of fish.

Fish that present with a history of tachypnea or gulping air at the water surface should have their gills examined. Common differentials for such cases include poor water quality, bacterial infections, and parasite infestations. Fish suffering from ammonia toxicity appear irritated, gasp at the water surface, and may rub against rocks in the enclosure as a result of the irritation caused by the toxin. Affected animals can die suddenly. Anytime a fish presents with breathing at the water surface, a thorough evaluation of the gills should be done.

A gill biopsy is a simple diagnostic test that can provide significant information regarding the patient's status. Fish should be anesthetized for a gill biopsy to provide appropriate sedation and analgesia, and MS-222 is the anesthetic of choice for this procedure. Once a fish is anesthetized, it should be removed from the anesthetic solution using gloved hands and placed onto a dechlorinated, moist paper towel. A pair of fine iris scissors should be inserted under the operculum and gently lifted, enabling the veterinarian to insert his or her thumb under the operculum to provide direct visualization of the gills. Iris scissors should be reinserted under the operculum, and 4–6 gill filaments should be collected

(Figure 8.8). The gill filaments should be placed onto a microscope slide with a drop of 0.9% saline or water from the fish's aquarium/recovery bucket, covered with a coverslip, and reviewed under a light microscope. Samples can also be stained to review the tissues for the presence of bacteria. Once the procedure has been completed, the animal should be recovered in dechlorinated, fresh water.

Fish that present with a history of scraping against materials in the aquarium, increased mucus production, hemorrhage on the skin, or loss of scales should have a skin scrape done to determine the underlying cause of disease. Common differentials for these types of cases include poor water quality, bacterial infections, and parasite infestations. A skin scrape is a simple diagnostic test that can be used to identify specific pathogens on the surface of a fish integument. Once again, the animal should be anesthetized to reduce stress. The animal can be restrained by hand or placed on a moistened paper towel. A microscope slide should be placed at a 45° angle on the skin at the site of the lesion(s) and gently dragged in a caudal direction (Figure 8.9). The material collected from the skin scrape should be placed on an additional

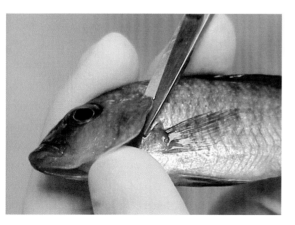

Figure 8.8 *A gill biopsy in a cichlid. To perform the procedure, insert your free thumb under the operculum and lift. Insert a pair of iris scissors under the operculum and clip 4 to 6 primary lamellae to examine.*

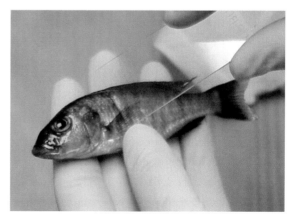

Figure 8.9 *A skin scrape in a cichlid. Place the microscope slide at a 45° angle to the skin at the site of the lesion and draw the slide caudally. Dragging the slide cranially will damage scales.*

microscope slide, a drop of 0.9% saline or water from the fish's aquarium/recovery bucket added to the mix, and the material covered with a coverslip. Additional slides can be made with Diff-Quik or Gram stains to look specifically at cell types and bacteria. A light microscope with the capacity of 1,000× magnification (10× eye pieces, plus a 100× immersion oil objective) will be required to screen the samples. The fish should be recovered in dechlorinated water.

Fish that present with a history of abnormal growths, discolorations, or ulcerations in their fins should receive a fin biopsy. Common differentials for these types of cases include poor water quality, trauma, water mold infections, bacterial infections, and parasite infestations. A fin biopsy can be especially useful in cases with ectoparasites, bacteria, or water molds, because these organisms can be seen on the cytologic review of the fin biopsy. A fish undergoing this procedure should be anesthetized. A pair of iris scissors should be used to cut a sample from an affected fin (Figure 8.10). Do not worry about cutting around fin rays, as the fins will heal rapidly once the inciting cause is treated. The sample should be placed on a microscope slide, mixed with a drop of 0.9% saline or water from the aquarium/recovery water, covered with a coverslip, and evaluated under a light microscope. The fish should be recovered in dechlorinated water.

The examination of blood samples (hematology and biochemistries) can provide insight into the general health of an animal that might not otherwise be obvious on physical examination. The volume of blood that can be collected from a fish has been estimated to be similar to that of mammals, approximately 0.8%–1.0% of the body weight.[6] Always preload the needle with heparin to prevent blood clotting. The primary sites of venipuncture in fish are the caudal tail vein and

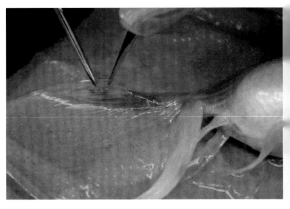

Figure 8.10 *A fin biopsy in a cichlid. Using a pair of iris scissors, remove a section of affected fin. Place the fin on a slide with a drop of 0.9% saline or water from the fish's aquarium and cover it with a coverslip. Review the slide under a light microscope.*

the heart. The caudal tail vein is located ventral to the vertebral column and runs parallel to the spine. A 3 ml syringe with a 25- to 30-gauge needle is recommended for sample collection. There are 2 approaches to the ventral tail vein: a lateral approach and a ventral approach. For the lateral approach, the needle should be gently inserted at a 45° angle (between scales) into the caudal peduncle at the level of the lateral line and walked off the ventral edge of the vertebral column until a flash of blood can be seen in the needle (Figure 8.11). For the ventral approach, the animal should be held in dorsal recumbency and the needle inserted into the ventral midline of the caudal peduncle at a 90° angle. The needle should be inserted to the level of the vertebral column and gently walked along the spine until a flash of blood is observed. The heart is located ventral and caudal to the gills/operculum. For cardiac blood samples, the operculum should be elevated (similar to the technique used for a gill biopsy) and a needle inserted caudally and ventrally at the level of the caudal isthmus (Figure 8.12). Once collected, samples should be placed immediately into their appropriate transport tubes. When working with tropical fish, many prefer using Microtainers (Becton Dickinson Corp., Franklin Lakes, NJ), because the sample volumes collected are typically small. These transport tubes have a dry anticoagulant, so there is no concern about sample dilution.

Red blood cell estimates are not typically done for fish unless there is a problem, because it is necessary to do manual counts and standard hematologic machines cannot count nucleated erythrocytes. Fortunately, most veterinarians are comfortable reviewing packed cell volumes (PCV) to get an appreciation of erythrocyte numbers; PCV values for fish are typically between 20% and 40%. When veterinary technicians read manual differentials for white blood cell counts, they should note what they see with the erythrocytes. Immature erythrocytes in fish, as in amphibians, reptiles, and birds, are smaller in size, have a higher nuclear to cytoplasmic ratio, and have a basophilic cytoplasm, compared with mature erythrocytes. When large differences (3–4+) are noted in color (polychromasia) or size (anisocytosis) of erythrocytes, it is important to document and consider when interpreting the overall erythrocyte status of a patient.

Complete blood counts in fish require special care. Because all of the blood cells are nucleated in fish, standard hematologic equipment cannot be used. Instead, manual counts must be done. To perform a manual count in a fish, start by making a high-quality blood smear. Make the blood smear using either standard microscope slides or coverslips. Blood cells in fish are more fragile than those found in mammals; therefore, it is important to use caution when making blood smears to minimize the likelihood of cell rupture ("smudgeocytes"). Premixing a blood sample with 22% bovine albumin (Gamma

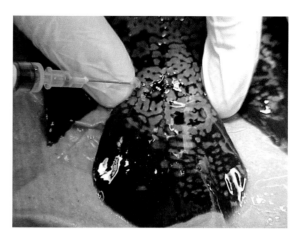

Figure 8.11 *Ventral tail vein venipuncture in an oscar.*

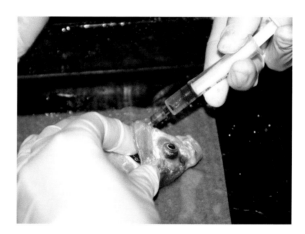

Figure 8.12 *Cardiac venipuncture in a goldfish.*

Biologics, Houston, TX) can stabilize the cells and minimize "smudgeocytes." To do this, add 1 drop of bovine albumin and 5 drops of whole blood to a test tube. Mix the solution by gently rotating/rocking it. Once it is mixed, use a hematocrit tube to collect some blood from the tube and make your smears using standard glass microscope slides. Blood smears can also be made using coverslips (without bovine albumin). In reptiles, no significant difference in the number of "smudgeocytes" has been noted between samples premixed with albumin and made with slides and those made with coverslips, although both of these techniques resulted in significantly fewer "smudgeocytes" than smears made only using glass slides (not pretreated with albumin).

Once the slides are made, estimating white blood cells and differential count is easiest if you do the following:

1. Count the number of white blood cells on 10 fields at 400× (10× eyepiece and 40× objective). The fields should represent a section of the blood smear where the cells fill (but don't overfill) the slide and are evenly distributed.

2. Divide the total number of white blood cells counted by 10 to get the average number of cells per field.

3. Multiply the average number of cells per field by 2,000 to get the estimated white blood cell count.

4. Perform a 100- or 200-cell differential to determine the proportions of white blood cells. The more cells counted (200 vs. 100), the tighter the results will be. These proportions can then be multiplied by the estimated white blood cell count (see step 3) to estimate absolute values of the different cell types.

Microbiology

Microbiologic samples can be collected from a fish during an antemortem or postmortem exam. Antemortem samples are routinely collected from specific lesions on the skin, fins, or eyes. Contamination is a significant concern in these cases, and results should be interpreted accordingly. A sterile swab can be rubbed over the affected area to collect the sample. The sample should be refrigerated until it is plated, which should occur within 24 hours.

Postmortem cultures routinely involve internal organs. To ensure sterility, the necropsy should be performed in a consistent manner. Seventy percent ethyl alcohol should be applied to the ventral surface of the fish and the area flamed. Once the alcohol has burned off, the fish should be opened using sterile scissors and forceps. After the coelomic cavity is exposed, samples can be collected using either a sterile swab or sterile biopsy techniques.

There are many opinions about the most appropriate culture media and incubation temperatures for isolating bacterial pathogens from fish. A standard blood agar plate can be used as the initial plate, or other specialized plates can be used if a specific pathogen is suspected. Salt should be supplemented to the plate when attempting to isolate pathogens from marine fish. Plates should be incubated at 25°C and 37°C. Although it is often argued that the 25°C incubation temperature is preferred because it mimics the temperature of the ectothermic host, bacteria can grow at a range of temperatures and most grow faster and more proficiently at higher temperatures (37°C). Exceptions to this are water molds and fungi. These organisms can be outcompeted at 37°C and tend to grow better at 20°–25°C. Culture plates should be evaluated for growth at 24- and 48-hour time periods. A Gram stain should be performed on any isolate. Biochemical identification of the organism should follow standard microbiologic protocol.

Radiology

Several case presentations require radiographic evaluation, including foreign body ingestion, neoplasia (Figure 8.13), internal abscesses, and swim bladder disease (Figure 8.14). Fish should be anesthetized during the procedure to prevent thrashing and damage to the mucous barrier and integument. Tricaine methane sulfonate is the anesthetic of choice. The fish should be recovered as soon as the procedure is completed. The techniques used to perform the radiographs will vary from machine to machine. High-detail films should be used to provide the best radiographic image.

Parasitology

Parasites are a common finding in fish. Although the majority of the parasites encountered with captive fish are found externally (e.g., skin and gills), there are certainly endoparasites (e.g., gastrointestinal, liver) reported in these species, too. As mentioned previously, screening for parasites should be done as a component of the general examination of a fish (see "Diagnostic Sampling"). Skin scrapes, fin biopsies, and gill biopsies are invaluable for evaluating fish for external parasites. Fecal examinations, both direct saline fecal smears and fecal flotations, can be used to screen fish for gastrointestinal parasites. Because fish serve as intermediate hosts for a variety of parasites (e.g., trematodes, nematodes), some parasites can be identified/confirmed only using histopathology at postmortem.

THERAPEUTICS

Therapeutics can be administered to fish in a water bath, orally, via intramuscular injection, via intracoelomic injection, or by intravenous route. Water bath treatment with certain drugs is of little value to freshwater fish, but have been used with success to treat marine fish. Marine fish actually drink water, so any medication placed in the water will be ingested. Freshwater fish do not drink water and are not likely to receive the same benefit. Carbon filters should be removed when a bath or immersion treatment is used.

Oral medications can also be placed in food and delivered to the fish during routine feedings. Unfortunately, many sick fish are anorexic and do not benefit from medicated food. Per os medica-

tions can also be administered via a stomach tube. A red rubber feeding tube can be used for this procedure. The distance from the mouth to just distal to the opercula should be measured and marked, thereby denoting the approximate location of the stomach. The tube should be inserted to the level of the mark, and the medication delivered. If the tube is not passed through the esophagus, it will be seen passing out one of the opercula.

Intramuscular injections are administered into the epaxial muscle surrounding the spine. The needle is inserted between scales. Irritating

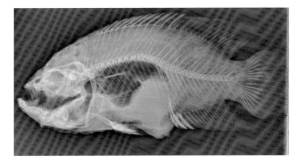

Figure 8.13 *A lateral survey radiograph of an oscar with a renal tumor.*

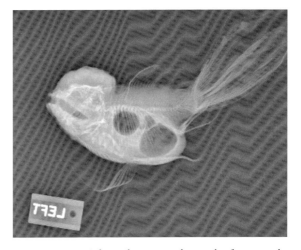

Figure 8.14 *A lateral survey radiograph of an oranda goldfish with a swim bladder problem. In this case, the fish had excess gas in the caudal chamber that displaced it ventrally.*

compounds should not be administered intramuscularly because they can lead to muscle necrosis.

Intracoelomic injections are routinely used to administer antibiotics to fish. The fish is held in dorsal recumbency, allowing gravity to drop the viscera, and the injection administered between the scales of the ventrum into the coelomic cavity (Figure 8.15). Again, irritating compounds should not be used.

Intravenous injections are not routinely used, but might be useful during emergency situations. Inappropriate use of antibiotics and antiparasitics can lead to development of resistant strains of bacteria and parasites.

SURGICAL AND ANESTHETIC ASSISTANCE

Surgical procedures are becoming routine with fish. The basic tenets of surgery in domestic species apply to fish surgery as well. Fish surgery can be performed in or out of water. The preferred method is out of water because it increases visualization of the surgical field. Tricaine methane sulfonate is the anesthetic of choice for surgical procedures. Surgical procedures should be performed using a recirculating anesthetic machine. Preparation of the surgical area should be done with a noninsulting disinfectant or saline. Avoid alcohol rinses for surgical preparation, because they increase heat loss. Many disinfectants cause chemical burns or are toxic and should be avoided. Microsurgical equipment should be used to perform surgeries in fish. Synthetic absorbable sutures are typically used for fish to ligate internal structures and for body wall closure. Although it is possible to use nylon to close the skin, most surgeons prefer not to use this suture material because they would need to renet the fish to remove the sutures. Clear drapes should be used to limit contamination of the surgical site, while retaining good overall visualization of the patient.

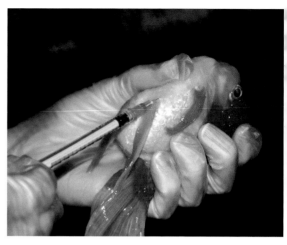

Figure 8.15 *Intracoelomic injections are an excellent way to provide essential medications to fish. Note how the fish is placed in dorsal recumbency to allow gravity to pull the viscera away from the injection site. Also, note how the needle and syringe are held parallel to the body to limit the potential for deep injection into the viscera.*

Historically, veterinarians working with lower vertebrates (e.g., fish, amphibians, and reptiles) have relied on "bruticaine" to restrain animals for physical examination and short surgical procedures. This technique is unacceptable, because there are a number of safe, reliable anesthetic agents that can be used to appropriately restrain or anesthetize a fish for different procedures.

A fish should be thoroughly evaluated prior to performing an anesthetic procedure. Fish that are stressed, maintained under inappropriate water temperatures, or have ingested a recent meal are not considered good anesthetic candidates. Prospective anesthetic candidates should be maintained in clean, dechlorinated, well-oxygenated water (5–10 ppm) under reduced lighting. Food should be withheld for a minimum of 6–8 hours to ensure that they do not regurgitate and contaminate the anesthetic solution.

Always wear a pair of examination gloves when handling fish to administer an anesthetic (e.g., intramuscular injection) or to perform a procedure. Fish that are mishandled might develop an injury to their integument, damaging their dermis (scale loss) and increasing their susceptibility to opportunistic pathogens. Gloves are also beneficial to handlers and will protect them from potentially zoonotic diseases such as *Mycobacterium* spp.

Monitoring fish during an anesthetic procedure can be difficult. In most cases, opercular movement, loss of equilibrium, sensitivity to painful stimuli, fin color, and gill color are used to assess the patient. In larger specimens, a pulse oximeter, EKG, or crystal Doppler can be used to monitor heart rate, although the heart of a fish can continue to pump for a period of time after the animal is dead. In the case of waterborne anesthetics, dechlorinated water can be used to irrigate the gills and "lighten" the plane of anesthesia.

The most widely used anesthetic agent for fish is tricaine methane sulfonate (MS-222). It is a benzocaine derivative with a sulfonate radical. Tricaine methane sulfonate is absorbed across the gill epithelium and biotransformed in the liver and possibly the kidney.[7] The drug and its metabolites are excreted primarily through the gills. The stock solutions are very acidic and should be buffered prior to being used. Sodium bicarbonate (baking soda) can be used to buffer the anesthesia water, and it should be added at an equal weight to the MS-222. Induction with MS-222 is generally accomplished with 100–150 ppm. For some larger fish, a higher dose (200 ppm) may be needed. Maintenance of anesthesia during a procedure can typically be done using 50–100 ppm MS-222.

For short anesthetic procedures, such as physical examination and basic diagnostics, anesthesia can be infused over the gills (through the mouth or under the opercula) via a syringe (Figure 8.16),

although for longer procedures animals should be maintained on a recirculating anesthetic system. A simple system consisting of a submersible electric pump, flexible tubing, and two reservoirs (one for anesthetic and one for recovery) can be used to maintain a fish during a surgical procedure (Figure 8.17). The tubing should be placed directly into the animal's mouth to irrigate the gills. The recirculating pump can be moved from the anesthetic solution to nonanesthetic solution as the depth of anesthesia varies.

Clove oil has been used for centuries by humans for a variety of ailments, including as a topical anesthesia for dental pain. Because MS-222 is regulated for food fish and there is a withdrawal period associated with it, aquaculturists have shown increased interest in clove oil as an unregulated anesthetic. The active component of clove oil is eugenol, which can provide surgical levels of anesthesia for fish; however, the duration and quality of anesthesia are not as good as those provided with MS-222. The safety index of this drug is also considered to be lower than that of MS-222.

Quinaldine sulfate is another water-based drug that can be used to anesthetize fish. Quinaldine sulfate, like MS-222, is strongly acidic in solution and should be buffered before use. The dose used for quinaldine sulfate is similar to that used for MS-222, although some consider quinaldine to have a lower margin of safety. Quinaldine is not metabolized by the fish and is excreted unchanged. Quinaldine can be used for many basic procedures, but is not recommended for surgical procedures that require total loss of movement.

Inhalant anesthetics have been used with variable success. An inhalant anesthetic, such as isoflurane, can be poured directly into the aquatic medium in the concentrated form or "aerated" in

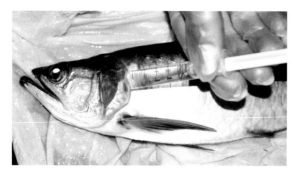

Figure 8.16 *This fish was anesthetized for its examination and diagnostic testing (venipuncture and radiographs). Because these are short procedures, anesthesia was maintained by flushing the gills with 50 ppm MS-222. Moistening the body during the procedure to prevent drying out is also recommended.*

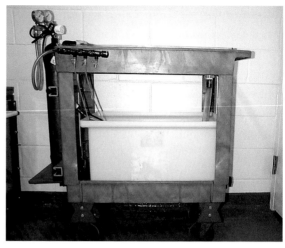

Figure 8.17 *A recirculating anesthesia machine for fish. Notice how the equipment was placed on the cart to make it portable. This system has a reservoir in the bottom to hold the anesthesia water. A power head within the reservoir drives the anesthesia water up to the fish. The tubing from the reservoir is placed in the fish's oral cavity. Anesthetic water that passes out of the opercula and mouth flows through a drain back to the reservoir. Note the valve to connect an air pump for oxygenating the anesthesia water.*

the form of a gas. Regulating the concentration of anesthetic in the water can be difficult. Incomplete distribution of the inhalant anesthetic in the water column can result in "pockets" of gas and variable anesthetic effects. The use of inhalants places additional risk on individuals performing the surgery; therefore, attempts should be made to scavenge the waste gas.

Reports in lay literature have suggested that carbon dioxide can be used as a fish anesthetic.[8] There are many different commercially available sources of CO_2, including Alka-Seltzer, carbon dioxide gas (used for aquatic plant aquariums), and sodium bicarbonate. Unfortunately, CO_2 is difficult to regulate, and if not monitored closely, will result in a rapid decrease in pH and death of the fish. With the availability of safe, effective anesthetics such as MS-222, there is no reason for veterinarians to use CO_2.

Injectable anesthetics are rarely used to anesthetize ornamental fish, because high doses of drug are required and incomplete anesthesia is achieved. Injectable anesthetics have proven effective in elasmobranchs, and recent research indicates that medetomidine and propofol can be used to effectively immobilize elasmobranchs.[9] Propofol has also been found to have value as an anesthetic in larger teleosts, in which it is possible to gain access to a blood vessel to deliver the anesthetic intravenously.

HEALTH MAINTENANCE AND DISEASE

Bacterial Diseases

Bacterial diseases are commonly reported in ornamental fish, and the majority of infections are caused by Gram-negative rods. Many of the opportunistic pathogens isolated from sick fish, such as *Aeromonas* spp. and *Pseudomonas* spp., are routinely isolated from the water column; therefore, it is important to minimize/restrict antibiotics in the water where resistance can develop. Many of these infections develop when there is damage to the animal's protective integument or immune system. Septicemia is a common finding and must be treated aggressively. In a number of these cases, the organisms isolated from the lesions are multidrug-resistant, similar to the "flesh-eating" bacteria isolated from humans (Figure 8.18). Bacterial infections should be diagnosed by culture and sensitivity. A therapeutic plan should follow the sensitivity results.

Viral Diseases

Viral diseases in ornamental fish are rare. The pathogenicity of viruses can vary with temperature. Most viral infections in fish are host-specific. In many cases, young, naive fishes become sick, and older animals become carriers. The most commonly reported virus in ornamental fish is lymphocystis, an iridovirus that infects fibroblasts.[10] Affected animals develop large coalescing nodules that can occur anywhere on the body. The virus is self-limiting. In most cases, the fish resolve spontaneously; however, in cases where the lesions affect the eyes or mouth (i.e., the vision or ability to eat), the animal may die. Lymphocystis can be diagnosed on gross examination or histopathology. There is no effective treatment, although the mass can be surgically debulked if the tumor affects the animal's ability to eat, see, or swim.

Parasites

Parasites are routinely identified on imported ornamental fish. When parasitized animals are added to an established aquarium, the parasites will soon spread to the other tank inhabitants. Both ectoparasites and endoparasites are reported in fish. The clinical signs associated with a parasite infestation will vary, depending upon the location of the parasite. Fish with gill (*Dactylogy-*

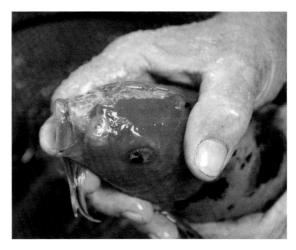

Figure 8.18 *Severe ulcerative dermatitis in a koi. The* Aeromonas salmonicida *isolated from this lesion was resistant to the majority of antibiotics it was screened against.*

rus spp.) flukes will become hypoxic, gulping air at the surface and coughing (Figure 8.19). Fish infested with skin parasites, such as ich (*Ichthyopthirius multifiliis*), rub against hard surfaces, lose scales, and hemorrhage in the area of parasite attachment. Fish with endoparasites are often anorexic, in poor condition, and fail to thrive. The diagnostic tests routinely used to identify ectoparasites include a skin scrape, fin biopsy, and gill clip. A fecal float and direct saline smear should be performed to evaluate a fish's endoparasite status.

Water Molds

Saprolegnia spp. is a common water mold isolated from tropical ornamental fish and cold-water aquaculture species. Water molds are primarily opportunists; they often infect open wounds, although primary infections are also possible. Affected fish generally present with white, cotton-like lesions on fins and skin. A skin scrape or biopsy of an affected area can be used to confirm a diagnosis of water molds, which are classified based on their branching nonseptate hyphae.

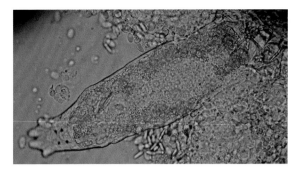

Figure 8.19 Dactylogyrus *spp. isolated from the gills of a goldfish. Note the characteristic eyespots of this parasite.*

Noninfectious Diseases

Elevated ammonia, nitrite, and chlorine, and highly variable water temperatures, dissolved oxygen, and pH, can cause clinical disease in fish. In most cases the fish respond similarly by being tachypneic, gulping for air at the surface of the water, producing excess mucus, and swimming in an agitated pattern. Routine water testing can prevent these problems because they can be identified early and corrected.

Swim bladder disease is being seen more frequently in goldfish, and most cases are associated with the "round belly"/fancy types (e.g., orandas, ryukins, black moors). In most cases, the fish float abnormally (e.g., like a fish bobber); however, in some cases the swim bladder disease causes the fish to be unable to get lift in the water (i.e., they present with always lying on the bottom of the aquarium). The former cases are typically associated with excess gas in the swim bladder, and the latter are associated with fluid in the swim bladder. Radiographs can be used to assess the swim bladder and give insight into the fish's status. Fine needle aspiration with cytology can be used to remove excess gas from the swim bladder and evaluate cell types within the bladder (e.g., epithelial, blood cells, bacteria). In some cases, deflating/

aspirating the swim bladder once or twice with a needle and syringe and correcting the diet (changing from floating to sinking foods and adding squashed cooked peas to the diet once weekly) are sufficient to treat this condition. In other cases, especially when there is infection, systemic antibiotics might be necessary. In some cases, surgery is needed to correct the swim bladder disease (Figure 8.20).

As fish live longer because of improved husbandry, the incidence of neoplasia is expected to increase. Anytime a mass is seen on a fish, neoplasia should be included in the differential. Neoplasia can show up in many different locations on fish, although integumentary (Figure 8.21) and visceral (Figure 8.22) tumors are the most common. In most cases, a surgical approach is taken for these cases. Chemotherapeutics and radiation therapy are not well studied in fish.

ZOONOTIC DISEASES

Humans can be exposed to fishborne diseases through ingestion of contaminated fish or water or through direct contact with fish or water. Zoonotic diseases attributed to ornamental fish are

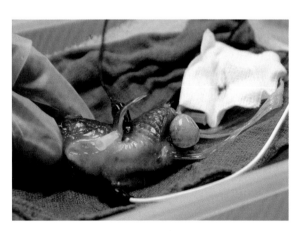

Figure 8.20 *This oranda goldfish was not responsive to several aspirations of the swim bladder, so the caudal chamber was amputated at surgery.*

routinely associated with contamination of open wounds or puncture wounds that occur during handling. Humans with a compromised immune system might be predisposed to opportunistic infection. Most cases of fishborne zoonotic diseases result in mild episodes of the disease.[11] A number of bacteria have been associated with human illness, including *Clostridium* spp., *Erysipelothrix rhusiopathiae, Mycobacterium* spp., *Staphylococcus* spp., and *Streptococcus iniae.* Several of these pathogens, including *Erysipelothrix rhusiopathiae, Mycobacterium fortuitum,* and *M. marinum,* have been associated with "fish handler's disease," which is characterized by lesions on the hands and arms (the areas we place our hands). Members of the family Enterobacteriaceae, including *Edwardsiella tarda, Klebsiella* spp., *Salmonella* spp., and *Yersinia* spp., are routinely isolated from aquatic environments and have also been associated with human illness. Increased numbers of multidrug-resistant *Aeromonas* spp. and *Pseudomonas* spp. are also being seen associated with tropical fish, especially koi, and special care should be taken in these cases because these organisms are opportunists in humans. Fish parasites and toxins have been found to cause human illness, but are generally associated with ingestion of the fish. To prevent the transmission of potentially zoonotic diseases, veterinary professionals should follow standard safety protocols and wear protective clothing.

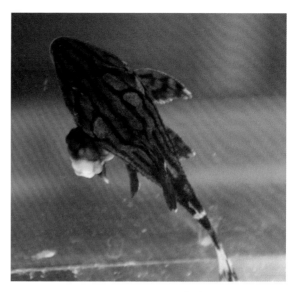

Figure 8.21 *An osteoma in a royal plecostamus associated with the pectoral fin.*

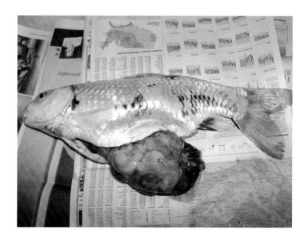

Figure 8.22 *An ovarian adenocarcinoma in a koi.*

SELF-STUDY QUESTIONS

1. What does mucus on the skin of a fish represent?

2. What are the primary functions of the gills of a fish?

3. What are the different types of filters that are available?

4. How does a biologic filter work?

5. What water chemistry parameters should be tested during a fish exam?

6. Why is untreated tap water fatal to fish?

7. What are common questions that should be included in an anamnesis for fish?

8. How do you anesthetize fish?

9. Describe a physical examination of a fish.

10. Where can you collect blood from a fish?

11. What diagnostic tests would you perform to evaluate a fish presenting for dyspnea and rubbing against materials in its aquarium?

12. How can you deliver medications to a fish patient?

13. What are some common infectious diseases of fish?

14. If a goldfish presents for "bobbing" at the water's surface, which anatomic structure is most likely affected?

15. Which group of pathogens is most commonly associated with zoonotic disease from tropical fish?

REFERENCES

1. Russo RC. Ammonia, nitrite, and nitrate. In: Rand GM, and Pertocelli SR, eds. *Fundamentals of aquatic toxicology*. New York: Hemisphere, 1985:455–71.
2. Emerson K, Russo RC, Lund RE, and Thurston RV. Aqueous ammonia equilibrium calculations: Effect of pH and temperature. *Journal of Fish Research Board of Canada* 1975;32: 2379–83.
3. Tucker CS. Water analysis. In: Stoskopf MK, ed. *Fish medicine*. Philadelphia: WB Saunders; 1993:166–97.
4. Piper RG, McElwain JB, Orne LE, McCraren JP, Fowler LG, and Leonard JR. Fish hatchery management. United States Department of Interior, Fish and Wildlife Service, Washington, DC; 1982.
5. Tomasso JR, Davis KB, Parker NC. Plasma corticosteroid and electrolyte dynamics of hybrid striped bass (white bass x striped bass) during netting and hauling stress. *Proceedings of the World Mariculture Society*, 1980; 11:303–10.

6. Stoskopf MK. Clinical pathology. In: Stoskopf MK, ed. *Fish medicine*. Philadelphia; WB Saunders; 1993:113–31.
7. Stoskopf MK: Anesthesia of pet fishes. In: Bonagura JD, ed. *Kirk's current veterinary therapy XII*. Philadelphia: WB Saunders; 1995:1365–69.
8. Gratzek JB. *Aquariology: The science of fish health management*. Morris Plains, NJ: Tetra Press; 1992:232.
9. Miller S, Mitchell MA, Heatley JJ, Wolf T, Lapuz F, Lafortune M, and Smith JA. Clinical and cardiorespiratory effects of propofol in the spotted bamboo shark (*Chylloscyllium plagiosum*). *J Zoo Wild Med* 2005; 36(4):673–76.
10. Dunbar CE, and Wolf K. The cytological course of experimental lymphocystis in the bluegill. *Journal of Infectious Disease* 1996; 116:466–72.
11. Nemetz TG, and Shotts EB. Zoonotic diseases. In: Stoskopf MK, ed. *Fish medicine*. Philadelphia: WB Saunders; 1993:214–20.

Index

nematode, 27
newspaper, 8
oral exposure, 75
parasite, 62
pasting, 17
physical examination, 12, 26, 26–27, 45, 124, 152
polymerase chain reaction testing, 100
sample, 8
soiling, 17
staining, 24, 88
strong-smelling, 111
Feeding, 112, 125, 128, 192, 203, 211
Feet, 18–19, 112
Feline infectious peritonitis (FIP), 104
Femoral vein, 56, 171
Femur, 92, 120, 125, 149, 172, 174, 185
Fenbendazole, 153, 174, 190
Ferret. *See also* specific topics on
    anatomy, 80–81
    anesthetics, 98–99
    cage, 81, 84
    diagnostic sampling, 89–94
    disease, 99–105
    health maintenance, 99–105
    history, 83–85
    husbandry, 81–83
    physical examination, 86–89
    restraint, 85–86
    surgical procedure, 98–99
    therapeutics, 95–97
Ferret-cell origin vaccine, 94
Fiber, 112, 113, 143
Fibia, 172
Fibroadenoma, 160
Fibroblast, 215
Fighting, 80, 112, 136, 167
Filter, 189, 205
    biologic, 196–198
    carbon, 211
    chemical, 196–199
    combination, 197
    mechanical, 196–197
    sand, 197
    water, 182
Fin, 205, 206, 208, 211, 213, 215
    types of, 191, 193
Fine needle aspiration, 88
Fipronil, 25
Fish. *See also* specific topics on
    anatomy, 190–194
    diagnostic sampling, 206–211
    disease, 214–216, 217
    health maintenance, 214–216
    history, 204–205
    husbandry, 194–204
    identification, 192
    physical examination, 205–206

restraint, 212
surgical and anesthetic assistance, 212–214
taxonomy, 190
therapeutics, 211–212
zoonotic disease, 216–217
"Fish handler's disease," 217
Fish tank, 81, 189, 194–196, 204
Fistula, 16
Flea, 94, 122, 123, 152–153, 173
Flora, 184
Fluid therapy, 125, 159
Fluke, 174
Fluoxetin, 187
Fly, 44, 94, 123–124
Fly-strike, 94, 112
Follicular stasis, 46
Food, 43–44, 126–127, 139. *See also* specific types of
    baby, 83
    brand, 84
    decaying, 199
    dry, 182
    leftover, 197–198
    live, 203
    medicated, 211
    moist, 182
Footpad, 100, 108, 109, 157, 171
Foraging, 6
Force-feeding, 159
Foreign body, 16, 32, 49, 82–83, 196, 210
    gastrointestinal tract, 49, 88, 99
    intestinal, 88
    physical examination, 99
    swallowing, 25
Fracture, 24, 87, 115, 117, 122
    pathologic, 185
    splinting pathologic, 69
    wings, 17
Free-roaming, 82, 83, 111
Freshwater coldwater species, 195
Freshwater system, 201–202
Frog, 45, 48–50, 64
Fruit, 5, 44, 45, 128, 168, 182
Fundic gland, 170
Fundus, 87
Fungus, 24, 29–31, 70, 73, 104, 175, 190

G

Gape, 49
Gas, 99, 191
Gastritis, 99
Gastroenteritis, 32, 129, 153, 158
Gastrointestinal (GI) tract, 81–82, 94, 96, 115. *See also* specific types of exotic animals

bacteria, 29–31, 129
delayed emptying, 96
disease, 99, 122, 187
disorder, 158
epithelium, 30
etoxicosis, 33
flora, 158
foreign body, 49, 99
gastric ulcer, 99
motility, 128
parasite, 211
stasis, 25, 127–128
ulcer, 82, 99, 104
Gastropod, 196
Gastrotomy, 99
Gecko, 44, 49
Genitalia, 108, 137
Genitourinary system, 103–104, 206
Gerbil. *See also* specific topics on
    cage, 142
    health maintenance and disease, 159–160
    parasite infestation, 153
    restraint, 145
Gill
    arch, 191
    biopsy, 207, 211, 215–216
    clip, 215
    color, 213
    epithelium, 213
    examination, 207
    filaments, 207
    fluke, 215
    plate, 191
Gingival disease, 83
Glass refraction, 42
Globe, 145, 159, 170
Glossitis, 72
Glottis, 16, 49, 63, 155, 157
Glucose, 82, 159
Goitrogen, 45
Gonopodium, 193
Gout, 70
Granuloma, 15
Grass, 112–113, 128
Gravel, 195–196
Grazing ark, 109
Greater wax moth larva, 44
Green beans, 44
Green iguana, 38, 42–43, 46–47, 51, 58. *See also* specific types topics on
Griseofulvin, 175
Grit, 4
Grooming, 98, 143, 180. *See also* specific types of exotic animals
Guinea pig. *See also* specific topics on
    anesthesia, 155, 158
    background information, 143–144

Ventricular septal defect, 17
Ventrum, 49, 51, 191
Vermin, 4, 12
Vertebrae, 17, 54–55, 124
Vinegar, 17, 198
Viral disease, 33, 215
Viral infection, 61
Viral isolation, 72
Virus, 70–73, 190. *See also* specific
    types of
Viscera, 46, 64, 70
Vision, 166
Vitamin A, 30, 69–70
Vitamin B, 112
Vitamin C, 136, 142, 144, 157–158
Vitamin D, 42, 69
Vitamin D$_3$, 185
Vitamin K, 112
Vitamins, 7, 30, 44–45, 83
Vivarium, 40
Vocalization, 18, 28
Voice box, 28
Vomiting, 81, 95, 99, 127
Vulva, 79, 88–89, 101, 103, 166

W

Walking, 82
"Walk the bone," 55
Walnut shell, 4, 168
Wart, 17
Waste, 196–197
Water. *See also* specific types of

alkalinity, 202
ammonia, 202
anesthetic, 213
automatic system, 12
balancing, 191
changing, 199, 199–200, 200, 203
chemistry of, 205
chlorinated, 182
dechlorination, 213
distilled, 48, 202
exposure, 75
hardness, 202
healthy, 196
mold, 215–216
monitoring, 203
municipal supply, 202
nitrate, 202
nitrite, 202
open system, 199
pH, 198–199, 201–202, 202
pressure, 192
quality, 191, 192, 199–203
sources, 84
temperature, 195, 198, 204
testing, 201–203
weight, 194
Water-circulating heat pads, 66
Waterfowl, 17, 24–25
Water-recirculating heating pad, 98, 174
Weakness, 102, 103, 176
Weaning, 113, 140
Weight, 72, 80, 115, 175
    body, 5, 7, 15, 147, 149, 183–185

fish tank, 194
water, 194
"Wet-tail," 158–159
Wheezing, 104
White blood cell (WBC), 52–54, 56,
    172, 194, 210
White-gray slime, 190
Wings
    feathers, 10
    fracture, 17
    joint integrity, 17
    physical examination, 17–18
    range of motion, 18
    towel, 14
    trimming, 32
Wire wheel, 168
Woodchips, 141, 168
"Wool block," 127–128
Wounds, 14, 67–69, 75

Y

Yawn, 85
Yogurt, 128, 158

Z

Zinc, 32, 81, 202
Zolazepam, 64
Zoonotic disease, 38, 69, 161–162. *See
also* specific types of exotic animals

About the Authors

Dr. Thomas N. Tully Jr. graduated from Louisiana State University in 1982 with a BS in animal science. After receiving his veterinary degree from the LSU School of Veterinary Medicine in 1986, he practiced as an associate veterinarian at veterinary hospitals in Florida and Louisiana.

Since 1987, he has been on the faculty at the LSU School of Veterinary Medicine, teaching in the Zoological Medicine Section of the Department of Veterinary Clinical Sciences. Currently Dr. Tully is a professor in the Veterinary Clinical Science Department and is hospital section chief of the Bird, Zoo, and Exotic Animal Service. He is a diplomate of the American Board of Veterinary Practitioners (Avian) and the European College of Zoological Medicine (Avian).

Dr. Tully has coedited four books, *Ratite Management, Medicine and Surgery*, two editions of *The Handbook of Avian Medicine*, and *Manual of Exotic Pet Medicine*; he has coedited two issues of *Veterinary Clinics of North America*, and coauthored the text *A Technician's Guide to Exotic Animal Care*. He has authored and coauthored numerous chapters in other veterinary medical texts. He is also coeditor in chief of the *Journal of Exotic Pet Medicine*.

Dr. Mark A. Mitchell graduated from the University of Illinois in 1990 with a BS in veterinary science. After receiving his veterinary degree from the U of I College of Veterinary Medicine in 1992, he practiced as an associate veterinarian in Champaign, Illinois, and worked on a Master of Science degree in wildlife epidemiology. He received his MS in 1997 from the University of Illinois. Dr. Mitchell continued his training in wildlife epidemiology at Louisiana State University and received a PhD in 2001. From 1996 to 2007, he was on the faculty at LSU, working alongside his friend and mentor Dr. Tom Tully.

In 2007, Dr. Mitchell returned to the U of I. Currently, he is a professor in the Veterinary Clinical Medicine Department and is chief of staff of the Small Animal Hospital and section head of Companion and Zoological Animal Medicine. He is a diplomate of the European College of Zoological Medicine (Herpetology).

Dr. Mitchell has coedited two books, *Manual of Exotic Pet Medicine* and *A Technician's Guide to Exotic Animal Care*. He has also authored and coauthored numerous book chapters, scientific articles, and abstracts. He is currently the editor in chief of the *Journal of Herpetological Medicine and Surgery* and coeditor in chief of the *Journal of Exotic Pet Medicine*.